ICU RECALL
2ND EDITION

RECALL SERIES EDITOR

LORNE H. BLACKBOURNE, M.D.
Senior Fellow, Trauma/Critical Care
Department of Surgery
University of Miami
Jackson Memorial Hospital
Miami, Florida

ICU RECALL
2ND EDITION

EDITOR

Nelson L. Thaemert, M.D.
Resident in Anesthesiology, Pain, and
Perioperative Medicine
Brigham and Women's Hospital
Harvard Medical School
Boston, Massachusetts

SENIOR EDITOR

Curtis G. Tribble, M.D.
Professor and Vice Chairman
Department of Surgery
Division of Thoracic and Cardiovascular Surgery
University of Virginia Health Sciences Center
Charlottesville, Virginia

First Edition Editor

Jeffrey T. Cope, M.D.

M. Brogan, R.N

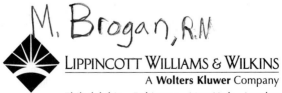

LIPPINCOTT WILLIAMS & WILKINS
A **Wolters Kluwer** Company
Philadelphia • Baltimore • New York • London
Buenos Aires • Hong Kong • Sydney • Tokyo

Editor: Neil Marquardt
Managing Editor: Emilie Linkins
Marketing Manager: Scott Lavine
Production Editor: Caroline Define

Designer: Doug Smock
Compositor: Lippincott Williams
& Wilkins
Printer: R.R. Donnelley & Sons

Library of Congress Cataloging-in-Publication Data
ICU recall/senior editor, Curtis G. Tribble ; editor, Nelson L. Thaemert.--2nd ed.
   p. ; cm. -- (Recall series)
Includes index.
ISBN 13: 978-0-7817-4589-5
ISBN 10: 0-7817-4589-6
   1. Critical care medicine--Examinations, questions, etc. I. Tribble, Curtis G. II. Thaemert, Nelson L. III. Series.
   [DNLM: 1. Intensive Care--Examination Questions. 2. Critical Care--Examination Questions. 3. Intensive Care Units--Examination Questions. WX 18.2 T822i 2004]
   RC86.9.I38 2004
   616.02′8′076--dc22

Dedication

We would like to dedicate this book to R. Scott Jones, our former Chairman and long-term mentor, friend, and role model.

During Dr. Jones' tenure at the University of Virginia one of his crowning accomplishments, in my opinion, was the creation of an environment in the Department of Surgery that was extremely friendly to learning. During this time the surgical interest society known as the Cabell Society was formed with support from the department. The Recall Series of books was proposed to and accepted by Lippincott Williams & Wilkins and became one of the fastest growing medical publication series in that company's history. In the recent years, the national average for students matching in general surgery has been 5%. At UVA that average has been nearly twice that. The resident who is considered by the graduating medical school class to have been their best teacher receives an award called the James Kindred Award. During Dr. Jones's tenure at UVA as Chairman, twelve residents won these awards in eighteen years. During his last six years as Chairman, general surgical residents won this award in five of those years. There are more than six hundred residents and fellows at the University of Virginia who are eligible for this award. The Dean had established a tradition in 1994 to award ten awards for teaching excellence of medical students by residents. Surgical residents have gotten, on average, two of those awards every year. Twice, three of our four chief residents have won these awards.

One of the most prestigious awards at the University of Virginia is called the All the University Award. One of our faculty members and five of our residents have won these awards during Dr. Jones' tenure as Chairman. The students at UVA choose one of the faculty members of the medical school as a baccalaureate speaker each year. Three times in the last ten years the baccalaureate speaker was a member of the department of surgery. The faculty member who is considered to be the best teacher by the graduating medical school class is given the Robley Dunglison Award. Two surgical faculty members have won this awards in the past ten years.

The medical student government at the University of Virginia is called the Mulholland Society. This student government established an award called the Mulholland Award for the best teaching department. Since this award was established in 1989, a few years after Dr. Jones came to the University of Virginia, the Department has won this award five times. In the last year of Dr. Jones' tenure as Chairman of the Department of

Surgery, at UVA one faculty member won the Dean's Award for teaching excellence, three of the four chiefs won the Dean's Award for teaching excellence, one faculty member was the baccalaureate speaker, one faculty member was the Robley Dunglison Award winner, one chief resident was the James Kindred Award winner, and the clerkship won the Mulholland Award.

Thus, these data support my feeling the Scott Jones created a culture friendly to learning, where education was a priority and where education was a product and not a by-product of our department, and, in my view, this saga shows how when the influence starts at the top, this type of culture can be created and maintained.

In the midst of winning all of these awards a faculty member from another department came to ask me what was going on in our department to allow this to happen. This was particularly troubling to this particular faculty member because the Department of Surgery in the past had not won any of these kinds of awards. This faculty member wanted to know what we did, what kind of food we brought if we were entertaining the students, and he wondered if it was the grades we gave them. I answered that "it" is not what we do but "it" is who we are, and I added that "who we are" is influenced by the extraordinary role model we have had as our department chairman.

Perhaps this can be best summarized with a quotation from Robert Graves' *Lawrence of Arabia*.

> The last and most that can be said. . . .is that he is a good man. This good is something that can be understood by a child or savage or any simple-minded person. It is just a feeling you get from him, the feeling that here is a man of great powers, a man that can make most men do for him exactly whatever he desired, but yet one who would never use his powers from respect for the other man's freedom.

It is because of the environment he created and because of the man that he was, and is, that we dedicate this book to our friend and colleague, Dr. Scott Jones.

Curtis G. Tribble, M.D.

Preface

ICU Recall, 2nd Edition, is an outgrowth of the earlier effort at the University of Virginia in writing *Surgical Recall* and *Advanced Surgical Recall.* Medical students, residents, and faculty members at the University of Virginia, allied with the Department of Surgery, wrote most of the questions used in the first edition.

Additional residents and faculty members, some of whom were previously affiliated with the University of Virginia, have contributed to the second edition to provide material that is both broader and deeper than before. Every chapter has had a comprehensive revision, and several new chapters have been added, including ICU Anatomy, Bedside Procedures, Head and Neck, Vascular Surgery Patients, and Pediatric Cardiology. In addition, over 40 illustrations have been included to aid in understanding the material. Our goal is to continue to provide young trainees with concise information and understanding about intensive care unit issues.

Curtis G. Tribble
Nelson L. Thaemert

ASSOCIATE EDITORS

Toby C. Campbell, M.D.
Resident in Medicine
University of Wisconsin—Madison School of Medicine
Madison, Wisconsin

Tae Chong, M.D.
Resident in Surgery
University of Virginia School of Medicine
Charlottesville, Virginia

Heather L. Evans, M.D.
Resident in Surgery
University of Virginia School of Medicine
Charlottesville, Virginia

Benjamin Peeler, M.D.
Assistant Professor of Surgery
University of Virginia School of Medicine
Charlottesville, Virginia

Reid B. Adams, M.D.
Associate Professor of Surgery
University of Virginia School of Medicine
Charlottesville, Virginia

Chardrick E. Denlinger, M.D.
Resident in Surgery
University of Virginia School of Medicine
Charlottesville, Virginia

Brendon M. Stiles, M.D.
Resident in Surgery
University of Virginia School of Medicine
Charlottesville, Virginia

Subinoy Das, M.D.
Resident in Otolaryngology
University of North Carolina—Chapel Hill
Chapel Hill, North Carolina

Aneesa M. Das, M.D.
Resident in Medicine
University of North Carolina—Chapel Hill
Chapel Hill, North Carolina

Thomas S. Maxey, M.D.
Resident in Surgery
University of South Florida College of Medicine
Tampa, Florida

CHAPTER EDITORS

Chapter 1 Introduction

Douglas S. Newburg
Lecturer
Department of Surgery
University of Virginia School of Medicine
Charlottesville, Virginia

Chapter 2 Ethical Issues in the ICU

Toby C. Campbell, M.D.
Resident in Medicine
University of Wisconsin—Madison School of Medicine
Madison, Wisconsin

Chapter 3 ICU Pharmacology

Ashley M. Shilling, M.D.
Resident in Anesthesiology
University of Virginia School of Medicine
Charlottesville, Virginia

Chapter 4 Anesthesia in the ICU

David R. Vaughn, M.D.
Resident in Anesthesiology
University of Virginia School of Medicine
Charlottesville, Virginia

Chapter 5 ICU Anatomy

Peter Ellman, M.D.
Resident in Surgery
University of Virginia School of Medicine
Charlottesville, Virginia

Chapter 6 ICU Radiology

Alan V. Padgett, M.D.
Resident in Radiology
University of Virginia School of Medicine
Charlottesville, Virginia

David J. Spinosa, M.D.
Associate Professor of Radiology
University of Virginia School of Medicine
Charlottesville, Virginia

Chapter 7 Monitoring

Brendon M. Stiles, M.D.
Resident in Surgery
University of Virginia School of Medicine
Charlottesville, Virginia

Chapter 8 Bedside Procedures

Thomas S. Maxey, M.D.
Resident in Surgery
University of South Florida College of Medicine
Tampa, Florida

Chapter 9 Central Nervous System

Philip Smith
Medical Student
University of Virginia School of Medicine
Charlottesville, Virginia

Michael L. Smith, M.D.
Resident in Neurosurgery
Hospital of the University of Pennsylvania
Philadelphia, Pennsylvania

Chapter 10 Head and Neck

Subinoy Das, M.D.
Resident in Otolaryngology
University of North Carolina—Chapel Hill
Chapel Hill, North Carolina

Chapter 11 Respiratory System

Aneesa M. Das, M.D.
Resident in Medicine
University of North Carolina—Chapel Hill
Chapel Hill, North Carolina

Chapter 12 Cardiac Arrhythmias

Tae Chong, M.D.
Resident in Surgery
University of Virginia School of Medicine
Charlottesville, Virginia

Chapter 13 Cardiovascular Pump Problems

Brett Reece, M.D.
Resident in Surgery
University of Virginia School of Medicine
Charlottesville, Virginia

James D. Bergin, M.D.
Associate Professor of Cardiology
University of Virginia School of Medicine
Charlottesville, Virginia

Chapter 14 Coronary Syndromes and Cardiac Arrest

David C. Isbell, M.D.
Fellow in Cardiology
University of Virginia School of Medicine
Charlottesville, Virginia

Chapter 15 Management of the Postcardiac Surgery Patient

Benjamin Peeler, M.D.
Assistant Professor of Surgery
University of Virginia School of Medicine
Charlottesville, Virginia

Chapter 16 Renal

Elizabeth C. McLemore, M.D.
Resident in Surgery
Mayo Clinic
Scottsdale, Arizona

Chapter 17 Fluids and Electrolytes

Eric Marderstein, M.D.
Resident in Surgery
University of Pittsburgh School of Medicine
Pittsburgh, Pennsylvania

Matthew J. O'Connor
Medical Student
University of Virginia School of Medicine
Charlottesville, Virginia

Chapter 18 Gastrointestinal System

Robert L. Smith, III, M.D.
Resident in Surgery
University of Virginia School of Medicine
Charlottesville, Virginia

Chapter 19 Obstetrics and Gynecology

Timothy Villegas, M.D.
Resident in Obstetrics and Gynecology
Captain, Medical Corps
United States Army
Fort Sam Houston, Texas

Chapter 20 Endocrine System

Heidi M. Farinholt
Medical Student
University of Virginia School of Medicine
Charlottesville, Virginia

Chapter 21 Hematology

Stefan Hura, M.D.
Resident in Radiology
Stanford University School of Medicine
Stanford, California

Chapter 22 Skin

Jodi M. Eisner MD
Resident in Dermatology
University of Virginia School of Medicine
Charlottesville, Virginia

Chapter 23 Musculoskeletal System

Christian D. Monson
Medical Student
University of Virginia School of Medicine
Charlottesville, Virginia

Chapter 24 Malnutrition

Joseph J. Dubose, M.D.
Resident in General Surgery
Captain, Medical Corps
United States Air Force
Keesler Air Force Base, Mississippi

John S. Minasi, M.D.
Chief Scientific Officer
Zassi Medical Evolutions
Fernandia Beach, Florida

Chapter 25 Infection

Heather L. Evans M.D.
Resident in Surgery
University of Virginia School of Medicine
Charlottesville, Virginia

Chapter 26 Immunosuppression

Gregory L. Livers
Medical Student
University of Virginia School of Medicine
Charlottesville, Virginia

Chapter 27 Neoplasia

Meghan L. Milburn
Medical Student
University of Virginia School of Medicine
Charlottesville, Virginia

Chapter 28 Pediatric Patients

David Lanning, M.D., Ph.D.
Fellow, Pediatric Surgery
Children's Hospital of Michigan
Wayne State University School of Medicine
Detroit, Michigan

Scott Langenburg, M.D.
Associate Professor of Surgery
Children's Hospital of Michigan
Wayne State University School of Medicine
Detroit, Michigan

Chapter 29 Pediatric Cardiology

Robert L. Hannan, M.D.
Cardiovascular Surgeon
Miami Children's Hospital
Miami, Florida

Anthony F. Rossi, M.D.
Director, Cardiac Intensive Care Unit
Miami Children's Hospital
Miami, Florida

David G. Nykanen, M.D.
Pediatric Cardiologist
Miami Children's Hospital
Miami, Florida

Chapter 30 Trauma Patients

Michael H. Lebow, M.D.
Resident in Surgery
Louisiana State University School of Medicine
New Orleans, Louisiana

Chapter 31 Burn Patients

Benjamin J. Schalet
Medical Student
University of Virginia School of Medicine
Charlottesville, Virginia

David B. Drake, M.D.
Associate Professor of Plastic Surgery
University of Virginia Medical Center
Charlottesville, Virginia

Chapter 32 Vascular Surgery Patients

David C. Cassada, M.D.
Vascular Surgeon
University of Tennessee Graduate School of Medicine
Knoxville, Tennessee

Chapter 33 Transplant Patients

Wesley Thayer, M.D., Ph.D.
Resident in Surgery
University of Virginia Medical Center
Charlottesville, Virginia

Contributors–the following contributed as medical students at the University of Virginia School of Medicine, Charlottesville, Virginia

David Dougherty
Elizabeth Robertson
Charles Robertson

The authors acknowledge the contributions of the following people to the first edition of this book:

Reid B. Adams, M.D.
James D. Bergin, M.D.
Eugene F. Foley, M.D.
Robert Hannan, M.D.
Michael Ishitani, M.D.
William Killinger, M.D.
Ryan Lesh, M.D.
George Leisure, M.D.
Alan Matsumoto, M.D.
Eugene D. McGahren, M.D.
Katherine Michael, Pharm.D.
John S. Minasi, M.D.
George Rich, M.D.
Karen Schwenzer, M.D.
Craig Slingluff, M.D.
Burkhard Spiekermann, M.D.
J. Benjamin Tribble, M.D.
David E. Tribble, M.D.
Reid W. Tribble, M.D.
Jeffrey S. Young, M.D.
Scott Arnold, M.D.
Christopher Bartels, M.D.
Joseph Bianchi, M.D.
Oliver Binns, M.D.
Lorne H. Blackbourne, M.D.
Osbert Blow, M.D.

Scott A. Buchanan, M.D.
Barry Chan, M.D.
Gerald Cephus, M.D.
John Connors, M.D.
Richard Earnhart, M.D.
Tim Edmiston, M.D.
Matt Edwards, M.D.
David Graham, M.D.
Nancy Harthun, M.D.
Ryan Herrington, M.D.
John Kern, M.D.
Steve Kim, M.D.
Christopher King, M.D.
Lisa King, M.D.
Michael C. Mauney, M.D.
Addison May, M.D.
Lynn Rosenlof, M.D.
Scott Ross, M.D.
Robert Sawyer, M.D.
Donald Schmit, M.D.
John Sperling, M.D.
Steve Thies, M.D.
Michael Towler, M.D.
Blake vanMeter, M.D.
Kent Weathers, M.D.

Table of Contents

Section 3 — Pathologic Processes

Section 4 — Special ICU Populations

Section 1

Overview and
Background ICU
Information

1   Introduction

WHY THE ICU?

In the movie *Good Will Hunting,* the community-college professor and counselor Sean McGuire, played by Robin Williams, confronts Matt Damon's character, Will Hunting, a natural mathematical genius who has read books on a vast array of subjects. Will thinks he knows everything because he is so well read. The truth, however, is that Will has never been out of Boston, whereas McGuire has fought in Vietnam, lost a wife to cancer, and questioned his own existence. McGuire questions what Will knows about love and loss as he relates his months in the hospital watching his wife die: "The doctors could see in my eyes that the term 'visiting hours' didn't mean anything to me." McGuire has lived what Will has only read about.

Students belong in the ICU for many reasons, one of which is to learn the technical aspects of patient care. Having said this, however, the best students—the best doctors—take this time to experience every facet of the ICU, to connect what they have read to real-life experience, experiences that will define the care of their future patients for the rest of their career.

Duke basketball coach Mike Krzyzewski said it best: "You have a chance for everybody to have ownership—that's the ultimate goal, that the team is owned by everyone on the team. It's always 'WE.' Psychology is the most important factor. What happens in sport—and it happens in business, too—people try to learn the business or they learn the sport, and the time they spend on that is disproportionate to the time they spend learning about people."

The ICU provides an opportunity to learn about people under dire circumstances. It is an opportunity to observe yourself, your teammates, and your patients. This is important because no matter what career you choose, what specialty you pursue, chances are good that some of your patients will spend time in the ICU. Your role might be to counsel a family who wants to talk, or you might need to communicate information to the ICU staff. Your experience of ICU situations will be as important as your medical expertise.

Most mistakes are made not from a lack of medical knowledge but from poor leadership, a lack of communication, or an absence of teamwork. These mistakes can be exacerbated by increased levels of stress. Bad outcomes are often the result of several small mistakes rather than a single, gross incident.

Students rotate through the ICU to increase their medical knowledge and their competencies in people skills (e.g., caring for a person, communicating with team members, leading a team, listening). This process requires as much participation and self-motivation as learning the book knowledge does. The major difference is that the books can be read and then read again, but the opportunity to experience the ICU might only come along once.

Doug Newburg
Sports psychologist

USING THIS STUDY GUIDE

This study guide is based on the premise that knowing the right questions is at least as important as knowing the answers and that people learn better when they are questioned rather than lectured. This approach dates back to Socrates, and it has been perpetuated in medicine as much as anywhere else in Western education. In fact, a case could be made that knowing the right questions is *more* important than knowing the answers. All medical students are taught that at least half of what they learn in medical school will be outdated within 5 years—if not sooner. However, it is the answers, not the questions, that change.

This guide can be used most effectively by covering the answers with the bookmark while posing the questions to yourself. The book is designed so that it can be carried around in your pocket, allowing you to take advantage of the scraps of time that inevitably accrue during a clinical day. Because each question is relatively self-contained, very small bits of time can be used efficiently in this way. Some readers have even found it useful to tear up these books into portions, making them even more portable. An electronic version to be stored on a personal digital assistant is also available.

ICU NOTES

Daily notes in the ICU are a comprehensive way of reviewing all the patient information that is presented on rounds. The generally accepted method is the "checklist approach." This is analogous to the use of a checklist by a pilot taking off in a commercial jetliner. Pilots are required to have a checklist that they review to make sure they have addressed each issue before takeoff. This methodical approach to ICU care ensures that all issues are addressed in a standardized manner. By nature, patients in the ICU are the sickest patients in the hospital, and caring for them requires the utmost diligence and thoroughness.

A sample checklist for ICU follows. It covers all basic organ systems and necessary considerations and, by convention, generally addresses the patient from head to toe. Feel free to add to and subtract from this list as you see fit.

Neuro
  Mental status, pain, pain relief
  Neuro checks, neuro deficits
  Psych, consults, meds
  EtOH, DT precautions
  Seizures, seizure meds
Respiratory
  Respiratory distress, ABGs, vent settings
  Exam, CXR
  Bronchodilators, meds, levels
CVS
  BP, P, rhythm, ectopy, EKGs
  CV meds, drips, levels, digoxin
  Cardiac enzymes
Renal
  Fluid status, UOP, wt, IVFs (type and rate)
  I&O, CVP, CXR fluid, BUN, Cr, Foley
  Lytes, Ca^{2+}, Mg^{2+}, PO_4
  Acid-base status
  Dialysis
GI
  Bowel fxn, gas, nausea, diet
  NGT, OBR, lactulose
  Liver fxn, LFTs, PT, bilirubin
  Panc fxn, amylase, panc enzymes
Endo
  DM: glc, insulin
  Thyroid, TFTs, synthroid
  Adrenals, steroids, adrenal insufficiency
Heme
  Hct, transfusions, blood in bank
  Clotting studies, vitK

ID
    Temp, Tmax, WBC
    Cultures, sensitivities, abx, abx levels
    CXR, UA, lines
Nutrition
    TPN, tube feedings, PO intake
    Lipids, trace elements, vitamins
    N_2 balance, wt increase, visceral proteins
Wounds
    Appearance of wounds, debridement
    Drains, dsg changes
    Review traumatic injuries of multiple-trauma victims
Prophylaxis
    Stress ulcer, DVT
Meds
    List
Path
    Reports of all tissues sent to path
Impression
    List all issues, problems, and impressions
Plan
    Have a plan that addresses each issue listed in your impression

COMMON ICU ABBREVIATIONS YOU SHOULD KNOW

2,3-DPG = 2,3-diphosphoglycerate
ABG = arterial blood gases
Abx = antibiotic
AC = assist control
ACh = acetylcholine
ACLS = advanced cardiac life support
ACS = acute coronary syndrome
ADH = antidiuretic hormone
ADP = adenosine diphosphate
Afib = arterial fibrillation
Aflutter = atrial flutter
ANP = atrial natriuretic peptide
AP = anteroposterior
ARDS = acute respiratory distress syndrome
ASA = aspirin
AV = atrioventricular
AVM = arteriovenous malformation
AVNRT = arteriovenous nodal reentry tachycardia

BID = twice a day
BDZ = benzodiazepines
BP = blood pressure
Bpm = beats per minute
BSA = body surface area
BUN = blood urea nitrogen

C# = cervical spine vertebra/nerve
Ca = calcium
cAMP = cyclic adenosine monophosphate
CBC = complete blood count
CBF = cerebral blood flow
CEA = carotid endarterectomy
CHF = congestive heart failure
CI = cardiac index
CN = cranial nerve
CNS = central nervous system
CO = cardiac output
CO_2 = carbon dioxide
CPAP = continuous positive airway pressure
CPP = cerebral perfusion pressure
CPR = cardiopulmonary resuscitation
Cr = creatinine
CSF = cerebrospinal fluid
Cspine = cervical spine
CT = computed tomography
CTA = computed tomographic angiogram
CTPA = computed tomographic pulmonary angiogram
CV = cardiovascular
CVP = central venous pressure
CXR = chest radiograph

DM = diabetes mellitus
DNI = do not intubate
DNR = do not resuscitate
DO_2 = oxygen delivery
DPL = diagnostic peritoneal lavage
Dsg = dressing
DT = delirium tremens
DVT = deep-vein thrombosis

ECG = electrocardiogram
ECMO = extracorporeal membrane oxygenation

EEG = electroencephalogram
ERV = expiratory reserve volume
ESV = end-systolic volume
ET = endotracheal
EtOH = alcohol
ETT = endotracheal tube

FiO_2 = delivered concentration of oxygen
FFP = fresh frozen plasma
FRC = functional residual capacity
Fxn = function

GCS = Glasgow coma scale
GI = gastrointestinal
Glc = glucose

Hct = hematocrit
Hgb = hemoglobin
HIT = heparin-induced thrombocytopenia
HOB = head of bed
HPV = hypoxic pulmonary vasoconstriction
HTN = hypertension

IABP = intra-aortic balloon pump
IC = intercostal
ICD = internal cardiac defibrillator
ICP = intracranial pressure
ICU = intensive care unit
ID = infectious diseases
IDDM = insulin-dependent diabetes mellitus
IJ = internal jugular
IM = intramuscular
IMV = intermittent mandatory ventilation
INR = international normalized ratio
I&O = ins and outs
IV = intravenous
IVF = intravenous fluids

J = joules

L# = lumbar vertebra/nerve
LBBB = left bundle branch block
LDH = lactate dehydrogenase

LFT = liver function test
LMW = low molecular weight
LOC = loss of consciousness
LP = lumbar puncture
LVEDP = left ventricular end-diastolic pressure
LVEDV = left ventricular end-diastolic volume
LVEF = left ventricular ejection fraction

MAP = mean arterial pressure
MAT = multifocal atrial tachycardia
MCA = middle cerebral artery
Meds = medications
Mg = magnesium
$MgSO_4$ = magnesium sulfate
MH = malignant hyperthermia
MI = myocardial infarction
MRA = magnetic resonance angiogram
MRI = magnetic resonance imaging

N_2 = nitrogen
NDMR = nondepolarizing muscle relaxant
NG = nasogastric
NGT = nasogastric tube
NMB = neuromuscular blockers
NSR = normal sinus rhythm
NTG = nitroglycerine

O_2 = oxygen
OBR = (orthopedic) bowel regimen
OG = orogastric
OR = operating room

PA = pulmonary artery
PAC = pulmonary artery catheter
PAD = pulmonary artery diastolic
Panc = pancreatic
PAS = pulmonary artery systolic
PAWP = pulmonary arterial wedge pressure
PC = pressure control
P_{CO_2} = partial pressure of carbon dioxide
PCWP = pulmonary capillary wedge pressure
PE = pulmonary embolism
PEA = pulseless electrical activity

PEEP = positive end-expiratory pressure
PEG = percutaneous endoscopic gastrostomy
PFO = patent foramen ovale
PIP = peak inspiratory pressure
PO = by mouth
PO_2 = partial pressure of oxygen
PO_4 = phosphate
POD = postoperative day
PRVC = pressure regulated volume control
PT = prothrombin time
PTCI = percutaneous transluminal coronary intervention
PTT = partial thromboplastin time
PVC = premature ventricular contraction
PVD = peripheral vascular disease
PVR = pulmonary vascular resistance
PVRI = pulmonary vascular resistance index

QD = once a day

RA = right atrial
RAP = right atrial pressure
RBC = red blood cells
RQ = respiratory quotient
RV = residual volume or right ventricular

S# = sacral spine nerve
SA = sinoatrial
SAH = subarachnoid hemorrhage
SaO_2 = arterial oxygen saturation
SBP = spontaneous bacterial peritonitis or systolic blood pressure
SCD = sequential compression device
SCh = succinylcholine or "sux"
SIMV = synchronized intermittent mandatory ventilation
$SmvO_2$ = mixed venous oxygen saturation
SNP = sodium nitroprusside
SQ = subcutaneous
Stat = immediately
SVC = superior vena cava
SvO_2 = venous oxygen saturation
SVR = systemic vascular resistance
SVRI = systemic vascular resistance index
SVT = supraventricular tachycardia

T# = thoracic spine vertebra/nerve
TFT = thyroid function test
TLC = total lung capacity
Tmax = maximum temperature
TPN = total parenteral nutrition
TV = tidal volume

UA = urine analysis
UOP = urine output

VC = vital capacity
Vfib = ventricular fibrillation
VitK = vitamin K
VO_2 = oxygen consumption
V/Q = ventilation-perfusion
Vtach = ventricular tachycardia

WBC = white blood cell
WPW = Wolff-Parkinson White (syndrome)
Wt = weight

WORKING IN THE ICU ENVIRONMENT

What should be your overall relationship with the rest of the health care team?

All professionals who work together caring for ICU patients form a team, and no teammate is unimportant. Team members may include respiratory therapists, nurses, and perfusionists, and all should function as colleagues.

What should be the role of the medical student in the care of an ICU patient?

Medical students should view themselves as the patient's primary doctor. Using the more senior members of the team as consultants, students should take responsibility for information-gathering and note writing as well as for communicating with families, reviewing studies, and participating in procedures.

What types of things are considered to be unimportant in the ICU?

No detail is unimportant. *Everything* matters. Nothing is neutral. Virtually everything that goes on in the ICU will either help or hinder your patient. Even things as subtle as the noise level, temperature, light, and music as well as the more obvious details of laboratory values, medicines, and procedures can be critical to a patient's outcome.

How do you determine an ICU patient's level of awareness?

Assume that patients will hear, see, and feel everything that is said about and done to them. This ethic must be carried from rounds to procedures to discussions with the family. Both the health care team and the family should be encouraged to talk to the patients as well. You can never be certain how much the patient will know at any given time, and you may be astonished by how much patients remember from their ICU experiences.

2

Ethical Issues in the ICU

DECISION-MAKING, COMPETENCY, AND CONSENT

Who makes decisions for ICU patients?

If the patients are awake, alert, and communicative, they make decisions for themselves. If they are sedated, unconscious, brain injured, or otherwise have an altered mental status, another person makes the decisions.

Who becomes a decision maker?

Patients may designate a health care proxy or appoint someone with medical power of attorney. Otherwise, family members make decisions on the patient's behalf.

Who can provide consent for an adult patient who is unable to consent for himself or herself?

When seeking consent, courts have determined the order in which relatives are given priority for surrogate decision-making. Many families choose to make joint decisions, but the technical order in which to proceed is:
1. The spouse
2. Adult children of the patient
3. A parent
4. An adult brother or sister
5. A legally appointed guardian of the patient at the time of consent

Can a legal surrogate be appointed by the court if a patient has no family or legal guardian?

Yes, the court can appoint a legal guardian to act as a decision maker. In this case, these are usually unrelated persons who have strict guidelines to follow when making decisions regarding health care.

Who can determine if a patient is legally competent?

Competency is a legal determination of an individual's ability to manage his or her own affairs and, as such, must be determined by a judge. Two physicians may agree that a patient is incapacitated or incapable of making decisions and, instead, may turn to a patient's decision maker.

What are the steps in assessing decision-making capacity?

To assess a patient's ability to make his or her own judgments, two physicians must evaluate the patient in three distinct aspects of decision-making. If the patient fails at any of the following tasks and the two physicians agree, the patient can be declared to be incapable of decision-making:
1. Ability to understand
2. Ability to evaluate
3. Ability to communicate

How can a physician test a patient in the three areas of decision-making?

Ability to understand:

Ask the patient to paraphrase the discussion, including the different treatment options and the major risks and benefits of each.

Ability to evaluate:

The observers must feel that the patient is able to deliberate the options, is rational in his or her choices, maintains a consistent choice over time, and makes a decision concordant with his or her own principles.

Ability to communicate:

Ask the patient to communicate his or her final decision.

Can a physician or group of physicians legally withdraw life support if the team has determined that continued medical treatment will be futile but the family or legal surrogate will not consent to this action?

No

What are the elements of informed consent?

Informed consent is often rushed through by a busy resident, and informed consent forms vary greatly. Informed consent, however, is vitally important to protect the patient and the health care team when complications or unsuccessful interventions occur. According to a Presidential Commission in 1982, the patient must have a clear understanding of:

1. The disease process (diagnosis in layman's terms)
2. The prognosis
3. The benefits and burdens of recommended treatment
4. The benefits and burdens of reasonable alternative treatments
5. The likely outcome of electing to receive no treatment

The patient must then voluntarily authorize the proposed treatment or intervention.

If the patient is unable to provide consent and no next-of-kin is available, what is needed to perform an emergency procedure?

A note must be written in the hospital chart that states the emergent need for a life-saving procedure and bearing the signature of two treating physicians.

ETHICAL DECISION-MAKING IN THE ICU

What is the single most important question you should ask when ethical concerns arise?

Is the benefit of the therapy worth the burden of the therapy in the context of the patient and his or her decision maker's wishes?

How do you decide when to continue or discontinue what may seem to be aggressive or even futile therapy?

These decisions should be made jointly by the entire health care team, the patient, and the patient's family.

Who should have the greatest say in what treatments are instituted or discontinued?	The patient. In the ICU, however, the patient's immediate wishes often cannot be discerned. In this case, the health care team and the family are obligated to determine what the patient would want. Sometimes written guidelines, such as a living will, exist. If they do not, the team should direct the decision maker to "allow" the patient to make the decision by imagining what he or she would want in this situation.

CARE OF THE PATIENT WITH A TERMINAL DISEASE

What are "comfort care measures"?	Interventions meant to decrease the pain and suffering of a patient by eliminating pain, controlling nausea, palliating dyspnea, and controlling fever or other uncomfortable symptoms of the dying process.
What are some typical comfort care measures?	1. Pain medications, such as narcotics or opiates 2. Anxiolytics, such as benzodiazepines or Haldol 3. Antiemetics 4. Antipyretics, such as acetaminophen 5. Humidified oxygen 6. Medications that decrease or eliminate dyspnea, such as morphine or Dilaudid
Ethically, is there any difference between withholding and withdrawing medical interventions?	No. Bioethicists agree that no ethical difference exists between these principles. Practically speaking, however, it is more difficult to convince family members to withdraw than it is to withhold treatments.
What do the acronyms DNR and DNI mean?	**D**o **N**ot **R**esuscitate and **D**o **N**ot **I**ntubate. Typically, this refers to the

actions involved in a "code": CPR, intubation, defibrillation, and pharmacologic resuscitation (i.e., vasopressors). These terms do not mean Do Not Treat, although this is a common misunderstanding by patients, families, and other hospital staff. Any DNR/DNI orders should be clearly explained to everyone involved with the patient.

What does the acronym AND stand for?

Allow **N**atural **D**eath. Many palliative care specialists use this term to describe the various treatment options available in caring for the terminally ill. The AND order encompasses antibiotics, tube feeding, intravenous hydration, ICU admissions, DNR/DNI, psychosocial care, and other aspects of holistic palliative care. Also, AND has a positive connotation, so it is better received by patients than the negative terminology of a DNR order.

BRAIN DEATH AND ORGAN TRANSPLANTATION

What are the criteria for determining brain death?

All of the following must be met:
1. Coma, unresponsive above the foramen magnum to stimuli. Peripheral reflexes may still be present.
2. Apnea off ventilator for a period sufficient to produce hypercarbic respiratory drive (usually defined as a $PaCO_2$ of 50–60 mm Hg).
3. Brainstem reflexes, including pupillary, corneal, oculocephalic (doll's eyes), oculovestibular (calorics), gag, and sucking, are absent.
4. Core body temperature is greater than 34°C.
5. The diagnosis is known to be irreversible and may be either metabolic or structural.

6. Drug intoxication must be excluded.
7. No improvement occurs in neurologic exam over 24 hours, and drug screen is negative.

What confirmatory diagnostic tests may be performed to determine brain death?

1. EEG
2. Cerebral perfusion studies by MRI, CT, or radioisotope scans
3. Brainstem-evoked potentials

Name 4 ways in which brainstem reflexes are tested.

1. Corneal: absent blink with corneal touch.
2. Oculovestibular: done with cold caloric stimulation. When cold water is instilled against the tympanic membrane, an intact reflex will cause a sustained deviation of both eyes toward the stimulation. The acronym **COWS** (**C**old-**O**pposite, **W**arm-**S**ame) refers to the fast movement of the nystagmus, which can occur during stimulation with either cold or warm water.
3. Oculocephalic: doll's eyes. When the oculocephalic reflex is intact (positive doll's eyes) and the patient's head is turned, the eyes do not move with the head and appear to be focused on a point.
4. Oropharyngeal: no gag reflex.

Who is absolutely qualified to determine brain death in a patient?

The attending neurologist or neurosurgeon. However, some states allow other doctors to determine brain death.

How can a patient become an organ donor?

Only consent is required to be considered for organ donation. However, multiple factors are considered before organs are accepted for transplant, including the cause of death, infections at the time of death, and previously known organ disease.

How should I approach a patient or family about organ donation?

Don't! Leave this to the hospital or state organ procurement coordinator. The likelihood of a family consenting to organ donation is much higher if they are approached by an outside, impartial source than by a well-meaning member of the team.

PERSISTENT VEGETATIVE STATE

What is a persistent vegetative state?

A total loss of cerebral function with a functioning brainstem. Colloquially, this is referred to as "being a vegetable."

What are some of its characteristics?

1. A deep sleep or coma for a few days to weeks, followed by eyes opening and sleep–wake cycles.
2. Many reflexes are still present. Infantile reflexes may manifest, and brainstem reflexes are intact.
3. Swallowing is impaired, and the patient must be tube fed.
4. Unintelligible grunts and screams that do not seem appropriate to stimulation. Patients may grimace or have chewing motions without clear purpose or intent. Gross involuntary or reflexive movements occur without purpose.
5. These patients have "eyes-open unconsciousness." They do not track but may orient briefly toward a sound (a primitive reflex). They are often described as being awake but unaware.
6. The patients usually are not on a ventilator.

How can it be diagnosed?

Unlike brain death, this is a clinical diagnosis and is not considered to be "death" by the courts. This can be devastating for families, who need lots of support and education to understand the patient's terminal condition.

What is the prognosis for these patients?

After 3 months, these patients have virtually no chance of recovery. Families will face the decision of withholding feedings or hydration because, if they are well cared for, these patients can remain in a vegetative state for many years.

WITHHOLDING/WITHDRAWING LIFE SUPPORT

What is considered to be basic life support?

Although some states define this, these definitions may be loose and ultimately depend on the practitioner. Typically, food, water, supplemental oxygen, and other noninvasive comfort cares are considered to be basic life support.

What is considered to be advanced life support?

Invasive, aggressive, or experimental treatments and life-saving techniques, such as mechanical ventilation, dialysis, vasopressive drugs, mechanical circulatory support, or invasive monitoring (e.g., Swan-Ganz catheters). In general, critical care medicine is advanced life support.

Is it ever appropriate to withhold basic life support?

Yes and no. Any patient should be provided with basic food and water by mouth if they desire it. Even terminally ill patients near the end of life should have ready access to nourishment and someone nearby to feed them if they desire it. Likewise, supplemental oxygen via a nasal cannula or face tent can be provided without bothering the patient or impeding communication, and this may improve the patient's mentation and appearance. However, for patients near the end of life, it is appropriate to withhold IV fluids or tube feedings because these may prolong the patient's suffering and indignity. By providing basic life support only in natural ways (orally), you are allowing the normal dying process to occur.

What percentage of patients undergoing CPR in the hospital survive to leave the hospital?

Approximately 13%

What percentage of patients who undergo CPR in the hospital survive the event?

Approximately 22%

What patient populations are the most likely to survive to discharge after a cardiac arrest?

Cardiac patients who are more likely to suffer from arrhythmias and to receive immediate defibrillation have the greatest chance of surviving the event, recovering, and leaving the hospital ($\approx$26%).

What patient populations are unlikely to survive to discharge after a cardiac arrest?

Patients with metastatic cancer, with renal failure (or on chronic hemo-dialysis), and with liver failure have a very poor chance of leaving the hospital after a cardiac arrest ($\approx$0%–3%). Patients with cancer without known metastasis also have a poor prognosis for survival to discharge after cardiac arrest ($\approx$3%–10%).

What 3 criteria help to determine medical futility?

1. The disease must be terminal.
2. The disease must be irreversible.
3. Death must be imminent.

When should you consider withdrawing advanced life support?

When the burden of treatment outweighs the potential benefit, or when the treatments are incongruous with the patient's expressed desires

LEGAL PRECEDENTS AND LEGISLATION

What case decided by the New Jersey Supreme Court in 1976 determined that "substituted judgments" by a family or legal surrogate were valid as consent for withdrawal of mechanical ventilation?

The Karen Ann Quinlan case

In which 1981 case were two California physicians found to be innocent of committing murder when they decided to withdraw basic life support from a terminally ill patient with the consent of the patient's family?

Barber v Superior Court

Which court decision mandated the ability of the patient or legal surrogate to refuse medical therapy necessary to sustain life against the wishes of the physician?

Bartling v Superior Court

What other important ruling was determined by the *Bartling v Superior Court* decision?

Mr. Bartling was deemed to be legally competent while on the ventilator.

What was the first case to reach the U.S. Supreme Court concerning withdrawing or withholding life support from a legally incompetent patient?

Cruzan v Harmo

What was the ruling in *Cruzan v Harmo*?

The U.S. Supreme Court supported the state of Missouri Supreme Court ruling, which prohibited families from withdrawing life support from an incompetent patient unless "clear and convincing" evidence existed that this was the patient's wish before he or she was incapacitated (living will).

What document allows a family or legal guardian to determine the type of health care a patient can receive if that patient is deemed to be incompetent?

An advanced directive or living will

What three types of living will legislation exist?

1. Generic living will
2. Natural death act directives
3. Durable Power of Attorney for Health Care

Which type of living will is most consistently recognized as valid by state legislatures?

The Durable Power of Attorney for Health Care

What does the Durable Power of Attorney for Health Care do?

It appoints an "attorney in fact" who is empowered to make medical decisions for the patient if that patient becomes legally incompetent.

Should an individual have both a health care power of attorney and a living will?

No. The two are redundant. Most health care providers prefer a power of attorney because this allows for a dialogue with the surrogate decision maker so that issues not explicitly covered in the living will can be addressed. For example, living wills typically limit care if a patient is in a vegetative state; thus, they are of limited use when a patient is incapacitated but not brain dead (e.g., in encephalopathy or sepsis).

What 1990 Act passed by the U.S. Congress supported the use of advance directives?

The Patient Self-Determination Act

What did the Patient Self-Determination Act require of health care providers?

1. To provide information to patients about advance directives at the time of admission
2. To document whether advanced directives had been executed
3. To educate the health care staff and community about advance directives

What are advance directives?

Documents stating the desires of the patient regarding specific treatments that should be either withheld or rendered in the event that patient becomes seriously ill.

3   ICU Pharmacology

PHARMACOKINETICS AND PHARMACODYNAMICS

Define and differentiate between pharmacokinetics and pharmacodynamics.

1. **Pharmacokinetics** is the absorption, distribution, metabolism, and elimination of a drug ("what the body does to the drug").
2. **Pharmacodynamics** is the concentration-related effect of the drug on the organism ("what the drug does to the body").

What major factors affect the pharmacokinetics of a drug?

1. Renal and hepatic function affect elimination and metabolism.
2. Protein binding and volume status affect distribution.

What parameter is most commonly used to estimate renal function?

Serum creatinine

What formula can be used to estimate creatinine clearance?

The Cockcroft-Gault equation:
Creatinine clearance (mL/min) =
$$\frac{(140 - \text{age}) \ (\text{wt in kg})}{72 \times \text{serum Cr (mg/dL)}}$$
Normal is greater than 100 mL/min

What factor other than renal function affects serum creatinine in ICU patients?

Patients with decreased muscle mass will have falsely low serum creatinine levels.

Are any laboratory parameters useful in estimating hepatic function?

There are no reliable indicators of metabolic capacity. Bilirubin, however, is an indication of the liver's ability to conjugate, and PT is a marker of the liver's synthetic capacity.

What role does the liver play in affecting the pharmacokinetics of orally dosed drugs?

First-pass metabolism. Orally administered drugs are absorbed into the portal circulation and partially metabolized by the liver before reaching the systemic circulation. First-pass metabolism can account for as much as a 100-fold difference between the oral and parenteral dose.

What are some possible factors that can cause poor oral and/or IM drug absorption in ICU patients?

Poor tissue perfusion of the GI tract and extremities, ileus, bowel wall edema

What is half-life ($t_{1/2}$)?

The time required for the serum concentration of a drug to decrease by half. Remember, this does not always correspond to the duration of therapeutic effect.

ANTIPLATELET DRUGS

Name 3 commonly used antiplatelet agents.

1. Clopidogrel (Plavix)
2. Ticlopidine (Ticlid)
3. Aspirin

What is the mechanism of action?

Inhibition of platelet aggregation by inhibiting the binding of ADP

What are the 4 main indications?

1. ACS
2. Poststenting procedures for revascularization
3. Thromboembolic stroke prophylaxis
4. PVD

THROMBOLYTIC AGENTS

How do thrombolytic agents work?

They activate plasminogen to plasmin, thus promoting fibrinolysis.

What are the 4 available thrombolytic agents?

1. Alteplase (rTPA)
2. Anistreplase (APSAC)
3. Urokinase (UK)

4. Tenecteplase (TNKase)

What are the indications?

1. Acute MI: greater than 2-mm ST elevation in 2 or more contiguous leads, or new left bundle branch block and history that is consistent with acute MI. Indicated if less than 12 hours into the event and patient younger than 75 years.
2. Ischemic cerebral event: may use systemically if within 3 hours of event; up to 6 hours intra-arterially.
3. Treatment of pulmonary embolus (PE).
4. Intra-arterial for occlusion of dialysis arteriovenous fistula.
5. Clearance of occluded infusion catheters.

What are the adverse reactions?

1. Bleeding
2. Hypotension
3. Anaphylaxis
4. Reperfusion arrhythmias
5. Reperfusion cerebral hemorrhagic strokes

What are 5 absolute contraindications?

1. Previous hemorrhagic stroke
2. Other strokes or cerebrovascular events within the past year
3. Known intracranial neoplasm
4. Active bleeding (not including menses)
5. Suspected aortic dissection

ANTIARRHYTHMIC AND RATE-CONTROLLING AGENTS

LIDOCAINE

What are the indications?

Vtach; prevention of recurrent Vfib after resuscitation

What is the mechanism of action?	Class IB antiarrhythmic. Decreases phase-4 depolarization, and decreases conduction in re-entry pathways.
What is the dosage?	1. Loading dose: 1.5 mg/kg total body weight; may repeat in 5 to 10 minutes for a total of 3 doses. 2. Infusion: 20 to 50 mg/kg/min.
What is the therapeutic serum concentration?	2 to 5 mg/L
What are the pharmacokinetics?	1. Plasma half-life: 90 minutes. 2. Metabolism: 90% hepatic, liver blood-flow dependent clearance (decreased clearance with CHF, MI, advanced age). Active metabolites may accumulate with renal dysfunction. 3. Protein binding: 70% bound to α_1-acid glycoprotein.
What are the adverse effects?	Dose-related CNS effects (paresthesias, psychosis, lethargy, seizures) and, at a higher dose, cardiac side effects (bradycardia, hypotension, sinus arrest)

PROCAINAMIDE

What are 3 indications?	1. Treatment of both atrial and ventricular dysrhythmias 2. Prevention of recurrences of Afib/Aflutter 3. Use in wide-complex tachycardia in which Vtach and SVT cannot be distinguished
What is the mechanism of action?	Class IA antiarrhythmic. Stabilizes membranes, and depresses phase-0 action potential.
What is the dosage?	1. Loading dose: 15 to 17 mg/kg IV at rate of 20 to 30 mg/min (usually 1-g load, maximum of 1.5 g) 2. Infusion: 1 to 4 mg/min IV

What is the therapeutic serum concentration?	4 to 12 mg/L
What are the pharmacokinetics?	1. Plasma half-life: 3 to 5 hours 2. Metabolism: hepatically metabolized to active metabolite
What are the adverse effects?	1. Cardiac effects: conduction disturbances, AV block, prolonged QT leading to torsades de pointes, hypotension 2. GI effects: nausea, vomiting, diarrhea 3. Lupus-like syndrome 4. Toxicity more common in renal failure patients

AMIODARONE

What are 4 indications?	1. Treatment of Vtach and Vfib 2. Wide-complex tachycardias 3. Afib/Aflutter 4. Antiarrhythmic of choice if cardiac function is impaired
What is the mechanism of action?	Class III antiarrhythmic. A sodium-, potassium-, and calcium-channel blocker, it prolongs phase-3 action potentials.
What is the dosage?	150 mg IV over 10 minutes, then 1 mg/min IV for 6 hours, then 0.5 mg/min IV for 18 hours
Where is amiodarone metabolized?	Liver
What are the adverse effects?	1. Arrhythmias, prolonged QT, bradycardia, sinus arrest 2. Hypotension 3. CHF 4. Pancreatitis 5. Interstitial pneumonitis/pulmonary fibrosis

6. Hyperthyroidism/hypothyroidism
7. Hepatic toxicity

ADENOSINE

What are 2 indications?

1. Rate control and/or conversion of SVT to sinus rhythm (including WPW syndrome)
2. Initial treatment/diagnosis of narrow-complex tachycardia of uncertain type

What is the mechanism of action?

Slows AV node conduction

What is the dosage?

6 mg rapid IV push followed immediately by a saline flush (administer centrally if possible because of rapid degradation); may repeat with 12-mg dose if needed.

What are the pharmacokinetics?

1. Plasma half-life: 5 to 10 seconds (clearance not influenced by renal or hepatic disease)
2. Metabolism: metabolized to inosine and adenosine monophosphate by erythrocytes and vascular endothelial cells

What are the adverse effects?

1. Transient facial flushing because of vasodilation.
2. Transient hypotension.
3. Bronchospasm.
4. May cause transient bradycardia or AV block, and can transiently cause asystole.
5. Contraindicated in second- or third-degree heart block.

β-BLOCKERS

What are the most common β-blockers used in the ICU?

Esmolol, metoprolol, labetolol, and propranolol

What β-blocker may be used as a continuous infusion?	Esmolol (Brevibloc)

What are 4 indications?

1. SVT
2. Afib with rapid ventricular response for rate control
3. Control of BP in patients with hypertensive emergency
4. During ACS

What are the severe adverse effects?

1. Hypotension
2. CHF
3. Bronchospasm

DIGOXIN

What are 2 indications?

1. Rate control in Afib and Aflutter if not related purely to catecholamine excess.
2. Positive inotropic effects.

What is the mechanism of action?

1. Inhibits Na/K-ATPase, leading to an increase in Na with an increase in intracellular Ca and a positive inotropic effect.
2. Increases vagal activity to decrease heart rate.

What is the dosage?

1. Loading dose: 15 to 20 μg/kg lean body weight (reduce 25% for uremic patients); divide loading dose into 2 to 4 doses, given 4 to 6 hours apart, to allow drug distribution to the myocardium and to assess therapeutic/adverse effects.
2. Maintenance dose: 0.125 to 0.25 mg/day (adjust for renal dysfunction).

What is the therapeutic serum concentration?

0.8 to 2.0 ng/ml (serum level does not correlate with effectiveness)

What are the pharmacokinetics?	1. Plasma half-life: 36 hours (longer with decreased renal function)
	2. Excretion: primarily by the kidneys (not cleared in dialysis)
What are 5 adverse effects?	1. Arrhythmias, conduction disturbances
	2. Anorexia, nausea/vomiting/diarrhea
	3. Visual disturbances
	4. Fatigue, weakness
	5. Maintain serum potassium greater than 3.5 mEq/mL to decrease toxicity risk
What are 4 agents that would cause drug interactions with digoxin?	Procainamide, quinidine, verapamil, and amiodarone (all increase digoxin serum concentration)
How is digoxin toxicity treated?	The antibody Digibind can be used to bind digoxin, and plasmapheresis will clear the antibody–digoxin complex.

DILTIAZEM

What are the indications?	Rate control in Afib/Aflutter and MAT
What is the mechanism of action?	Calcium-channel blocker
What is the dosage?	1. Loading dose: 0.25 mg/kg IV push over 2 minutes; may repeat at 0.35 mg/kg in 15 minutes if inadequate response.
	2. Maintenance infusion: 5 to 15 mg/hr.
What are the dosage conversion rates to oral therapy?	5 mg/hr equals 180 mg/day, 7 mg/hr equals 240 mg/day, and 11 mg/hr equals 360 mg/day
What are the pharmacokinetics?	1. Plasma half-life: 3 to 4 hours; rapid decline in serum concentration after IV bolus

	2. Metabolism: hepatically metabolized to inactive metabolites
List 4 adverse reactions.	1. Hypotension, bradycardias. 2. Flushing, headache, nausea, dizziness. 3. May exacerbate CHF in patients with decreased left ventricular function, particularly with β-blockers. 4. Contraindicated in WPW syndrome.
What is another cardiac selective calcium-channel blocker?	Verapamil
What are 2 common examples of dihydropyridine calcium-channel blockers?	Amlodipine and nifedipine
Do dihydropyridines have an effect on the heart?	No. Dihydropyridines affect blood vessels.

DRUGS USED IN ADVANCED CARDIAC LIFE SUPPORT

EPINEPHRINE

What is the mechanism of action?	α- and β-adrenergic agonist, causing vasoconstriction and inotropic effects
What are the indications?	Vfib, pulseless Vtach, and PEA
What is the dosage?	For a pulseless situation, 1 mg IV every 3 to 5 minutes for maximum of 3 to 5 mg; if the patient fails to respond, new ACLS guidelines suggests use of vasopressin or another drug.
What is the route of administration?	1. Central administration is preferred. For peripheral administration, flush well with 10 to 20 mL, and elevate the extremity.

2. May be given down an ETT in a dose of 2- to 2.5-fold the IV dose (dilute in 10 mL).
3. Can be given by the intracardiac route at 0.1 to 1 mg.

What are the adverse effects?

Arrhythmias, palpitations, HTN, tissue necrosis if extravasated

ATROPINE

What is the mechanism of action?

Inhibition of muscarinic action of ACh, resulting in increased heart rate and faster AV nodal conduction

What are 2 indications?

1. Symptomatic bradycardia
2. Ventricular asystole

What is the dosage?

0.4 to 1 mg IV push every 3 to 5 minutes, up to a maximum of 3 mg

What is the route of administration?

1. Central administration is preferred. For peripheral administration, flush well with 10 to 20 mL, and elevate the extremity.
2. May be given down an ETT in a dose of 2- to 2.5-fold the IV dose (dilute in 10 mL).

What are 3 adverse effects?

1. Paradoxical bradycardia with a dose less than 0.5 mg.
2. Anticholinergic effects (dry mouth, tachycardia, urinary retention).
3. May precipitate ventricular arrhythmias in patients with myocardial ischemia.

AMIODARONE

(See "Amiodarone" under **"Antiarrhythmic and Rate-Controlling Agents"**)

What is the dosage in a code situation?

300 mg IV; may give second dose of 150 mg IV.

LIDOCAINE

(See "Lidocaine" under **"Antiarrhythmic and Rate-Controlling Agents"**)

What is the dosage in a code situation?	1 to 1.5 mg/kg IV; may repeat in 3 to 5 minutes.

MAGNESIUM SULFATE

What is the mechanism of action?	Intracellular cation. Deficiency is linked to arrhythmias.
What are the indications?	Torsades de pointes Vtach; Vfib/Vtach unresponsive to lidocaine
What is the dosage?	1 to 2 g IV push over 1 to 2 minutes
What are the adverse effects if given too quickly?	Hypotension, heart block, asystole, muscle weakness, and hyporeflexia

SODIUM BICARBONATE

What is the mechanism of action?	Increases sodium bicarbonate, and increases pH.
What is the indication?	Metabolic acidosis
What are 3 adverse effects?	1. Metabolic alkalosis 2. Cardiac arrest 3. Extravasation cellulitis
What is the dosage?	1 mEq/kg IV

INOTROPIC AGENTS

DOPAMINE

What is the dosage of "low-dose" dopamine?	1 to 2 μg/kg/min
What are the sites of action for low-dose dopamine?	Dopaminergic (D_1 and D_2)-receptor activation, resulting in renal and mesenteric vasodilation, which causes increased renal and mesenteric blood

flow, respectively. This is known as "renal-dose dopamine," and the net effect is diuresis.

What is the "intermediate" dose of dopamine?

3 to 10 μg/kg/min

What are the sites of action by intermediate-dose dopamine, and what is its use?

α_1- And β_1-receptor activation, resulting in increased inotropy and chronotropy. The net result is increased cardiac output as well as possible dysrhythmias.

What is the dosage of "high-dose" dopamine?

10 to 20 μg/kg/min

What are the sites of action of high-dose dopamine?

α_1-Receptor activation: causes significant increase in arterial vasoconstriction; also activates dopaminergic and β-adrenergic receptors.

DOBUTAMINE (DOBUTREX)

What are the sites of action?

β_1- And β_2-receptors

What are the effects?

1. Increased inotropy (β_1 effect)
2. Decreased afterload and peripheral vascular resistance (β_2 effect)
3. Mildly increased chronotropy (B_1 effect) that can lead to tachycardia and increased myocardial oxygen demand

What is the dosage?

2 to 20 μg/kg/min; tolerance may develop after 72 hours because of downregulation of receptors.

MILRINONE (PRIMACOR)

What is the mechanism of action?

Phosphodiesterase III inhibitor, which inhibits the breakdown of cAMP and, therefore, increases intracellular cAMP and intracellular calcium

What are the effects?	1. Increased inotropy 2. Decreased afterload 3. Minimal to no increase in chronotropy 4. Mild pulmonary vasodilation
What is the dosage?	1. Loading dose: 50 to 75 µg/kg over 10 minutes 2. Maintenance dose: 0.375 to 0.75 µg/kg/min

EPINEPHRINE (ADRENALINE)

What are the sites of action?	α_1-, α_2-, β_1-, And β_2-receptors
What are the effects of an epinephrine infusion?	1. Increased inotropy. 2. Increased chronotropy. 3. Little effect in BP at low doses (0.005–0.02 mg/kg/min) because of peripheral vasodilation, but may have marked increases in BP at higher doses.
What is the dosage?	1. Loading dose: 0.25 to 1 mg. 2. Maintenance dose: 1 to 4 µg/min

NOREPINEPHRINE (LEVOPHED)

Where are the sites of action?	α_1-, α_2-, And β_1-receptors
What are 3 side effects?	1. Increased inotropy 2. Increased chronotropy 3. Marked increase in BP
What is the dosage?	0.5 to 1 µg/min, and titrate to a maximum of 8 to 12 µg/min.

PHENYLEPHRINE (NEO-SYNEPHRINE)

What are the sites of action?	Predominantly α_1-adrenergic receptor

What are the effects?	Marked increase in BP and systemic vascular resistance because of vasoconstriction
What is the dosage?	0.25 to 1 μg/kg/min

VASOPRESSIN (PITRESSIN)

What is the mechanism of action?	Stimulates smooth muscle V_1-receptors; also acts like ADH.
What is the net effect?	Vasoconstriction; particularly useful in shock
What is the dosage?	0.01–0.1 U/min

USES AND INDICATIONS

What pressors are typically used for cardiogenic shock?	Dopamine and dobutamine
What pressor is particularly useful in cardiogenic shock with pulmonary edema?	Milrinone
What pressors are commonly used for septic shock?	Norepinephrine and vasopressin

INTRAVENOUS ANTIHYPERTENSIVE AGENTS

NITROGLYCERINE

What are the effects?	1. Primarily venodilation with mild arterial dilation 2. Inhibition of platelet aggregation
What is the dosage?	5 to 300 μg/min IV
What are the uses?	Increases myocardial oxygen supply, and decreases demand. Decreases BP.

SODIUM NITROPRUSSIDE (NIPRIDE)

What are the effects?
1. Venodilation.
2. Arterial dilation.
3. Equally dilates venous and arterial tone to allow for BP titration.

What is the dosage?
0.25 to 10 μg/kg/min IV

What are 3 major side effects?
1. Hypotension and possible intracoronary steal
2. Cyanide toxicity and methemoglobinemia; more common if the dose is greater than 5 μg/kg/min
3. Increased ICP

HYDRALAZINE

What is the mechanism of action?
Arterial smooth muscle dilation through guanylyl cyclase

What is the dosage?
10 to 20 mg IV per dose, or 10 to 50 mg IM

What are 3 side effects?
1. Reflex tachycardia
2. Headaches
3. Lupus-like syndrome

FENOLDOPAM

What is the mechanism of action?
Vasodilation by activating D_1-dopamine receptors, as well as questionable α_2-receptor activation

What is the dosage?
0.01 to 1.6 μg/kg/min

What are the clinical effects?
Decreased systolic and diastolic BP, reflex tachycardia, and increased renal blood flow

What are the adverse effects?
Increased intraocular pressure and anaphylactic reactions

DIURETICS

What are the most commonly used loop diuretics in the ICU?	Furosemide (Lasix) and bumetanide (Bumex)
What are 4 common indications for loop diuretics?	1. Acute pulmonary edema 2. CHF 3. Peripheral edema 4. HTN
What are 3 common side effects of Lasix?	1. Hypokalemic hypochloremic metabolic alkalosis 2. Sensorineural hearing loss 3. Weakness/muscle cramps
What is a commonly used osmotic diuretic?	Mannitol
What are 3 indications for mannitol?	1. Reduction of increased ICP 2. Prevention and treatment of oliguria 3. Diuresis effect
What are 2 adverse effects of mannitol?	1. Initial increase in intravascular volume, leading to pulmonary edema 2. Hyponatremia and hyperkalemia (transient)
Why are loop diuretics sometimes given in conjunction with mannitol?	To help excrete the increased intravascular volume
What is a commonly used oral aldosterone antagonist?	Spironolactone (Aldactone)
What is the common indication for spironolactone?	Fluid overload in patients with secondary hyperaldosteronism; particularly useful in cirrhotic patients

ATRIAL NATRIURETIC PEPTIDE (NESIRITIDE)

What is the function of ANP?	Increase in sodium and water excretion, suppression of renin and aldosterone, and venous/arterial dilation
When is it beneficial?	In patients with decompensated CHF
What are 4 adverse effects?	1. Hypotension 2. Headache 3. Back pain 4. Nausea

MUSCLE RELAXANTS

What are the sedative or analgesic properties of NMBs?	There are no sedative/analgesic properties. Patients can be paralyzed and still aware of their surroundings.
What are the 2 classes of NMB?	1. Depolarizing 2. Nondepolarizing
What is the class, onset, and duration of SCh?	Class: depolarizing Onset: approximately 45 seconds to 1 minute Duration of action: 5 to 10 minutes
What is the primary indication for SCh?	Rapid muscle relaxation for endotracheal intubation or to treat laryngospasm. (See Chapter 4, "Anesthesia in the ICU," for further information on SCh.)
How do NDMRs work?	By blocking nicotinic ACh receptors
Name 1 example each of a short-acting, intermediate-acting, and long-acting NDMR.	Short-acting: mivacurium Intermediate-acting: atracurium, vecuronium, rocuronium Long-acting: pancuronium, D-tubocurarine (Curare)

Which NDMR also has antimuscarinic activity?	Pancuronium
What NDMRs are safe to use in renal-failure patients?	Cisatracurium, atracurium, and mivacurium
What is the advantage of rocuronium?	Rapid onset, which gives adequate muscle relaxation for rapid-sequence intubation in patients with a contraindication to SCh
What drugs are used to reverse the effect of NDMRs?	Anticholinesterases (neostigmine, edrophonium, pyridostigmine)
What drugs should be used with the above agents when reversing the effect of NDMRs, and why?	Antimuscarinic drugs, either atropine or glycopyrolate, are given to counteract the profound vagal stimulation evoked by anticholinesterases and to prevent bradycardia.

BARBITURATES

What are 3 barbiturates commonly used in the ICU?	1. Thiopental 2. Methohexital 3. Phenobarbital
What are 2 major uses?	1. Anesthesia induction 2. Anticonvulsant
What barbiturate is used commonly as an anticonvulsant?	Phenobarbital
What is the effect on cerebral blood flow?	Constriction of cerebral vasculature, resulting in decreased ICP and cerebral oxygen consumption
What are 3 adverse effects?	1. Respiratory depressant 2. Hypotension and tachycardia 3. Tissue necrosis with SQ injection

OPIATES

What 4 opiates are commonly used in the ICU?	1. Morphine 2. Hydromorphone 3. Fentanyl 4. Sufentanyl
What are the primary therapeutic effects of the opiates?	Analgesia and sedation
What are the major side effects?	Decreased respiratory rate, cardiac depression including decreased heart rate and contractility, constipation.
Which opiate is known for its histamine release?	Morphine
Which opiates should be avoided in patients with renal failure?	Morphine and meperidine (morphine 6-glucuronide and normeperidine are active metabolites and excreted by the kidney)
What drug can be used as a narcotic antagonist?	Naloxone
Morphine, 10 mg IV, is equivalent to what dose of the following medications?	
Hydromorphone	1.5 mg
Fentanyl	100 μg
Codeine	120 mg

BENZODIAZEPINES

What are the 3 BDZs most commonly used in the ICU?	1. Midazolam (Versed) 2. Diazepam (Valium) 3. Lorazepam (Ativan)
What are the clinical effects of BDZs?	Anxiolytics, hypnosis, sedation, and anticonvulsion

What are the durations of action of the follow medications?

    Midazolam   2 to 5 hours

    Lorazepam   10 to 20 hours

    Diazepam   20 to 50 hours

How are BDZs metabolized, and what is the significance?

The BDZs are hepatically metabolized. Therefore, patients with liver failure and geriatric patients have prolonged duration of action.

Which BDZ is not primarily metabolized hepatically?

Oxazepam (Serax)

What is the BDZ antagonist?

Flumazenil

MISCELLANEOUS SEDATIVE AGENTS

PROPOFOL

What is the therapeutic effect?

Generalized CNS depression; likely analgesic effects

What are 7 advantages of propofol over barbiturates?

1. Propofol may be used as a continuous infusion, resulting in rapid changes in level of sedation.
2. Rapid recovery, usually within 10 to 15 minutes of bolus of infusion.
3. Antiemetic properties.
4. Anticonvulsant properties (also seen in barbiturates).
5. Not habit-forming.
6. Antipruritic properties.
7. Anxiolytic effects.

What are 5 major adverse effects?

1. Cardiac depression, particularly vasodilation.
2. Pain on injection.

3. Excitatory seizure-like activity is associated with injection.
4. Respiratory depressant.
5. Expensive drug.

KETAMINE

What are the uses?

Anesthesia and analgesia

What are the routes of administration?

1. IV
2. IM (good for an uncooperative patient)

What are the advantages over other induction agents?

1. Sympathomimetic effects prevent cardiovascular depression.
2. Causes bronchodilation, and can be helpful in patients with reactive airway disease.
3. Does not cause respiratory depression.
4. Has analgesic properties.
5. Can be given IM.

What are 5 major adverse effects?

1. Increases secretions (may be treated with anticholinergics).
2. May cause emergence reactions and hallucinations.
3. May cause jerky movements and myoclonus.
4. Increases intraocular pressure and ICP.
5. Has the potential for abuse.

ETOMIDATE

What is the use?

Induction of anesthesia

What is the advantage over propofol and barbiturates?

Less cardiac depression; useful in patients with decreased ventricular function and in hypovolemic patients

PROPHYLACTIC AGENTS IN THE ICU

What are 4 indications for stress ulcer prophylaxis?

1. Prolonged mechanical ventilation (>48 hours)

2. Steroid therapy
3. Severe burns or trauma
4. Prolonged ICU stay (>48 hours)

What 4 classes of medications can be used for stress ulcer prophylaxis?

1. Antacids
2. H_2-blockers
3. Cytologic barrier (e.g., sucralfate)
4. Proton-pump inhibitors (e.g., omeprazole, rabeprazole)

What 3 interventions are most commonly used as DVT and PE prophylaxis?

1. SCDs or Venodynes on lower extremities
2. SQ heparin injections (usually 5,000 U SQ every 12 hours)
3. LMW heparins (enoxaparin and dalteparin)

What is the mechanism of action by LMW heparin?

Binds antithrombin III, and inhibits Factor X and thrombin

In what 4 patient populations is LMW heparin contraindicated?

1. Patients with renal insufficiency (creatinine clearance <30 mL/min)
2. Patients with active bleeding, indwelling epidural catheters
3. Patients with history of HIT
4. Relatively contraindicated in patients with GI bleed history, hemorrhagic stroke history

What are the treatment steps of DVT/PE?

1. Heparin bolus, 80 U/kg IV, or enoxaparin, 1 mg/kg SQ every 12 hours
2. Heparin infusion starting at 18 U/kg to maintain heparin PTT at approximately 1.5- to 2-fold control
3. Warfarin (Coumadin) therapy beginning approximately 24 to 48 hours after PTT at therapeutic levels
4. Anticoagulation a PT INR of 2 to 3
5. Maintenance of anticoagulation for 3 months for DVT, 6 months for PE

POWER REVIEW

LIVER DISEASE

What medications are used to treat and prevent hepatic encephalopathy?	Lactulose; Less commonly, neomycin and metronidazole
What class of medications is typically used for empiric treatment of spontaneous bacterial peritonitis?	Third-generation cephalosporins, such as ceftriaxone or cefotaxime
What medication decreases the incidence of hepato-renal syndrome in patients who develop spontaneous bacterial peritonitis?	Albumin, given at 1.5 mg/kg on day 1 and 1 mg/kg on day 3 of treatment
What medications are commonly used to treat portal HTN and GI bleeds?	Propranolol and octreotide

SEPSIS

What emerging drug has shown benefit in severe septic shock?	Activated protein C
What class of drugs may be of benefit in patients with sepsis and shock?	Corticosteroids, at "stress doses"

RESPIRATORY DISTRESS AND FAILURES

What class of medications can be used to treat airway constriction?	β-Agonists, such as albuterol, or anticholinergic agents, such as ipratropium bromide
What classes of medications are the mainstays of treating an exacerbation of chronic obstructive pulmonary disease?	Steroids and antibiotics in combination

RENAL DISEASE

In patients with renal failure and anemia, what drug may help to correct the anemia?	Erythropoietin
What are 3 emergency drug treatments for hyperkalemia?	1. Insulin and glucose 2. Sodium bicarbonate 3. Kayexalate
What drug can be used to stabilize cardiac arrhythmias in hyperkalemia?	Calcium gluconate
Calcium gluconate is contraindicated in patients on what heart medication?	Digoxin, which increases the risk of arrhythmia

CENTRAL NERVOUS SYSTEM INJURY

What drugs are used to temporarily treat elevated ICP?	Osmotic diuretics, such as mannitol or urea
What other 2 methods can lower ICP?	1. Hyperventilation 2. Surgery

SHOCK

What medication is used in anaphylactic shock?	Epinephrine, either SQ (mild shock) or IV (severe shock)
What medications can be used to increase the BP of patients in shock?	Vasopressors, such as dopamine, dobutamine, phenylephrine, vasopressin, and norepinephrine
Which pressor has the least tachycardiac effect?	Phenylephrine

Why are pressors typically given centrally rather than peripherally?

The arterial constrictive effects can often cause infiltration of the IV line, with extravasation of the pressor and local necrosis.

OVERDOSE TREATMENT

For each of the following drugs, name the antidote for an overdose.

    Morphine, dilaudid, and fentanyl

Naloxone (Narcan)

    Lorazepam, midazolam, and diazepam

Flumazenil

    Acetominophen (Tylenol)

Acetylcysteine

    Warfarin (Coumadin)

Vitamin K, FFP

    Ethylene glycol, methanol, and isopropyl alcohol

Ethanol (and, for ethylene glycol ingestion, fomepizole)

    Tricyclic antidepressants

Supportive care

4

Anesthesia in the ICU

What is the single most important principle regarding the use of anesthetic agents in the ICU?

Be sure that anesthetic medicines do not lead to respiratory and hemodynamic compromise. No one dies of acute pain, but patients die when they lose control of their airway, quit breathing, or suffer cardiac depression from the inappropriate use of some medications.

AIRWAY

How low should your threshold be for intubating an ICU patient?

Extremely low. By the time you have thought about this question more than once, you have probably waited too long to intubate your patient.

What are 3 indications for intubation? (Think 40-60-60.)

1. Respiratory rate greater than **40** respirations/min, especially if progressive
2. PCO_2 greater than **60,** especially if progressive
3. PO_2 less than **60** (remember, this is $\approx 90\%$ saturation), especially if progressive and unresponsive to non-rebreather ($FIO_2 \approx 100\%$).

What are 5 other more general indications for intubation?

1. Impending loss of airway because of swelling or excessive secretions
2. Obtundation
3. Head injury
4. ARDS
5. The need for general anesthesia

When intubating the trachea, what is the most reliable way to determine correct tube placement?

Detection of end-tidal CO_2 (the most rapid and reliable indicator of proper tube placement, if this technique is available)

What are 2 ways to determine tube placement via a stethoscope?

1. Presence of equal, bilateral breath sounds. (It can be very hard to hear good breath sounds in many patients. You should, however, be able to tell if they are reasonably equal.)
2. Absence of breath sounds over abdomen

What are 4 other ways to determine tube placement?

1. Seeing humidity in the tube on exhalation. Hold something dark behind the tube to best see the fog of expiration.
2. Maintenance of oxygen saturation on monitor. It might take a healthy, thin, nonsmoker at least 3 (if not 5) minutes to begin to desaturate.
3. A good view of the vocal cords on direct laryngoscopy clearly defines tracheal placement.
4. Confirmation by CXR. This would be to assess mainstem intubation.

In the ICU, who is responsible for managing the airway and administering anesthetic medications?

This is the responsibility of the primary health care team, not of the anesthesiologist based in the OR. If Anesthesia is consulted for an intubation, however, the induction meds and doses are their responsibility.

How does the Mallampati classification predict difficult intubation?

A higher grade means a greater likelihood of difficult intubation. Intubation is all about visualizing the cords to get the tube through; a high Mallampati grade means a lower likelihood that you will be able to displace tongue and see directly to the cords.

What 3 other predictors might suggest difficult intubation?

1. Short distance (less than three finger breadths) from the thyroid cartilage to the genial tubercle on the underside of the chin
2. Inability to open the mouth by less than three finger breadths (very important)
3. Prominent incisors

Should you pay much attention to these predictors?

Yes. The inability to intubate may result in anoxic brain injury, and if you can tell ahead of time that intubation will be difficult, you can get an anesthesiologist to do it. Surgeons may be capable of intubating an easy airway, but anesthesiologists should handle difficult airways.

NEUROMUSCULAR BLOCKERS

NONDEPOLARIZING MUSCULAR BLOCKADE

Name several commonly used NDMR agents.

Pancuronium, vecuronium, rocuronium, atracurium, cisatracurium, and mivacurium

Prolonged neuromuscular blockade after the administration of an NDMR may be caused by the failure of what system?

Hepatic or renal disease that precludes metabolism or elimination of the drug(s)

What further physiologic disturbances can prolong blockade?

1. Hypothermia
2. Electrolyte abnormalities, such as hypokalemia, hypocalcemia, and hypermagnesemia
3. Undiagnosed nerve or muscle pathology, such as myasthenia gravis (oculobulbar myasthenics are notorious), amyotrophic lateral sclerosis, lupus, and polymyositis
4. Concomitant administration of other drugs, such as aminoglycoside

antibiotics or magnesium sulfate, which act to prolong the blockade

5. Acidosis

What are likely culprits for prolonged block in severe renal insufficiency?

Pancuronium and vecuronium

What are likely culprits for prolonged block in severe hepatic disease?

Pancuronium and rocuronium

Which nondepolarizing relaxants in current use do not require either hepatic metabolism or renal excretion for termination of their effect?

1. Atracurium and *cis*-atracurium (elimination by spontaneous Hoffman degradation in the plasma)
2. Mivacurium (metabolized by plasma cholinesterase)

Do muscle relaxants have any general anesthetic properties?

No

TRAIN-OF-FOUR SIMULATION AND ASSESSMENT OF RETURN OF MUSCLE FUNCTION

With which tool can you evaluate residual muscle paralysis?

A peripheral nerve stimulator

What muscle functions do you test with a nerve stimulator?

Remember, in an awake patient, these hurt:
1. Train-of-four stimulation: muscular twitches to four brief stimulator bursts
2. Tetanic stimulation: muscular contraction to a sustained electrical stimulus

What indicates residual blockade?

Any of the following suggest some degree of residual paralysis that is likely to be clinically significant:

1. Decrement in the intensity from first through fourth twitch during train-of-four testing
2. Muscle tension that fades over several seconds of tetanus
3. More intense train-of-four twitches after you tried the tetanus test (posttetanic potentiation)

If you do not have the above signs, are you guaranteed muscle strength to sustain ventilation?

Not necessarily. Even if you see full tetanus without fade, you can still have 50% of acetylcholine receptors occupied, and this could mean the patient needs reversal before being able to ventilate or oxygenate adequately.

How can you assess blockade without a nerve stimulator?

See if the patient can sustain lifting his or her head off the pillow for 5 seconds. A successful response correlates well with adequate return of pharyngeal and laryngeal protective reflexes as well as with return of muscle strength best correlated with being able to oxygenate and ventilate effectively.

Must muscle relaxants be reversed after cardiac surgery?

No. In general, by the time the patient is awake enough to be extubated after such surgery, the muscle relaxants have worn off.

DEPOLARIZING MUSCLE RELAXATION: SUCCINYLCHOLINE

When is SCh, or "sux," indicated?

Rapid onset of muscular paralysis for intubation

Use of SCh can be life-threatening by creating which electrolyte abnormality?

Hyperkalemia, with resulting cardiac conduction abnormalities

How much can SCh raise serum K^+ on average?

Use of SCh will increase serum K^+ by approximately 0.5.

Name 8 groups of patients who are at risk for hyperkalemia if SCh is administered.

1. Patients with existing hyperkalemia, such as those with renal failure. Check labs for the current day.
2. Patients having a peripheral neuropathy with clinically significant weakness.
3. Denervated patients, such as hemiparetics or paraplegics. Risk peaks 7 to 10 days from injury, but the duration of risk is unknown.
4. Patients with undiagnosed myopathy. (Note, however, that SCh should not be given to children because of several cases of Vtach death from hyperkalemia after inadvertent administration to children with undiagnosed myopathy.)
5. Patients with prolonged immobility (caution if > 2 weeks in-house immobile).
6. Trauma patients (massive crush injury). This would be most likely in patients with a high serum K^+ on initial trauma labs.
7. Burn patients. This group is prone to hyperkalemia from tissue injury during the first 24 hours (rare). This group is also prone to hyperkalemia after 48 hours from up-regulation of acetylcholine receptors.
8. Patients with closed-head injury because of risk of increasing intracranial pressure.

Is the above list worth referring to before you administer SCh?

Yes. Succinylcholine can kill, and it will be your fault.

How would you acutely treat symptomatic hyperkalemia?

Calcium chloride stat, one or two amps, preferably through central line

MALIGNANT HYPERTHERMIA

What is MH?	A genetic (autosomal dominant with variable penetrance) skeletal muscle abnormality that results in a hypermetabolic state from increased intracellular calcium in skeletal muscle
Is MH a common occurrence?	No. The incidence is approximately 1/40,000 adults. It is frequently fatal but responds to appropriate treatment 70% to 95% of the time.
What agents trigger MH?	1. Volatile anesthetic agents 2. SCh It can happen intraoperatively or postoperatively, and a history of previous uneventful anesthetics with volatile agents and/or SCh does not guarantee that a patient will not develop this.
What are the physical manifestations of MH?	1. Trismus/masseter muscle spasm or other skeletal muscle rigidity 2. Tachypnea
What might the monitors show in a case of MH?	1. Hypercapnia because of increased carbon dioxide production (early and sensitive) 2. Tachycardia/arrhythmias 3. Hypertension 4. Hyperthermia (can be a late and inconsistent sign, so use of this term in the name of this condition is not particularly accurate)
What 3 findings might the labs show?	1. Metabolic acidosis 2. Myoglobinuria 3. Disseminated intravascular coagulation
What are the 3 primary treatments for MH?	1. Discontinue any possible triggering agents.

2. Administer dantrolene sodium (2–3 mg/kg IV bolus).
3. Cool the patient, and provide supportive measures.

Sepsis and MH have several signs that overlap. How could you distinguish the two?

MH has the following:
1. Increasing minute ventilation requirements
2. Respiratory (not lactic) acidosis
3. Tissue breakdown products, consistent with rhabdomyolysis
4. Closer proximity to SCh or volatile agent (POD 1–2)

What would you, as an ICU resident, be expected to do if MH happened in your ICU?

Recognize the possibility, support vital signs, and call your supervisor and an anesthesia consult stat. You will need help from someone who has managed this life-threatening emergency before.

NARCOTICS AND RESPIRATORY DEPRESSION

What are the hemodynamic effects of sufentanil and fentanyl?

Bradycardia with minimal hypotension because of their vagotonic effects and depression of central sympathetic drive

What hemodynamic effect does morphine cause that fentanyl and sufentanil do not?

More significant hypotension. Morphine causes histamine release, leading to vasodilation.

What effects do narcotics have on ventilation?

Narcotics suppress ventilation in a dose-dependent manner. They blunt the normal response to a rise in CO_2 by depressing the respiratory centers in the brainstem. Fentanyl has a stronger effect than morphine.

Anesthesia for cardiac surgery is often based on the administration of large doses of opiate drugs, such as morphine, fentanyl, or sufentanil. Why?

Opiates provide adequate surgical analgesia with negligible direct myocardial depression when used with muscle relaxants and oxygen. Remember that the dosing here is thousands of micrograms of fentanyl.

Even so, this method of anesthesia carries risk for awareness, so in the OR, an amnestic (versed, valium, or scopolamine) is commonly added.

CONSCIOUS SEDATION FOR PROCEDURES

What two medicines are frequently used for conscious sedation?

Fentanyl and midazolam (some also employ Benadryl)

Why is conscious sedation dangerous?

Narcotics and sedatives have synergistic effects on respiratory depression, so you risk apnea or airway obstruction. Recall this chapter's first statement: "No one dies of acute pain, but patients die when they lose control of their airway, quit breathing, or suffer cardiac depression from the inappropriate use of some medications."

What doses are commonly used?

1. Fentanyl, 50 μg initially, then repeat twice. Remember, this is like giving approximately 5 mg of MSO_4 three times.
2. Midazolam, 1 to 2 mg.

What measures can be taken to minimize the risk of complications?

1. Document what you give to keep track of dosing.
2. Watch the patient. This sounds simple, but it is critical that you monitor respiratory status, O_2 saturation, and blood pressure during the procedure.

If respiratory compromise should occur, what steps can be taken?

Have the skills and the equipment to do the following *before* respiratory compromise occurs:
1. Perform a jaw thrust to open the airway. This is painful and may arouse the patient.
2. Insert an oral airway.
3. Bag the patient with O_2 and mask.
4. Intubate if necessary.

5

ICU Anatomy

AIRWAY AND BREATHING ANATOMY

ANATOMY OF THE MOUTH AND LARYNX

What is the Mallampati airway classification?

A method of airway assessment that correlates the difficulty of intubation with the extent to which the base of the tongue masks the pharyngeal structures

Describe the Mallampati airway classification.

Class I

Uvula, faucial pillars, and soft palate are visible.

Class II

Faucial pillars and soft palate are visible.

Class III

Only the soft palate is visible.

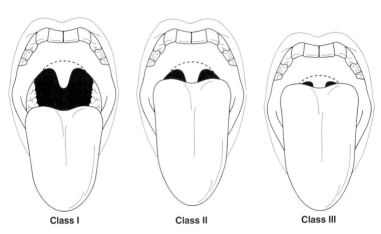

| Class I | Class II | Class III |

From Blackbourne LH. Advanced Surgical Recall. 2nd Ed. Philadelphia: Lippincott Williams & Wilkins, 2004:166–167.

What are the grades of glottic view during intubation?

Grade I	The entire glottis is seen.
Grade II	Only the posterior structures of the glottis are seen.
Grade III	Only the epiglottis is seen.
Grade IV	Even the epiglottis is not seen.

Where should the tip of a curved laryngoscope blade be placed?

In the vallecula (the space in between the tongue and the epiglottis)

Where should the tip of a straight laryngoscope blade be placed?

Under the epiglottis

How many types of cartilage are in the larynx?

9 (3 paired and 3 unpaired)

Name the 3 types of unpaired cartilage in the larynx.

1. Thyroid
2. Cricoid
3. Epiglottic

Name the 3 types of paired cartilage in the larynx.

1. Arytenoid cartilage
2. Corniculate cartilage
3. Cuneiform cartilage

Identify the following labeled structures:

A. Epiglottic tubercle
B. Vestibular fold (false chord)
C. Ventricle of the larynx
D. Vocal fold
E. Rima glottidis
F. Corniculate tubercle
G. Cuneiform tubercle
H. Piriform recess
I. Aryepiglottic fold
J. Greater horn of the hyoid bone

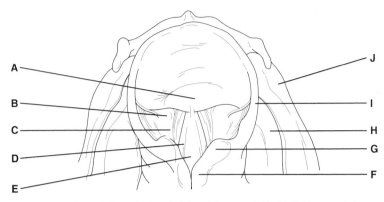

Adapted from Agur AMR, et al. Grant's Atlas of Anatomy. 10th Ed. Baltimore: Lippincott Williams & Wilkins, 1999.

What is the only complete cartilaginous ring in the larynx and trachea?	The cricothyroid cartilage
What important structure attaches the cricoid cartilage to the thyroid cartilage?	The cricothyroid membrane
How is an emergent airway obtained?	By performing a cricothryoidotomy (see Chapter 8, Bedside Procedures)

ANATOMY OF THE TRACHEA

Where does the trachea begin in relation to the spinal column?	Immediately below the cricoid cartilage (C6)
Where does the trachea end in relation to the spinal column?	At the carina (T5)
Why are right mainstem intubations much more common than left mainstem intubations?	The right mainstem is wider and comes off at a much straighter angle in relation to the trachea. This is also why aspirated objects are likely to lodge in the right middle or inferior bronchi.

Suppose you insert a bronchoscope and see the anatomy illustrated below at the carina. Which is the left mainstem bronchus, and which is the right mainstem bronchus?

A: right; B: left. Orientation is derived from the shape of the cartilaginous tracheal rings. They are incomplete posteriorly.

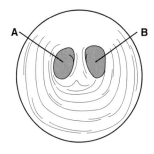

Describe the path of the innominate artery.

The innominate artery arises as the first major branch of the aorta, deep to the manubrium, and lies just anterior to the trachea and posterior to the left brachiocephalic vein.

Suppose a large arterial hemorrhage occurs around a cuffed tracheostomy tube that has been in for 3 weeks. What event has occurred?

Tracheo-innominate fistula

What should you attempt first to save the life of a person with a tracheo-innominate fistula?

Try to overinflate the tracheal cuff. Often, this can successfully tamponade the artery and act as a temporizing measure until the problem can be dealt with definitively.

What if overinflating the tracheal cuff is unsuccessful?

Reintubate the patient through the mouth, and apply digital pressure through the tracheostomy site, pulling the trachea up against the sternum to tamponade the artery.

ANATOMY OF THE BRONCHI

Name the 3 right upper lobe bronchi.	1. Apical segmental bronchus 2. Posterior segmental bronchus 3. Anterior segmental bronchus
Name the 2 right middle lobe bronchi.	1. Lateral segmental bronchus 2. Medial segmental bronchus
Name the 5 right lower lobe bronchi	1. Superior segmental bronchus (also called the apical lower bronchus) 2. Anterior basal segmental bronchus 3. Medial basal segmental bronchus 4. Posterior basal segmental bronchus 5. Lateral basal segmental bronchus
Name the 2 left upper lobe bronchi.	1. Apical posterior segmental bronchus 2. Anterior segmental bronchus
Name the 2 lingular bronchi.	1. Superior lingular segmental bronchus 2. Inferior lingular segmental bronchus
Name the 4 left inferior lobe bronchi.	1. Superior segmental bronchus (also called the apical lower bronchus) 2. Anteromedial basal bronchus 3. Posterior basal bronchus 4. Lateral basal bronchus

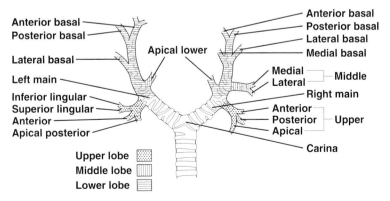

Adapted from Kaiser LR, et al. Mastery of Cardiothoracic Surgery. Baltimore: Lippincott Williams & Wilkins, 1997:5.

What is the lingula?

A small extension of the left upper lobe. It can be thought of as the left-sided equivalent of a middle lobe.

ANATOMY OF THE THORAX

Where is the costal line of pleural reflection in the following?

    Anteriorly?

Passes obliquely across the 8th rib.

    At the mid-axillary line?

Approximately the 10th rib

    Posteriorly?

Approximately at the 12th rib

Where does the neurovascular bundle run along the rib?

In the costal groove, in the inferior aspect of the rib. Therefore, when getting into the pleural space while performing tube thoracostomy or a thoracentesis, always go over the top of the rib.

In the setting of tension pneumothorax, where should one place the needle for decompression?

2nd intercostal space in the midclavicular line

ANATOMY FOR CIRCULATION AND VASCULAR ACCESS

ANATOMY OF THE NECK

Which small, U-shaped bone at the level of the body of vertebra C3 and just below the mandible serves as an attachment site for many neck muscles?

The hyoid bone

List the 7 neck muscles that insert on the hyoid bone.

1. Mylohyoid
2. Geniohyoid
3. Stylohyoid
4. Digastric
5. Omohyoid
6. Sternohyoid
7. Thyrohyoid

Which structures delineate the anterior triangle of the neck?

Anterior: the median line of the neck
Posterior: the anterior border of the sternocleidomastoid muscle
Base: the inferior mandible
Apex: the jugular notch

Which structures delineate the posterior triangle of the neck?

Anterior: the posterior border of the sternocleidomastoid muscle
Posterior: the anterior border of the trapezius muscle
Base: the middle third of the clavicle
Apex: the point where the sternocleido-mastoid and the trapezius muscles meet on the occipital bone

Identify the following labeled structures:

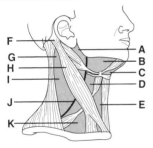

A. Parotid region
B. Digastric (submandibular) triangle
C. Submental triangle
D. Carotid triangle
E. Muscular triangle
F. Mastoid process
G. Apex of the posterior triangle
H. Sternocleidomastoid muscle
I. Occipital triangle
J. Cranial nerve (CN) XI: spinal accessory nerve
K. Supraclavicular triangle

What 3 structures run within the carotid sheath?

1. Carotid artery
2. Internal jugular vein
3. Vagus nerve

How does the internal jugular vein lie relative to the carotid artery?

Lateral to the carotid artery

What anatomical landmark can be used as a guide for the insertion point when performing an internal jugular stick?

The apex of the triangle formed by the sternal and clavicular heads of the sternocleidomastoid muscle

When performing an internal jugular stick, toward which nipple should you aim?

The ipsilateral nipple

Identify the following labeled structures:

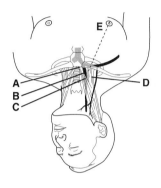

A. Clavicular head of the sternocleidomastoid muscle.
B. Internal jugular vein.
C. Apex of heads formed by sternal and clavicular heads of the sternocleidomastoid muscle (anatomic landmark for internal jugular stick).
D. Clavicular head of sternocleidomastoid muscle.
E. Dotted line depicting the direction of aspiration. This should be toward the ipsilateral nipple, holding the needle and syringe at a 45° angle to the neck.

SUBCLAVICULAR ANATOMY

What important clinical structure passes anterior to the anterior scalene muscle?

The subclavian vein

What important structure passes posterior to the anterior scalene muscle?

The subclavian artery

What is the anatomic relationship between the subclavian vein and the subclavian artery?

The subclavian vein is **anterior** and **inferior** to the subclavian artery.

Name the following labeled structures:

A. Sternal notch
B. Manubrium
C. First rib
D. Subclavian vein
E. Clavicle

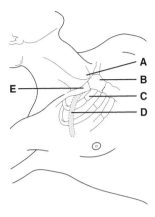

FEMORAL TRIANGLE

Describe the boundaries of the femoral triangle in the following areas:

    Superiorly?

The inguinal ligament

    Medially?

The medial border of the adductor longus muscle

    Laterally?

The medial border of the sartorius muscle

What forms the floor of the femoral triangle?

The adductor longus muscle, the pectineus muscle, and the iliopsoas muscle

What forms the roof of the femoral triangle?

The fascia lata

Name the 4 structures with the femoral triangle.

1. Femoral nerve
2. Femoral artery
3. Femoral vein
4. Lymphatics (contained within an empty space)

How can you remember these structures, thinking from *lateral* to *medial*?

Mnemonic: **NAVEL**
Nerve
Artery
Vein
Empty space containing
Lymphatics

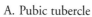

Identify the following labeled structures:

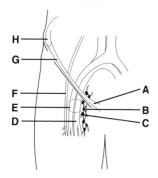

A. Pubic tubercle
B. Lymphatics
C. Empty space
D. Vein
E. Artery
F. Nerve
G. Inguinal ligament
H. Anterior superior iliac spine

Using surface anatomy, how would one locate the femoral artery?

The femoral artery can be found approximately 2 finger-breadths below the midpoint between the anterior superior iliac spine and the pubic tubercle.

When is the ability to locate the femoral artery particularly helpful?

When a pulse cannot be palpated

ANATOMY OF THE EXTREMITIES

ANATOMY OF THE LEG

Identify the following labeled arteries in the leg:

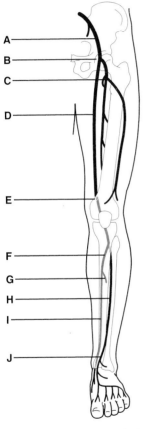

A. External iliac artery
B. Common femoral artery
C. Deep femoral artery
D. Superficial femoral artery
E. Popliteal artery
F. Tibial peroneal trunk
G. Peroneal artery
H. Anterior tibial artery
I. Posterior tibial artery
J. Dorsalis pedis artery

Adapted from Gay SB, et al. Radiology Recall. Baltimore: Lippincott Williams & Wilkins, 2000:202.

Identify the following labeled veins in the leg:

A. Plantar venous arch
B. Posterior tibial veins
C. Peroneal veins
D. Anterior tibial veins
E. Popliteal vein
F. Femoral vein
G. Deep femoral vein
H. Common femoral vein

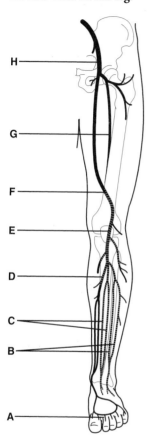

Adapted from Gay SB, et al. Radiology Recall. Baltimore: Lippincott Williams & Wilkins, 2000:204.

ANATOMY OF THE ARM AND HAND

What is the cubital fossa?	The hollow area on the anterior surface of the elbow
What is the lateral vein that runs along the forearm and eventually crosses over the shoulder through the deltopectoral groove?	The cephalic vein
What is the medial vein that runs along the forearm and eventually becomes the axillary vein?	The basilic vein
Which vein forms a communication between the basilic and cephalic veins in the cubital fossa?	The median cubital vein

Identify the following labeled structures:

A. Median cubital vein
B. Basilic vein
C. Cephalic vein
D. Brachial vein
E. Axillary vein
F. Subclavian vein
G. External jugular vein
H. Internal jugular vein
I. Brachiocephalic vein
J. Superior vena cava

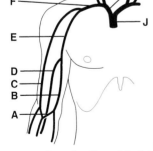

Adapted from Gay SB, et al. Radiology Recall. Baltimore: Lippincott Williams & Wilkins, 2000:200.

Identify the following labeled structures:

A. Thyrocervical trunk
B. Subclavian artery
C. Thoracoacromial artery
D. Axillary artery
E. Deep brachial artery
F. Brachial artery
G. Radial recurrent artery
H. Radial artery
I. Interosseous artery
J. Ulnar recurrent artery
K. Ulnar artery
L. Superficial palmar arch
M. Deep palmar arch
N. Common digital arteries

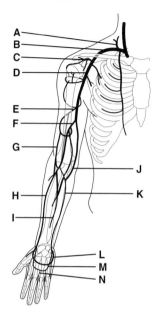

Adapted from Gay SB, et al. Radiology Recall. Baltimore: Lippincott Williams &Wilkins, 2000:199.

Identify the nerve that innervates each of the following regions:

A. Radial nerve
B. Median nerve
C. Ulnar nerve
D. Ulnar nerve
E. Radial nerve
F. Median nerve

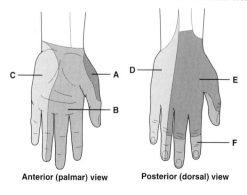

Anterior (palmar) view   Posterior (dorsal) view

Adapted from Blackbourne LH, et al. Anatomy Recall. Baltimore: Lippincott Williams &Wilkins, 2000:190.

ANATOMY OF THE HEAD AND BACK

ANATOMY OF THE SCALP AND SKULL

How can you remember the 5 layers that cover the scalp?	Mnemonic: **SCALP** **S**kin **C**onnective tissue **A**poneurosis **L**oose connective tissue **P**ericranium
What 8 bones make up the neurocranium?	Frontal bone Parietal bones (2) Temporal bones (2) Occipital bone Sphenoid bone Ethmoid bone
What are Kocher's point and Keen's point used for?	These are the anatomic sites used for performing a ventriculostomy.
Where is Kocher's point?	2 to 3 cm from the midline and 1 cm anterior to the coronal suture
How is a ventriculostomy performed at Kocher's point?	After making a burr hole at this site, a catheter is introduced approximately in the coronal plane and angled toward the medial canthus approximately 4 to 5 cm.
Where is Keen's point?	2.5 to 3 cm superior to and 2.5 to 3 cm posterior to the superior aspect of the pinna
Why would a ventriculostomy be performed at Keen's point?	This allows drainage from the trigone of the ventricle.

ANATOMY OF THE BRAIN

What are meninges?	Protective coverings over the surface of the brain

What are the 3 meningeal layers, from superficial to deep?	1. Dura mater 2. Arachnoid mater 3. Pia mater
What potential space is found between the dura mater and the arachnoid mater?	The subdural space
What causes a subdural hematoma?	Rupture of the cerebral veins as they pass from the brain surface into the venous (dural) sinuses
What artery provides the major blood supply to the dura mater?	The middle meningeal artery
The middle meningeal artery is a branch of which artery?	The maxillary artery
Damage to which artery causes an epidural hematoma?	The middle meningeal artery (most often damaged in fractures of the temporal bone)
Between what 2 layers does the blood collect in an epidural hematoma?	Between the dura and the skull
Between what 2 layers does the blood collect in a subdural hematoma?	Between the dura and the arachnoid
What is Battle's sign?	Bruising behind the ear; suggestive of a basal skull fracture

ANATOMY OF THE CRANIAL NERVES

What is the mnemonic to remember if the 12 nerves are sensory, motor, or both?	(CN I–XII) **S**ome **S**ay **M**arry **M**oney, **B**ut **M**y **B**rother **S**ays **B**ig **B**rains **M**atter **M**ore.

What is the function of CN I (olfactory nerve)?

Sense of smell

What is the function of CN II (optic nerve)?

Vision

What is the function of CN III (oculomotor nerve)?

Somatic motor fibers innervate the medial, inferior, and superior recti muscles; the inferior oblique muscle; and the levator palpebrae superioris muscle. Visceral motor fibers innervate the pupillary sphincter as well as the ciliary muscles.

What is the function of CN IV (trochlear nerve)?

Motor innervation of the superior oblique muscle, which moves the eye inferiorly and laterally in isolation and inferiorly in conjunction with the inferior rectus muscle

What is the function of CN V (trigeminal nerve)?

It supplies the muscles of mastication and tensors for the tympanic membrane and palate as well as afferent sensory fibers for the face and the anterior part of the scalp.

What is the function of CN VI (abducens nerve)?

Motor innervation to the lateral rectus muscle of the eye (abducts the eye)

What are the *motor* functions of CN VII (facial nerve)?

The muscles of facial expression, the stapedius muscle, the stylohyoid muscle, and the posterior belly of the digastric muscle

How can you remember the branches of CN VII?

To **Z**anzibar **B**y **M**otor **C**ar (from superior to inferior: temporal, zygomatic, buccal, mandibular, and cervical)

What are the *sensory* functions of CN VII?

Taste by the anterior 2/3 of the tongue, sensory innervation of the soft and hard palates, and the auricle and skin behind the ear

What is the function of CN VIII (vestibulocochlear nerve)?	Hearing and balance
What are the *motor* functions of CN IX (glossopharyngeal nerve)?	Innervation of the stylopharyngeus muscle (elevates the pharynx during swallowing and speech); innervation of the otic ganglion (secretomotor fibers to the parotid gland)
What are the *sensory* functions of CN IX?	Sensation to upper pharynx, tonsils, posterior 1/3 of tongue and taste, skin of external ear, portion of tympanic membrane; afferent input from the carotid body and sinus
What are the *motor* functions of CN X (vagus nerve)?	Innervation of some of the striated muscles of the pharynx and larynx; smooth muscle innervation of some of the thorax and abdominal viscera
What are the *sensory* functions of CN X?	Somatic innervation of the skin on the back of the ear, the external auditory meatus, the external tympanic membrane, and the pharynx; visceral innervation of the larynx, trachea, esophagus, thoracic and abdominal viscera, stretch receptors of the aortic arch, and chemoreceptors in the aortic bodies
What is the function of CN XI (spinal accessory nerve)?	Motor innervation to the sternocleidomastoid and trapezius muscles as well as motor innervation of the larynx and pharynx via the recurrent laryngeal and pharyngeal branches of CN X
What is the function of CN XII (hypoglossal nerve)?	All extrinsic and intrinsic muscles of the tongue, except for the palatoglossus (CN X)

ANATOMY OF THE SPINAL CORD

What are the 5 regions of the vertebral column, and how many vertebrae comprise each?

1. Cervical: 7 vertebrae
2. Thoracic: 12 vertebrae
3. Lumbar: 5 vertebrae
4. Sacral: 5 vertebrae
5. Coccygeal: 4 vertebrae

What is the distribution of the 31 pairs of spinal nerves that leave the spinal cord via the intervertebral foramina?

Cervical: 8 pairs
Thoracic: 12 pairs
Lumbar: 5 pairs
Sacral: 5 pairs
Coccygeal: 1 pair

How do the *cervical* spinal nerves exit the spinal canal relative to their corresponding vertebra (e.g., 2nd cervical nerve relative to the 2nd cervical vertebra)?

Above

How do the *thoracic* spinal nerves exit the spinal canal relative to their corresponding vertebra?

Below

Explain this phenomenon!

There are 8 cervical spinal nerves and only 7 cervical vertebra. Consequently, spinal nerve C8 exits below vertebra C7 and above vertebra T1. In turn, spinal nerve T1 exits below vertebra T1, and so on.

At what vertebral level should a lumbar puncture be performed?

L3-4 or L4-5, which is approximately midline between the iliac crests

What tissues, in order, are pierced?

After piercing the skin and superficial fascia, the needle passes through the supraspinous ligament and the ligamentum flavum before the dura mater and arachnoid mater to reach the CSF.

What are the most common contraindications to lumbar puncture?

Coagulation disorder (either endogenous or iatrogenic) and high CSF pressure (risk of fatal cerebellar or tentoral herniation; if there is any index of suspicion for increased CSF pressure, perform CT or MRI before proceeding)

Describe the location of the sensory dermatome associated with each of the following dorsal roots:

C6

Radial forearm and thumb ("six-shooter")

T4

Nipple

T10

Umbilicus

S3

Genitoanal region

Which muscles are supplied by ventral roots from:

C3 through C5

The diaphragm ("C3, 4, and 5 keep the diaphragm alive")

C8 through T1

Muscles of the hand

S1 through S2

Ankle plantar flexors

S3 through S5

Muscles of the bladder, anal sphincter, and genitals

6

ICU Radiology

GENERAL CONCERNS

Whose responsibility is it to interpret all films and studies done on an ICU patient?

You, the primary doctor, and your health care team have this responsibility. Review these studies with a more knowledgeable physician if you are not sure how to interpret them.

What is the single most important radiologic study in the ICU?

The CXR

What other imaging modalities are available to ICU patients?

Portable bedside evaluations include x-ray, ultrasound, and echocardiography. If the patient is stable for transport elsewhere in the hospital, helpful studies also include CT, MRI, nuclear imaging, and angiography.

ULTRASOUND

What are some uses for ultrasound examinations in the ICU?

Evaluating the gallbladder, kidneys, bladder, veins, and fluid collections

Does ultrasound have any other important uses in the ICU?

Ultrasound-guided aspiration of fluid collections, especially in the pleural space, can be very useful.

COMPUTED TOMOGRAPHY

What are 6 ways that CT scans may be used in critically ill patients?

1. Delineation of the state of the pulmonary parenchyma
2. Examination of the pleural spaces

3. Evaluation of perfusion of various organs
4. Examination of fluid collections and areas where free air has collected
5. Evaluation of contrast in various organs, such as the ureters and bowel
6. Detection of pulmonary embolism (CTPA)

Can a CT scan be dangerous to an ICU patient?

Yes

What are the 2 major reasons for this danger?

1. Any exam that requires a critically ill patient to leave the ICU can put that patient in danger. Unstable patients should be accompanied by you or another member of the health care team.
2. Any study requiring administration of IV or intra-arterial iodinated contrast material poses a risk of renal failure in patients with renal insufficiency (a common problem in ICU patients).

CONTRAST REACTIONS

What are *relative* contraindications to intravascular administration of contrast during a radiographic examination?

1. Previous allergic reaction to iodinated contrast material
2. Renal insufficiency

What kinds of allergic reactions to iodinated contrast material can occur?

Rash, hives, bronchospasm, or cardiac arrest

In a patient with previous allergic reactions to iodinated contrast, what can be done to reduce the risk of another allergic reaction?

Administer corticosteroids 2 hours before the procedure, or use nonionic contrast material.

What may happen to patients with chronic renal insufficiency if they are exposed to iodinated contrast?	Contrast-induced acute renal failure
How can the risk of contrast-induced acute renal failure be minimized?	Administer *N*-acetylcysteine before and after the contrast load, and aggressively hydrate the patient before administration of intravascular contrast.

CHEST RADIOGRAPHY

When should CXR be obtained for ICU patients?	Daily for most ICU patients, especially if the patient is intubated and has central lines, chest tubes, and other devices in place. A CXR should also be obtained every time a procedural change is made to a central line or chest tube (rewiring a line, water-sealing a tube, etc.)
What information can be gathered from a CXR?	A lot! Just to name a few: Tube, line, and device positions Rib and clavicle fractures Heart size and position Aortic arch shape Pulmonary artery fullness Pulmonary infiltrates (alveolar process) Pleural effusion Pneumothorax Peritoneal free air Gastric and upper abdominal bowel gas
Why are pleural effusions, pneumothoraces, and free air in the abdomen often difficult to discern on films taken in the ICU?	Most ICU films are exposed with the patient in the supine position.
What can be done if your suspicion for these pathologies is high?	Obtain either upright, lateral, or decubitus films. This will allow gas and fluid collections to "layer" against tissue

boundaries in a fashion that allows easy detection.

VERIFYING LINES AND TUBES

What lines and tubes should be visualized and identified on a portable CXR?

ETT, central line, Swan-Ganz (pulmonary artery) catheter, intra-aortic balloon pump, chest tube, NG suction tube, and feeding tube

Where should the ETT be located in an intubated patient?

Approximately 5 cm above the carina when the head and neck of an adult are in the neutral position

How much can this location vary with flexion or extension of the head and neck from a neutral position?

Approximately 2 cm in a caudad or cephalad position, respectively

What is the desired position for the tip of a central venous catheter inserted from a subclavian or internal jugular vein approach?

In the superior vena cava, with the tip positioned so that it lies in a parallel course with the lateral walls of the superior vena cava

Where is this identified on a frontal CXR?

Approximately 1 vertebral body caudal to the adjacent carina

What is the desired location for the tip of a Swan-Ganz catheter for hemodynamic monitoring?

Within the right or left main pulmonary artery. A more peripheral location can lead to pulmonary infarction, and a more central location can lead to cardiac arrhythmias and the inability to obtain satisfactory pulmonary capillary wedge pressures.

What is the desired location for the proximal tip of an intra-aortic balloon pump?

Just caudal to the left subclavian artery

Where is this identified on a frontal CXR?	Slightly cephalad to the adjacent carina
What is the desired position for the tip of an NG suction tube?	Ideally, beyond the inferior border of the CXR! If the stomach *can* be seen well, 10 cm of the tube should be past the gastroesophageal junction.
Where is the gastroesophageal junction located on a frontal CXR?	At the level of the left cardiophrenic angle
True or False: Inadvertent intubation of the trachea with an NG or feeding tube is prevented by a cuffed ETT.	False. Tracheal intubation is possible, and there may be no cuff leak. This is particularly true of feeding tubes. As a result, all tubes should have their positions verified radiographically before instilling material into them.
True or False: Patients are unable to talk if the trachea is intubated with a feeding tube.	False. Although patients may have some difficulty talking or have a weak voice, these are not reliable findings.

IMAGING PULMONARY PATHOLOGY

What is a pulmonary infiltrate?	A generic radiographic term that describes a white, poorly marginated density in the lung field that results from material that has permeated or infiltrated into the alveoli or adjacent tissues of the lung parenchyma
What are the potential causes of an infiltrate?	Pus, blood, or fluid
What is the differential diagnosis of a patient with acute respiratory insufficiency and a CXR demonstrating an alveolar process?	1. Atelectasis 2. Pulmonary edema 3. ARDS 4. Pneumonia (do not forget aspiration) 5. Contusion 6. Pulmonary hemorrhage

ATELECTASIS

What is the most common CXR abnormality in the ICU patient?

Atelectasis

What is atelectasis?

Collapse of a portion of the lung that results from incomplete alveolar distension. It can involve an entire lung or small peripheral pulmonary subdivisions. It is a common cause of fever in all patients.

Where is atelectasis most frequently seen in the ICU setting?

The left lung base

Describe the radiographic appearance of atelectasis.

With minimal atelectasis, the CXR is normal. More pronounced atelectasis produces consolidation and volume loss, predominantly in the bases of the lungs, obscuring the diaphragm and cardiac silhouette. Mediastinal shifting can occur toward the side of atelectasis.

What are the 5 most typical CXR findings of left lower lobe atelectasis?

1. Silhouetting of the diaphragm and the descending thoracic aorta: loss of definition of the margin of the left hemidiaphragm and the lateral border of the descending aorta
2. Increased density in the retrocardiac region on the lateral view
3. Depression of the left hilar structures
4. Shift of the mediastinum to the left hemithorax
5. Hyperlucency to the left upper lobe as it overexpands to compensate for the collapsed left lower lobe

PULMONARY EDEMA

What is pulmonary edema?	An abnormal amount of fluid in the extravascular tissues of the lung

What are some causes of pulmonary edema?

Use the mnemonic "A,B,C,D,E,F,G,H,I,J,K,L,M":
Aspiration of liquids (near drowning)
Brain injury/neurogenic causes
Cardiac decompensation (CHF)
Drug reaction (allergic reaction to drug)
Emboli (posttraumatic, fat emboli, PE)
Fluid overload
Gas inhalation
High altitude
Injury to the thorax
Junkie (IV drugs)
Kidney failure with fluid overload
Left atrial tumor obstructing pulmonary venous return
Miscellaneous (blood transfusion, rapid re-expansion of the lung)

What are the 7 characteristic CXR findings of pulmonary edema secondary to CHF?

Pulmonary edema produces:
1. Pulmonary vascular congestion (ill-defined vessels)
2. Cephalization (if patient is upright)
3. Peribronchial cuffing (thickening of the bronchial wall)
4. Increased interstitial marking (starts in the perihilar region)
5. Kerley B lines (pleural-based, horizontal interstitial lines)
6. Fluffy alveolar opacities
7. Pleural effusions

ACUTE RESPIRATORY DISTRESS SYNDROME

What are the radiographic features of ARDS as it develops?

1. The CXR is usually normal for 12 to 24 hours after the initiating insult.

2. After 24 hours, bilateral perihilar haze develops, followed by ill-defined linear opacities extending from the hilum consistent with interstitial edema.
3. By 36 hours, a diffuse, patchy pattern of alveolar edema is present.
4. Subsequently, little radiographic change occurs, unless the patient develops pneumonia.

PNEUMONIA

How is the diagnosis of pneumonia established radiographically in an ICU patient?

Radiographic findings are nonspecific but include:
1. Nondescript infiltrates
2. Acinar shadows
3. Air bronchograms
4. Segmental consolidation and asymmetric consolidation

PULMONARY CONTUSION

What are the radiographic characteristics of traumatic pulmonary contusion?

The CXR is usually abnormal on admission, but abnormalities can be delayed for up to 6 hours. Areas of contusion are frequently adjacent to solid structures. Opacities may appear as homogeneous air-space consolidation or as an irregular, coarse interstitial form.

When do these findings resolve?

They begin to resolve by 24 to 48 hours and are complete by 1 week.

PULMONARY EMBOLISM

Can PE be detected on a plain film?

Almost never. Rarely, a unilateral loss of pulmonary vasculature can be seen.

What 3 diagnostic tests are used to confirm a PE?

1. Pulmonary arteriogram: the gold standard, but invasive.

2. CTPA: can diagnose not only PE but also other causes of shortness of breath. It can reliably detect PE to the level of the segmental pulmonary artery but requires IV contrast.
3. V/Q scintigraphy: results are given as low, medium, and high probability. High probability scans usually indicate a PE.

What is an additional benefit of angiography?

You have the option to place an inferior vena cava (IVC) filter if the patient has a contraindication to anticoagulation.

What can limit accuracy of a V/Q scan?

Abnormalities on the CXR, such as atelectasis, effusion, and pneumonia

What are the benefits of a V/Q scan?

It can be used in patients with renal insufficiency and contrast allergies.

FAT EMBOLISM

What are the radiographic characteristics of fat embolism syndrome?

The CXR findings are nonspecific but usually normal early in the course. Patchy opacities subsequently develop that usually become diffuse within 72 hours. As in pulmonary edema, there is usually perihilar and basilar predominance with sparing of the apices.

How long does it take for these findings to resolve?

Usually 7 to 10 days

PNEUMOTHORAX

What are the findings of a pneumothorax on a CXR?

A thin, smooth, well-defined visceral pleural line outlined by air in the pleural cavity on one side and the lung parenchyma on the other side. No pulmonary markings can be detected peripheral to this line.

What radiographic "tricks" may be used to facilitate detection of a pneumothorax?	Either an upright CXR or a contralateral lateral decubitus film (i.e., left lateral decubitus CXR to rule out a right-sided pneumothorax) during expiration to facilitate detection of the pneumothorax. A CT scan of the chest is very useful in detecting a pneumothorax but requires a trip out of the ICU to radiology.

PLEURAL EFFUSION

What is a pleural effusion?	Fluid within the pleural cavity. It may be simple, as seen with CHF, or complex, as seen with infections (pus) or trauma (blood).
How can one determine whether a pleural effusion is free-flowing?	A decubitus CXR with the affected side dependent. If the fluid is free-flowing, there will be redistribution and layering of the fluid to the dependent portion of the pleural cavity.

IMAGING CARDIAC AND PERICARDIAL PATHOLOGY

What noninvasive imaging modalities are available to assess cardiac function, myocardial perfusion, and myocardial infarction.	1. Echocardiography 2. Multiple-gated acquisition study (MUGA) 3. Myocardial perfusion imaging
What can be assessed with echocardiography?	Chamber size, ejection fraction, wall thickening, segmental motion abnormalities, presence of mural thrombi, presence of ventricular aneurysm, and valve motion
What are the limitations of echocardiography?	The study is user dependent, and quality can frequently be limited by body habitus.
What does a MUGA study assess?	Utilizing ^{99m}Tc-labeled red cells and gated radioisotopic imaging during

diastole and systole, MUGA assesses ejection fraction, contractility, and segmental motion abnormalities.

How does myocardial perfusion imaging work?

Thallium-201 chloride is treated similarly to potassium by myocardial cells. It requires an intact Na^+/K^+-ATPase for uptake. Viable ischemic cells will demonstrate uptake after resolution of ischemia and thus provide the basis for stress thallium imaging.

What radiographic findings on CXR suggest the presence of a pericardial effusion that could cause pericardial tamponade?

1. The cardiac silhouette is triangular, globular, or flask-shaped.
2. Normal indentations of the cardiac border are lost.
3. Hilar shadows may be obscured.
4. Lateral CXR shows encroachment of the retrosternal space.
5. The pericardial stripe is widened to greater than 2 mm.
6. Separation of the epicardial and anterior mediastinal fat planes is visible on lateral projection (reported to be the most reliable sign and present in approximately half of cases).

What diagnostic test may be used to confirm the presence of a pericardial effusion if tamponade is suspected clinically?

1. Echocardiography: the preferred initial test
2. CT scan: if visualization is inadequate by echocardiography or more precise resolution is needed
3. Subxiphoid pericardial aspiration: for unstable patients

IMAGING AORTIC PATHOLOGY

List the CXR findings that suggest traumatic aortic transection.

1. Widened mediastinum
2. Tracheal deviation to the right (left wall of trachea to the right of T4 spinous process)

3. Deviation of the NG tube to the right (across T4 spinous process)
4. Loss of a distinct aortic knob or the lateral wall of the descending aorta
5. Left apical cap
6. Displacement of left and right paraspinal interfaces
7. Depression of left mainstem bronchus
8. Thickening of the right paratracheal strip
9. Left hemothorax

What is the usual location of injury in traumatic transection of the aorta?

At the aortic isthmus in the vast majority of cases (site of attachment of ligamentum arteriosum)

Do isolated first and second rib fractures correlate with traumatic aortic transection?

No. Although previously thought to indicate increased risk, such fractures are no longer used as an indication for arteriography.

If traumatic aortic transection is suspected, what is the diagnostic test of choice?

Aortography remains the study of choice; however, the role of CTA is expanding for this indication.

What role does CTA play in the diagnosis of aortic transection?

The role of CTA is in evolution. Some physicians recommend its use when the CXR is negative or equivocal. Any indication of aortic injury or mediastinal hematoma is an indication for aortography; this study is still considered to be the "gold standard." A CTA is a CT angiogram timed to film CT images showing maximum opacification of large arteries or veins.

What is the current study of choice to diagnose aortic dissection (as opposed to traumatic aortic transection)?

CTA or MRA

What is an MRA?	An MRA study is an MR angiogram timed to film MR images showing maximum opacification of large arteries or veins, depending on the indications.
How does MRA differ from CTA?	Besides the obvious difference of MRI versus CT modalities, MRA studies are performed with IV administration of gadolinium contrast material, a contrast agent that is safer in patients with renal insufficiency. Also, MRA studies are subject to more motion distortion, because they take longer to obtain than CTAs.

GASTROINTESTINAL AND ABDOMINAL RADIOGRAPHY

GASTRIC AND FEEDING TUBE PLACEMENT

How can you verify the position of a gastric or feeding tube?	By CXR (as described in above section) or, if specifically to look for the position of the tube, abdominal radiography.
Where should the tip of an NG tube be seen?	At least 10 cm caudal to the location of the gastroesophageal junction. Some NG tubes are fenestrated and have proximal sideholes. All sideholes of the NG tube should be positioned within the stomach.
Where should the tip of a postpyloric feeding tube be seen?	At least 10 to 12 cm into the small bowel
What should you do if you have any doubt about the location of the feeding tube?	You should not use the tube until you can confirm its location in the stomach or duodenum.

ABDOMINAL FREE AIR

What is the significance of free air (pneumoperitoneum) on chest or abdominal films?	Free air suggests perforation of a hollow viscus.

What are the best views to visualize free air?

Upright chest and/or left decubitus

What would an upright CXR demonstrate?

Free air accumulating underneath the diaphragm. This can be visualized as a translucent collection of air limited by the thin, curvilinear density of the diaphragm.

When is a left lateral decubitus film indicated?

When the patient is unable to sit upright

What would this study demonstrate?

Air between the right lobe of the liver and the abdominal wall

How long can free air be visualized on abdominal films after laparotomy?

Free air is usually absorbed by 7 to 10 days and is rare after 14 days.

EVALUATING ABDOMINAL FLUID AND ABSCESSES

What is the best study to determine the presence of free intraperitoneal fluid?

An ultrasound of the abdomen and pelvis is the preferred study, because it can be done portably in critically ill patients. A CT scan can demonstrate the presence of free intraperitoneal fluid but is more costly and requires the patient to make a trip to the radiology department.

What is the best study to evaluate for intra-abdominal abscess?

The best study is CT of the abdomen and pelvis with IV and oral contrast. This can be used to diagnose and treat with percutaneous drainage.

BOWEL OBSTRUCTION VERSUS ILEUS

What markings help to distinguish the small from the large bowel?

1. Valvulae conniventes (also called plicae circulares), which are thin, regular circumferential markings, are present in the small bowel and are described as a "stack of coins."

2. Haustra, which are thick, less regular markings that are not circumferential, are present in the large bowel.

What two clinical entities most commonly produce bowel distension?

Bowel obstruction and adynamic ileus

How can ileus and obstruction be differentiated on plain radiographs?

1. Ileus produces generalized distension of the entire intra-abdominal portion of the GI tract, with gas present from the stomach to the rectum. Localized inflammatory processes can produce a localized ileus with short segments of distended bowel.
2. Obstruction produces distension proximally with relative decompression distally.

What radiographs should be obtained when there is concern for small bowel obstruction?

Supine and upright or left lateral decubitus radiographs of the abdomen

What are the plain-film findings of small bowel obstruction of the abdomen?

1. Supine film: distended loops of small bowel arranged in a ladder-like configuration.
2. Upright or decubitus film: multiple small bowel air fluid levels, with the fluid level in one end of the loop differing in height from that in the other end of the loop. With a complete small bowel obstruction, there is usually an absence of gas within the colon and rectum.

If small bowel obstruction is suggested by plain radiographs, what should be determined, if possible, about the nature of the obstruction?

Partial small bowel obstruction should be distinguished from complete obstruction and from a closed-loop obstruction. Whereas partial small bowel obstruction may respond to NG decompression, complete and closed-loop obstruction can rapidly progress to bowel ischemia and necrosis.

Do normal films rule out small bowel obstruction?

No. Distended loops may be filled with fluid and may not be visualized on plain radiographs. Closed-loop obstruction in particular may not be distended with gas and may progress rapidly to necrosis.

What other radiographic studies may be useful in establishing the diagnosis of small bowel obstruction?

1. CT: may be useful if closed-loop obstruction is suspected. Bowel necrosis and the potential cause of obstruction may be identified.
2. Oral barium studies: may be useful in selected cases when differentiation of partial versus complete obstruction is difficult.
3. Enteroclysis: can be used instead of a routine follow-through to determine the level of obstruction and may actually relieve partial small bowel obstruction caused by adhesions.

When should barium be avoided?

If colonic obstruction cannot be excluded

What is enteroclysis?

A type of small bowel follow-through in which the barium is injected into the duodenum instead of taken orally. This study can identify well points of small bowel obstruction.

With colonic dilatation, either from obstruction or from ileus, what cecal diameter should raise the possibility of perforation?

When the diameter reaches 14 cm, the risk of perforation increases rapidly, and decompression must be undertaken.

In colonic obstruction, what radiographic test should be performed to identify the obstruction?

Water soluble enema. This test should be avoided, however, if in patients with signs of acute inflammation or perforation.

INTESTINAL ISCHEMIA

What plain radiographic findings suggest intestinal ischemia?	Findings are nonspecific but include: 1. General or localized distension 2. Thumbprinting (because of mucosal edema) 3. Bowel wall thickening 4. Pneumatosis intestinalis 5. Portal air

CHOLECYSTITIS

What is the initial radiographic study of choice when cholecystitis is suspected?	Ultrasound
What is the accuracy of ultrasound in the diagnosis of calculous cholecystitis?	Better than 90%
What ultrasound findings indicate calculous cholecystitis?	1. Stones in the gallbladder or biliary system 2. Sonographic Murphy's sign (pain from direct pressure of the transducer on the gallbladder) 3. Gallbladder distension 4. Sludge 5. Subserosal edema 6. Intraluminal membranes or debris 7. Pericholecystic fluid Both stones in the gallbladder or biliary system and sonographic Murphy's sign are very specific for cholecystitis!
When is radionuclide cholescintography useful in the diagnosis of cholescystitis?	In equivocal cases of calculous cholecystitis because of cystic duct obstruction or in cases of acalculous cholecystitis
What are some causes of falsely positive biliary scintigraphy scans?	Any condition that produces stasis and distension of the gallbladder, such as prolonged illness, hyperalimentation, recent postoperative state, and

hypoperfusion. In addition, hepatocellular dysfunction can produce false-positive scans.

How is the diagnosis of acalculous cholecystitis established?

Although the diagnosis is frequently based on clinical findings, serial sonograms demonstrating progressive changes in the gallbladder wall, especially the development of subserosal edema, are suggestive. Other findings may include intraluminal membranes, asymmetric wall thickening, and pericholecystic fluid.

What is the upper limit for the normal diameter of the common bile duct?

6 mm, unless the gallbladder has been removed or the patient is older than 60 years.

PANCREATITIS

What is the imaging study of choice in severe pancreatitis?

Dynamic CT. Bolus IV contrast is given while images are taken through the pancreas. This imaging study can identify pancreatic edema, fluid collections, areas of necrosis, and pseudoaneurysms.

GASTROINTESTINAL BLEEDING

What radiographic tests may be used to localize GI bleeding?

1. Angiography (with large amount of bleeding, ≈1 mL/min) for upper and lower GI bleeding
2. ^{99m}Tc-labeled RBC scan and ^{99m}Tc sulfur colloid scan (with intermediate or low levels of bleeding, ≈0.1 mL/min) for lower GI bleeding

How can common causes of upper GI bleeding be treated by angiographic intervention?

Bleeding ulcers, gastritis, and Mallory-Weiss tears may be treated with arterial embolization. Bleeding varices can be treated with a transjugular intrahepatic portal-caval shunt (TIPS) procedure.

IMAGING VEINS FOR DEEP-VEIN THROMBOSIS

How do you diagnose DVT? | Venography is considered to be the "gold standard," but duplex ultrasound is the initial study of choice.

Why is venography rarely performed? | Venography is invasive, requires contrast, involves radiation, can induce DVT, and is difficult to perform in an immobile ICU patient.

What is duplex ultrasound? | Duplex ultrasound is an ultrasound study that incorporates both "real-time" images and Doppler analysis in one study.

How accurate is duplex ultrasound for the diagnosis of acute DVT? | Duplex ultrasound has a high sensitivity and specificity (>90%) for diagnosing acute DVT in patients with unilateral, acute symptoms suspicious for DVT.

When is ultrasound less reliable in detecting DVT? | Iliac and pelvic thrombosis, asymptomatic patients, screening in orthopedic patients, and chronic DVT

7

Monitoring

BASICS OF HEMODYNAMIC MONITORING

What is the purpose of hemodynamic monitoring?

To assess volume status and CO

How reliable is an experienced physician's estimate of volume status based on examination of the patient?

About as reliable as flipping a coin. Studies have shown that even very experienced physicians are hardly better than 50% accurate in assessing a patient's volume status. Thus, invasive monitoring is needed if a patient's fluid status must be known.

What are 6 possible clinical indicators of poor perfusion?

1. Low urine output (probably the best clinical indicator of poor perfusion)
2. Low BP or decrease in arterial pressure with ventilator-delivered breaths
3. Cool extremities/sluggish capillary refill (>1 second)
4. Mental status changes (patients in the ICU have been sedated, making this assessment difficult)
5. Tachycardia
6. Dry mucous membranes/poor skin turgor

How much urine should a well-perfused adult produce?

0.5 to 1 mL/kg/hr

List 6 of the most fundamental monitoring devices for invasive and noninvasive monitoring.

1. BP cuffs
2. Oxygen saturation monitors
3. Arterial lines
4. Central venous lines
5. Swan-Ganz catheters (PACs)
6. The end-tidal CO_2 monitor

Name 3 possible sources of error in measuring BP with a sphygmomanometer.

1. Cuff size: using a cuff that is too small leads to falsely elevated pressures.
2. Low-flow states: leads to underestimation of BP.
3. Observer variability and error.

What is the proper size of a BP cuff bladder?

Length: 80% of the upper arm circumference
Width: 40% of the upper arm circumference

Are indirect measurements reliable in a hemodynamically unstable patient?

No. Every attempt should be made to establish direct intravascular recordings.

How reliable are the monitors used in the ICU?

The reliability of these monitors is far from perfect. Their reliability is determined partly by how well they were set up initially, including how well the lines and catheters are positioned and maintained. If some data do not fit with the other available information, then these data must be either disregarded or obtained in some other way to corroborate a finding that is an "outlier."

What are 3 sources of error when measuring pressures with a fluid-filled catheter (e.g., arterial line, Swan-Ganz catheter)?

1. Deterioration in frequency response: check for air or clot in the catheter/transducer.
2. Catheter whip: as the catheter is hit by the pulse wave, motion is generated, which increases systolic pressures and lowers diastolic pressures (i.e., the mean pressure is unaltered).
3. Catheter impact: caused by a valve hitting the catheter.

How do you test for catheter whip?

By inflating a BP cuff proximal to the line. As the cuff is deflated, the pressure that corresponds to the first pressure wave recorded on the arterial line is the true systolic pressure.

What 3 monitoring issues could arise that would kill your patient in the next 24 hours?

1. Access complications
2. PAC-induced arrhythmias
3. PA rupture caused by PAC

ARTERIAL BLOOD PRESSURE

What are the differences between arterial pressure measurements taken in the peripheral versus the central position?

The systolic pressure increases but narrows as the pressure wave moves toward the periphery. MAP remains relatively unchanged.

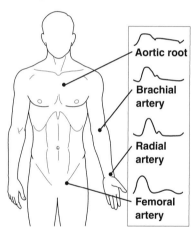

Aortic root

Brachial artery

Radial artery

Femoral artery

Adapted from Marino PM. The ICU Book. 2nd Ed. Philadelphia: Lippincott Williams & Wilkins, 1998:148.

What are 6 common locations for arterial lines?

1. Radial artery: most common, fairly safe and easy to maintain, small size
2. Femoral artery: second most common site, probably the safest
3. Brachial artery: most dangerous because of the risk of arm ischemia
4. Axillary artery: uncommon but occasionally useful, relatively safe

5. Temporal artery: uncommon and unsafe
6. Dorsalis pedis artery: uncommon but relatively safe

What are 5 possible complications associated with arterial lines?

1. Infection: very uncommon.
2. Distal embolization: relatively uncommon.
3. Occlusion of the artery: more common in smaller arteries.
4. Bleeding: be especially vigilant after a failed attempt at line placement, especially after femoral cannulation.
5. Air embolism.

What is purpose of the Allen's test?

To detect adequate collateral ulnar circulation before placing a radial arterial line. Normal response is 7 seconds or less.

Is the Allen's test useful?

In the absence of peripheral vascular disease, it is not an accurate predictor of hand ischemia. In fact, the results may be abnormal in approximately 3% of young, healthy individuals.

What is the pulse pressure?

Systolic BP - diastolic BP

What 5 conditions are associated with a wide pulse pressure?

1. Aortic regurgitation
2. Sepsis
3. Thyrotoxicosis
4. Arteriovenous fistula
5. Any high-output state

What condition is associated with a narrowed pulse pressure?

Hypovolemic shock

What is the MAP?

Diastolic BP + $\frac{1}{3}$ (systolic BP - diastolic BP)

Why is the MAP useful?

It is the true driving pressure of blood flow.

When measuring BP invasively, at what level should the transducer be placed?

At the level of the left atrium

What happens to the BP measurement if the transducer is not at heart level?

A transducer below heart level will falsely elevate the BP measurement. A transducer placed too high will falsely lower the BP measurement.

If one cannot maintain an arterial line in a patient, what are 3 alternative, less invasive techniques that can give information similar to that from the arterial line?

1. Mechanical BP cuff that cycles on a regular basis
2. Oxygen saturation monitor
3. End-tidal volume CO_2 monitor (if the patient is intubated), which can give a very good approximation of the arterial P_{CO_2} (the end-tidal CO_2 is usually $\sim$5 mm Hg lower than the arterial CO_2)

PULSE OXIMETRY

What does a pulse oximeter measure?

Peripheral arterial blood oxygen saturation

What 4 advantages does pulse oximetry have over conventional arterial blood gases?

1. Continuous monitoring
2. Noninvasive
3. Less morbid
4. Less expensive

How does a pulse oximeter work?

It measures the reflections of light of alternating intensities (arterial blood) at two different wavelengths. Oxygenated and deoxygenated Hgb reflect light more effectively at lower and higher wavelengths, respectively.

What 6 conditions can lead to erroneous recordings of pulse oximetry?

1. Significant hypoxemia
2. Dyshemoglobinemias
3. Hypotension
4. Anemia
5. Dark skin pigmentation
6. Use of fingernail polish

How do the following affect the affinity of oxygen for Hgb?

All will favor decreased oxygen affinity and increased oxygen delivery. Thus, all shift the oxygen dissociation curve to the right.

    Decreased pH

    Increased temperature

    Increased 2,3-DPG

    Increased P_{CO_2}

INTRACRANIAL PRESSURE MONITORING

What is CPP, and what does it measure?

Cerebral perfusion pressure (MAP - ICP). Represents the pressure gradient driving cerebral blood flow.

What is the optimal level for CPP, and why is it important?

CPP should be maintained at greater than 70 to 80 mm Hg. This significantly reduces mortality after severe head injury.

How can ICP be monitored, and what is the normal value?

With an ICP monitor, otherwise known as a "bolt." Normal values are from 0 to 10 mm Hg.

What are two indications for ICP monitoring?

1. Severe head injury (GCS = 3–8; see Chapter 9 for a full description of the GCS)
2. Moderate head injury (GCS = 9–12) with abnormal CT scan or unable to follow with serial neurological examinations (anesthetized or sedated)

CENTRAL VENOUS PRESSURE AND ACCESS

What are the 2 functions of central venous lines?

1. CVP monitoring
2. Administration of hypertonic or vasoactive substances that cannot be administered safely in peripheral veins, such as parenteral alimentation and vasoconstrictors (dopamine)

How is the CVP value useful?

As a rough estimate of volume status

What is the normal range of CVP?

0 to 8 mm Hg

How should CVP be measured in patients breathing spontaneously versus patients on ventilators?

The higher pressure should be used in patients who are spontaneously breathing, while the lower pressure should be used in patients who are on mechanical ventilation, because these values correspond with end expiration.

What is the significance of end expiration?

End expiration is when extravascular pressures are closest to zero. Remember that in a spontaneously breathing patient, inspiration is generated by negative intrathoracic pressure, whereas in a patient on mechanical ventilation, breaths are delivered though positive pressure.

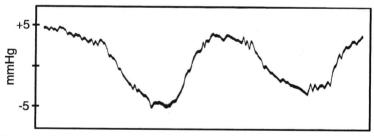

Respiratory variation in central venous pressure. From Marino PM. The ICU Book. 2nd Ed. Philadelphia: Lippincott Williams & Wilkins, 1998:167.

What are 4 locations in which one can gain access to the central venous circulation?

1. Internal jugular vein: commonly used for monitoring
2. Subclavian vein: most commonly used for parenteral alimentation
3. Femoral vein: most commonly used in code situations or states of hypovolemia

4. Supraclavicular subclavian vein: an uncommonly used but very reliable line

List the 4 potential central venous access points, from safest to most dangerous, during the acute phase of placement.

1. Femoral vein (safest)
2. Supraclavicular subclavian vein
3. Internal jugular vein
4. Infraclavicular subclavian vein (most dangerous)

What are 8 complications associated with central line placement?

1. Pneumothorax
2. Inadvertent arterial puncture
3. Bleeding from venous puncture sites
4. Vein thrombosis
5. Malposition of catheters
6. Infection
7. Mediastinal hemorrhage from great vessel injury
8. Venous air embolism

Which is the only central line that should be used in states of significant hypovolemia, such as trauma and code situations?

The femoral venous line

Describe the 2 main types of catheters that can be placed for central venous access.

1. Multilumen catheter (triple-lumen): has 3 channels, usually 16- to 18-gauge, that can be used for different infusate solutions.
2. Introducer catheter (cordis): large-bore (8- to 9-French) catheters with side-arm infusion ports; can be used to introduce smaller catheters (triple-lumen) or for infusion at rapid rates.

SWAN-GANZ CATHETERS

What is the ultimate indicator of volume status?

LVEDP

What is the best means to estimate LVEDP in the ICU?

Via a Swan-Ganz catheter that estimates left-sided pressures by right heart catheterization

What is a Swan-Ganz catheter?

A PAC with a balloon on the tip to allow the blood flow to carry it from the superior vena cava through the heart to the PA. It has ports for pressure measurements and blood sampling from the right atrium and the PA.

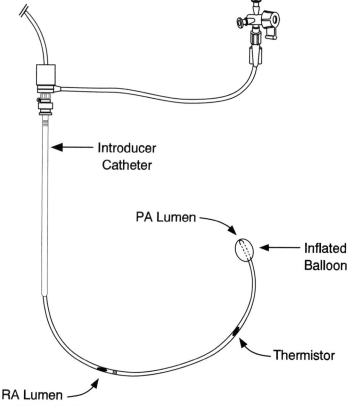

From Marino PM. The ICU Book. 2nd Ed. Philadelphia: Lippincott Williams & Wilkins, 1998:155.

Describe the 5 different ports and connections of a Swan-Ganz catheter.

1. Distal injection port: for PA pressure measurements and aspiration of blood for mixed venous oxygen measurements.
2. Balloon inflation valve: used to inflate and deflate the balloon.
3. Proximal injection port: used for CVP monitoring and fluid infusion.
4. Extra injection port: present on some models for continuous infusion of fluids.
5. Thermistor connector: plugs into bedside CO monitor.

What 5 measurements can be directly obtained with the Swan-Ganz catheter?

1. Central venous RAP
2. PA pressures
3. PCWP (left atrial approximation)
4. CO (via the thermodilution [TD] technique)
5. Mixed venous oxygen saturation

What are the 3 indications for placement of a Swan-Ganz catheter?

1. Uncertainty regarding fluid status, especially when either the heart or the kidneys are not working optimally
2. When right-sided cardiac pressures do not correlate with left-sided cardiac pressures
3. To assess left ventricular function when this function is unknown

List 4 situations in which right-sided cardiac pressures do not correlate with left-sided pressures.

1. Left ventricular dysfunction
2. Pulmonary hypertension
3. Right heart failure
4. Cardiac valvular dysfunction

Describe the characteristic pressure waveforms encountered on insertion of a Swan-Ganz catheter and the distances on the Swan.

RA: CVP tracing with baseline pressure oscillations at approximately 5 to 25 cm

RV: pulsatile ventricular systolic waveform with baseline diastolic waveform close to zero at approximately 25 cm

PA: elevated diastolic pressure (6–12 mm Hg) with a notch representing the PA valve closure in the waveform at approximately 35 cm

Wedge: dampened waveform with elevated baseline at approximately 40 cm

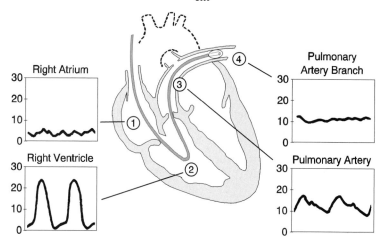

Pressure waveforms encountered during insertion of pulmonary artery catheter. From Marino PM. The ICU Book. 2nd ed. Philadelphia: Lippincott Williams & Wilkins, 1998:157.

What does it mean to "wedge" a Swan-Ganz catheter?	The catheter has been advanced until the balloon occludes the PA segment and a downstream PCWP is obtained.
What is the normal (mean) RAP (CVP)?	0 to 8 mm Hg, venous
What is the normal RV pressure?	15 to 30 (systolic)/0 to 8 (diastolic) mm Hg
What is the normal PA pressure?	15 to 30 (systolic)/3 to 12 (diastolic) mm Hg
What is the normal (mean) PCWP?	3 to 12 mm Hg

What is the characteristic Swan-Ganz tracing in acute mitral regurgitation?	A V-wave in the wedge tracing, representing regurgitant flow into the left atrium
What is the characteristic finding in acute ventricular septal rupture?	An oxygen saturation step-up in the PA as compared with the right atrium
What Swan-Ganz tracings are suggestive of a hemo-dynamically significant pulmonary embolus?	Elevated right heart pressures (CVP, PAS, PAD) with normal wedge pressure
What pressure profile is seen in cardiac tamponade?	Equalization of all central pressures (CVP, PAD, PCWP); high value = 30 cm H_2O
What 4 complications may occur with a Swan-Ganz catheter?	1. Ventricular ectopy: caused by irritation of the bundle of His fibers at the RV outflow tract during placement. 2. PA rupture: most common presenting symptom is acute hemoptysis; high mortality rate. 3. Pulmonary infarction. 4. Right bundle branch block: may cause complete heart block in the presence of pre-existing LBBB.
How do you decrease the likelihood of PAC-induced arrhythmias?	Consider use of a pacing catheter if LBBB is present. Do not let the PAC remain in the right ventricle.
How can you decrease the likelihood of PA rupture and pulmonary infarction?	Advance the catheter only with the balloon inflated. Avoid wedging the catheter frequently. Avoid balloon hyperinflation (no more than 1.5 mL). Do not leave the balloon inflated after wedging. Do not wedge if not necessary.

Do not wedge while on cardiopulmonary bypass (catheter is cold and stiff).

Do not leave the catheter sitting outside the mediastinal shadow on CXR.

What 4 factors predispose patients to PA rupture with placement of a PA (Swan-Ganz) catheter?

1. Pulmonary hypertension: difficult to obtain wedge.
2. Advanced age.
3. Coagulation at the catheter tip: difficult to obtain good wedge tracing.
4. Cardiac operations: catheter gets pushed in further during manipulation of the heart and becomes stiff during systemic cooling.

If the Swan-Ganz catheter does not wedge, what can be used to approximate the LVEDP?

PAD pressure

When does PAD not correlate with the wedge pressure?

In severe lung disease with pulmonary vascular changes

How do you calculate the SVRI?

$$SVRI = \frac{(MAP - CVP)}{CI} \times 80$$

Remember Ohm's law: resistance = pressure/flow.

What is the PCWP?

The downstream pressure against the tip of the catheter once it has been "wedged" in place in the distal PA. The wedge pressure reflects the left atrial pressure and, therefore, the LVEDP (i.e., the filling pressures of the left side of the heart).

How is the PCWP useful?

It helps to determine the volume status of the patient (i.e., PCWP > 12 represents volume overload, PCWP < 3 represents volume depletion).

List 3 situations when the PCWP not a good indicator of left heart filling pressures?

1. Mitral valve dysfunction: stenosis, regurgitation
2. High PEEP
3. Pulmonary veno-occlusive disease

How do PCWP, CO, and SVR change in various situations involving shock?

See Table 7-1.

Table 7-1

	PCWP	**CO**	**SVR**
Septic shock	Down	Up	Down
Hypovolemic shock	Down	Down	Up
Neurogenic shock	Down	Down	Down
Cardiogenic shock	Up	Down	Up

How does the Swan-Ganz catheter help to detect early myocardial ischemia?

Myocardial ischemia causes a decrease in left ventricular compliance. Consequently, an elevated PCWP or development of prominent A or V waves on the PCWP tracing may be early signs of ischemia.

A Swan-Ganz catheter is placed via the right subclavian vein. All pressure measurements are satisfactory, but the PA pulse-wave recording is continuously dampened. What might one find on CXR to explain this annoying problem?

The right angle turn at the junction of the right subclavian vein with the superior vena cava often produces a kink in the Swan-Ganz catheter at this point, producing a dampened waveform on the monitor.

METHODS TO DETERMINE CARDIAC OUTPUT

Name the 5 determinants of CO.

1. Heart rate (HR) and rhythm
2. Preload
3. Afterload
4. Contractility
5. Compliance

What is the CI?

Cardiac index: CO/BSA (m²); normal CI is 2.5 to 4 L/min/m².

Why is the CI used?

To normalize CO for different body sizes

What is the TD method of measuring CO?

Injecting a known quantity/temperature of fluid into the RA and measuring the bolus transit time

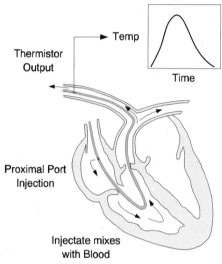

Measuring cardiac output using thermodilution. From Marino PM. The ICU Book. 2nd Ed. Philadelphia: Lippincott Williams & Wilkins, 1998:179.

When determining CO by the TD technique, what does the area under the curve represent?

The change in temperature of the injectate over time. There is an inverse relationship between the area under the curve and the output (i.e., a larger area indicates a lower output).

What are 6 pitfalls of the TD method?

1. Overestimation with low output states: tricuspid regurgitation (outputs < 2.5 L/min average a 35% overestimation)
2. Improper technique: slow injection, incorrect volume

3. Intracardiac shunts (ventricular septal defect), extracardiac shunts (arteriovenous fistula)
4. Cold patients
5. Distal tip of the catheter in the main PA
6. Changes in blood viscosity: anemia or polycythemia

How does the injectate volume affect the CO as measurement by the TD technique?

The fundamental idea is that a higher CO will dilute the cold injectate more than a low CO will. Injection of the wrong volume will produce an abnormal curve. For example, a lower volume than programmed will produce a falsely elevated CO, and a larger volume will produce a falsely low measurement.

For a postoperative cardiac patient, what CI indicates a severe reduction in cardiac function?

Less than 2.0 L/min/m²

What valvular lesions will produce errors in CO determination?

Tricuspid and pulmonic valvular regurgitation (will falsely increase the area under the curve, thus providing a falsely decreased CO)

What is the Fick equation?

A technique to estimate CO when a PAC is not present. The equation itself is:

$$CO = \frac{V_{O_2}}{8.5\,(Ca_{O_2} - Cv_{O_2})}$$

where Ca_{O_2} is arterial oxygen content and Cv_{O_2} is mixed venous oxygen content.

Name 3 pitfalls in estimating CO with the Fick equation

1. Intracardiac shunts.
2. Oxygen consumption is difficult to measure (generally estimated at 125 mL/min).
3. Incorrect data (e.g., estimated arterial partial pressure of oxygen

[PaO$_2$] vs. measured): this is a problem with some blood gas machines that estimate the saturation based on a nomogram for arterial blood.

What indicator does the Fick principle use?	Oxygen consumption

ICU FORMULAS AND NORMAL VALUES

VO$_2$?	$= CO \times 13.4 \times Hgb \times (SaO_2 - SmvO_2)$
Normal range of VO$_2$?	250 mL/min. Add 13% for each 1°C increase in temperature. Remember: coefficients of oxygen utilization range in various vascular beds from 0.6% to 0.85% of delivered oxygen. Hence, a minimal oxygen delivery of 500 mL/min is required for a 70-kg patient with a basal oxygen consumption of 250 mL/min and an additional 50 mL/min because of stress (i.e., $300 = 0.6 \times 500$).
DO$_2$?	$= CO \times 13.4 \times Hgb \times SaO_2$
Normal range of DO$_2$?	900 to 1,100 mL/min
Arteriovenous oxygen difference?	$CaO_2 - CvO_2 = (1.34 \times [Hgb] \times SaO_2 + 0.0031 \times PaO_2) - (1.34 \times [Hgb] + SvO_2 + 0.0031 \times PvO_2)$
CO?	$= \dfrac{VO_2}{8.5\,(CaO_2 - CvO_2)}$ (i.e., Fick equation) $= HR \times$ stroke volume $= HR \times$ (end-diastolic volume $-$ end-systolic volume)
Normal range of CO?	4 to 6 L/min
Normal range of CI? (CO/BSA)	2.5 to 4.5 L/min/m^2

MAP?

Diastolic BP + $\frac{1}{3}$ (systolic BP − diastolic BP)

Normal range of MAP?

60 to 95 mm Hg

Stroke work?

Stroke volume (SV) × MAP

SVR?

Remember Ohm's law:
Resistance = pressure/flow

$$\text{hence, SVR} = \frac{80 \; (\text{MAP} - \text{CVP})}{\text{CO}}$$

Normal range of SVR?

$1{,}200 \pm 300 \text{ dyne} \cdot \text{sec} \cdot \text{cm}^{-5}$

Normal range of SVRI?

$2{,}100 \pm 500 \text{ dyne} \cdot \text{sec} \cdot \text{cm}^{-5} \cdot \text{m}^{2}$

PVR?

80 × (mean PA pressure − mean left atrial pressure)/CO

Normal range of PVR?

$100 \pm 50 \text{ dyne} \cdot \text{sec} \cdot \text{cm}^{-5}$

What is the normal PVRI?

$170 \pm 70 \text{ dyne} \cdot \text{sec} \cdot \text{cm}^{-5} \cdot \text{m}^{2}$

What are Wood units?

Used in heart transplant evaluations:

$$\frac{\text{PA (mean)} - \text{PCWP (mean)}}{\text{CO (normal} < 4)}$$

Remember, the SVR, PVR, and so on are calculated numbers; that is, errors in pressure or CO measurements will affect these numbers. For example, a patient with a normal CO of 3.0 L/min and significant tricuspid regurgitation may have a measured CO of 6.0 L/min. This would halve the calculated SVRI and may result in inappropriate treatment.

8   Bedside Procedures

GENERAL PROCEDURES

SKIN CLEANSING

What is the difference between antiseptics and disinfectants?

Antiseptics are agents that reduce microflora on the skin; **disinfectants** are agents that reduce microflora on inanimate objects.

What are some commonly used antiseptic agents?

Alcohol (50%–90% ethyl alcohol) or isopropyl alcohol
Iodine (tincture) or povidone-iodine (Betadine)
Chlorhexidine gluconate (Hibiclens)
Hexachlorophene (pHisoHex)

How long should Betadine be left on the skin?

2 minutes. Iodophor is a water-soluble complex of iodine and a carrier molecule. The iodine is released slowly from the carrier molecule.

Why is Betadine no longer used in some institutions?

Betadine skin prep is associated with more bloodstream infections than chlorhexidine prep. Bacteria has even been cultured in Betadine, and allergy and irritation are common.

What is the disadvantage of an alcohol scrub?

An alcohol scrub has no detergent action and therefore does not work well on dirty skin, which is common in trauma patients

Should one shave the procedure site before cleansing?

No! Shaving abrades the skin and actually increases bacterial colonization. Use clippers if necessary.

LOCAL ANESTHETICS

What are the benefits of local anesthesia?

Analgesia/anesthesia without the risk of general anesthesia

Name 3 methods of administering local anesthetics.

1. Spinal
2. Regional
3. Locally administered

Name 5 commonly used local anesthetics and their maximum dose.

1. Procaine: 14 mg/kg
2. Lidocaine: 7 mg/kg
3. Mepivacaine: 7 mg/kg
4. Tetracaine: 1.5 mg/kg
5. Bupivacaine: 3 mg/kg

What local anesthetic is sufficient for most bedside procedures?

0.5% to 1.0% lidocaine

What techniques can be used to limit unwanted side effects?

Add a vasoconstrictor to slow absorption, and avoid inadvertent vascular injection by preinjection aspiration.

What 4 areas should never be injected with solutions containing epinephrine?

1. Digits
2. Ears
3. Tip of the nose
4. Penis
May cause local ischemic necrosis.

VASCULAR ACCESS

SELDINGER TECHNIQUE

Describe the 5 steps involved in the Seldinger technique of central venous or arterial cannulation.

    Step 1

A small-bore needle (20 gauge) is introduced percutaneously into a patent vessel.

    Step 2

A thin, flexible wire (J-wire) is introduced into the hub of the needle, and the needle is backed out over the wire.

Step 3	A dilator or series of dilators are passed over the guide wire and into the vessel.
Step 4	The vascular catheter is placed over the guide wire.
Step 5	The guide wire is removed and the catheter is secured into place.
Which of the 5 steps in the Seldinger technique has the potential for disaster?	All 5 can cause serious morbidity and even mortality.

CENTRAL VENOUS CATHETERIZATION

What are the 2 most common central venous access sites?	The IJ and subclavian veins
Which of these 2 vessels usually has the larger diameter?	The subclavian vein
What are the 3 most common complications associated with central venous cannulation through either of these sites?	1. Pneumothorax 2. Hemothorax 3. Arterial puncture
Which route of access is the shortest path to the atriocaval junction?	The right IJ vein (~12 cm)
Which route of access is the longest path to the atriocaval junction?	The left subclavian vein (~16 cm)
Describe the landmarks used and the path taken by the needle in the infraclavicular subclavian vein cannulation.	1. The probing needle is inserted into the skin (bevel up) approximately 2 cm caudal to the medial and middle third of the clavicle. 2. With the opposite hand, march the needle just beneath the clavicle in a plane parallel to the anterior chest wall.

3. Aiming toward the sternal notch, slowly advance the needle while gently withdrawing the syringe plunger.

Why does one need to be aware of the bevel position?

After the vein is cannulated, the bevel is turned down 90° to allow the guide wire to head down the SVC.

How can you know the location of the bevel once you have punctured the skin?

By aligning the bevel of the needle with the numbers on the syringe before you start the procedure. Once the vein is entered, the numbers on the syringe can be turned toward the patient's feet.

What is the relationship between the IJ vein and the carotid artery within the carotid sheath?

The IJ vein runs posterior and lateral to the carotid artery until it crosses anterior to the artery near its termination into the brachiocephalic vein.

Describe the landmarks used and the path taken by the finder needle during IJ vein central cannulation.

1. Palpate the carotid artery, and gently retract it medially.
2. Insert the finder needle at the apex of the triangle created by the two heads of the sternocleidomastoid (SCM) attaching to the clavicle.
3. Direct the needle inferior and lateral to the medial aspect of the clavicular head, aiming toward the ipsilateral nipple.

How deep should one pass the finder needle before withdrawing?

3 to 4 cm. If you do not encounter venous blood at this depth, you are in the wrong plane. Remove the needle, reassess the landmarks, and start over.

What should be done if the wire does not pass smoothly into the vein?

BEWARE! The wire must pass with minimal resistance over its entire length; otherwise, improper placement is likely. **Never advance the wire under resistance.** Remove the wire completely, and attempt recannulation.

If the wire is bent or deformed in any way that may prevent its passage through the needle or catheter, open a new kit, and use a new wire.

Why should your patient be on a cardiac monitor during central venous cannulation?

The guide wire may cause ectopy if it touches the heart.

When threading your catheter, what must you remember about the wire?

Never let go of it! Either hold it at the entrance to the skin, or once the catheter tip has passed, hold the distal wire end.

Once the catheter is thought to be in place, what should be done to confirm the procedure?

CXR

What do you look for with CXR in this setting?

Correct catheter placement. The tip of the venous catheter should be in the SVC at the cavoatrial junction. Also, inspect the film closely for evidence of pneumothorax.

When placing a venous cannula, how can the clinician ensure proper placement in the vein and not the artery?

1. The blood returning should be dark, without evidence of pulsatile flow.
2. The cannula can be transduced to monitor the venous waveform.
3. An ABG can be performed on the sample.

What should you do if you encounter arterial blood during an attempted venous cannulation?

Remove the needle immediately, apply **gentle** pressure for 10 minutes, and observe for signs of hemodynamic compromise.

What is the most common early complication of subclavian or IJ central venous line insertion?

Pneumothorax

What study should be obtained in every patient after subclavian or IJ central venous line insertion?

CXR. Because it is often impossible to obtain upright films in ICU patients, however, pleural air may not collect in the apex of the lung. Also, check the film along the anteromedial border of the mediastinum and in the subpulmonic recess.

You place a central venous line via the right subclavian vein. The guide wire and catheter seem to pass correctly, but slight resistance is encountered at approximately the 15-cm mark on the catheter. Venous blood is easily aspirated from it, however. The patient reports pain in the region of the right ear. What malposition of the venous catheter might be noted on CXR?

Passage of the venous line cephalad into the right IJ vein

How can this problem be corrected?

By trying to rewire the line with use of fluoroscopy, by holding pressure on the neck while advancing the wire, or most commonly, by inserting the line elsewhere

What is a potential complication of even briefly disconnecting a large-bore central venous line?

Air embolism

What can be done if a venous air embolism is suspected?

Place the patient left-side down, and attempt to aspirate the air from the venous line.

What rhythm disturbance may ensue if a newly placed central venous line extends into the right ventricle?

Ventricular tachycardia

When a central venous line must be replaced because of suspected infection and no new site is available, what procedure might be used?

A new catheter can be placed at the same site over a guide wire passed through the lumen of the old catheter.

How do you avoid septic complications from central lines?

1. Follow strict sterile procedure when placing lines.
2. Do not allow lines with dextrose (sugar water) in them to be violated.
3. If infection is a concern, rewire the lines, culture the tips, and rotate sites if these tips grow bacteria.
4. Always consider the line as a potential source when the patient is becoming septic (confused, febrile, etc.).

What should you do if air is aspirated during venous cannulation?

Terminate the procedure, and get a CXR to rule out pneumothorax before making further attempts.

Should you attempt cannulation of the contralateral side while waiting for a CXR?

NEVER! This is a recipe for disaster.

What do you do with a patient who becomes acutely, hemodynamically labile following central line placement?

Assume tension pneumothorax, and treat as such. Perform needle decompression, and do not wait on CXR.

What is the big deal about the Trendelenburg position?

The "head-down" position is thought to increase the venous pressure and, therefore, the diameter in the subclavian and jugular veins. This position also allows one to prevent and/or treat the dreaded venous air embolism.

What is the pathophysiology of venous air embolism?

Negative intrathoracic pressure can suck air into an unoccluded catheter port. As little as 5 mL of air can obstruct the pulmonary outflow tract and cause cardiac arrest.

What are the 3 steps in managing a patient in cardiac arrest with suspected air embolism?

1. Steep Trendelenburg and left lateral decubitus position to trap the air in the RV apex.
2. Aspirate while advancing the catheter into the right ventricle. A precordial thump may dislodge air trapped in pulmonary outflow tract. Maintain the patient in the same position until the air is dissolved into the blood.
3. Document by serial CXR.

What is a last-ditch resort for the hemodynamically labile patient with suspected air embolism?

Thoracotomy and open cardiac message to force air from the outflow tract. Needle aspiration of the RV apex may aid in the recovery of air.

Catheter Pearls

What is the difference between polyurethane and silicone catheters?

Polyurethane catheters are more rigid and more thrombogenic, and they are intended for short-term use. Silicone catheters (Hickman and Broviacs) are very flexible and less thrombogenic, and they are not routinely placed at the bedside in the ICU.

Do heparin-bonded catheters reduce the incidence of thrombosis?

No. They can cause heparin-induced thrombocytopenia, however, and typically should not be used in the ICU setting.

When sizing catheters, what does "French" mean?

French is a unit of measure commonly used for tube and catheters. It is the outer circumference in millimeters, or approximately the outside diameter multiplied by 3.

Is there a mathematical conversion between gauge and French?

No. They are inversely related: the bigger the French, the smaller the gauge.

What is the formula for Poisseuille's law?

$Q = \pi r^4 / 8\ \mu L$

How does Poisseuille's law apply to catheter size?

The radius of the tube (not the length) more directly influences the flow rate. Therefore, large, short tubes allow rapid flow rates.

What is the difference between a multilumen catheter and an introducer catheter?

Multilumen catheters (double or triple lumen) are commonly used as infusion ports for ICU patients. They are long (often 30 cm) and are usually 6.9 French. Introducer sheaths (Cordis) are large-bore catheters that can be used as a conduit for the insertion and removal of smaller catheters. These devices are short and have a large diameter.

TRIPLE-LUMEN CATHETER

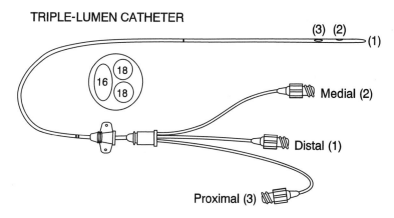

INTRODUCER CATHETER : 8-9 French

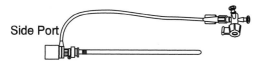

From Marino PM. The ICU Book. 2nd Ed. Philadelphia: Lippincott Williams & Wilkins, 1998:60.

Do triple-lumen catheters have higher rates of infection or thrombosis compared to single-lumen catheters?	No
Can introducer catheters be used as infusion devices?	Yes. Their large bore and short length make them ideal for rapid infusion, particularly in the trauma setting.

PULMONARY ARTERY CATHETERS

What is the purpose of a PAC?	Continuous hemodynamic monitoring in an unstable patient using CVP, PA pressures, and PAWP to optimize cardiac function. The indications are numerous and, sometimes, controversial.
What sort of monitoring should the patient have in preparation for a PAC?	Continuous ECG and a functioning IV
What is the purpose of the continuous ECG and functioning IV?	To diagnose and treat dysrhythmias
Describe the 8 steps in placing a PAC.	1. Place a large drape over the patient to ensure sterility of the long PAC. 2. Cannulate the IJ or subclavian vein using the Seldinger technique, and insert the introducer sheath. 3. Ensure that the catheter flushes easily, the balloon inflates, and a tracing can be generated on the screen by gently whipping the catheter in the air. 4. Thread the catheter through the sterile sleeve. 5. With the balloon down, insert the PAC in the introducer to a depth of 20 cm. 6. Inflate the balloon, and slowly advance the catheter, observing the

pressure tracing and any dysrhythmias until the characteristic PA waveform becomes dampened.

7. Deflate the balloon, and insure the return of PA systolic and diastolic tracing.

8. Note the catheter depth, and document in the chart the CXR to verify catheter position and rule out pneumothorax.

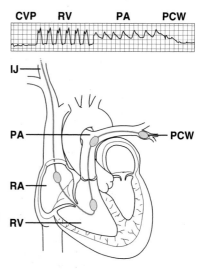

Pressure tracing and balloon position during insertion of pulmonary artery catheter. From Hurford WE, et al. Critical Care Handbook of the Masschusetts General Hospital. 3rd Ed. Baltimore: Lippincott Williams & Wilkins, 2000:20.

What are 10 potential complications associated with PAC placement?

1. Dysrhythmias
2. Pulmonary hemorrhage
3. PA rupture
4. Pulmonary infarction
5. Catheter entanglement
6. Cardiac perforation
7. Valvular damage
8. Air embolus
9. Endocarditis
10. Sepsis

When might a PA rupture occur?

If the catheter migrates beyond the original wedge position and overzealous attempts to inflate the balloon are made. Always use the syringe that is provided with the kit to inflate the balloon. Never a 10-mL syringe!

When might a pulmonary infarction occur?

When the balloon is left inflated for a prolonged period

What might happen when trying to float a PAC in a patient with a left bundle branch block?

Complete heart block

What are 5 contraindica- tions to PAC placement?

1. Pulmonic or tricuspid stenosis
2. Prosthetic pulmonic or tricuspid valves
3. Right heart masses or thrombus
4. Tetralogy of Fallot
5. Previous pneumonectomy

PAC Pearls

Where should the tip of the catheter be seen on CXR?

The main branch of the PA

What should be done if the catheter is more than 5 cm from the mediastinum?

Pull back (with the balloon deflated) to prevent PA rupture.

What do the black tic marks on the catheter indicate?

Each thin black line corresponds to 10 cm. A thick black line represents 50 cm.

At what insertion depth should an RV tracing appear?

28 to 32 cm

At what insertion depth should a wedge occur?

45 to 52 cm

What does it mean when you encounter a continuous CVP tracing at 30 cm?

The PAC has floated past the right atrium to the IVC.

What can help to resolve this problem?	Position the patient right-side down to allow the balloon to float "up" into the atrium.
Describe the correct status of the balloon while advancing and withdrawing the catheter.	The balloon is always inflated when the catheter is advanced forward. The balloon is always deflated when the catheter is pulled back.
What other options are available for difficult PAC placement?	Fluoroscopy
What does it mean when the PAWP is greater than the PA diastolic pressure?	A calibration error has occurred. The wedge cannot be higher than the PA diastolic pressure, because the blood will flow backward.

ARTERIAL CATHETERIZATION

What are 6 indications for arterial catheterization?	1. Continuous monitoring of arterial pressure 2. Hypertensive crisis 3. Shock 4. Hemodynamic lability 5. Administration of vasoactive or inotropic agents 6. Positive-pressure ventilation
What is the Allen test?	Assessment of collateral circulation to the hand
How is the Allen test performed?	Occlude the radial and ulnar arteries simultaneously until the hand blanches. Release the ulnar artery, and watch for reperfusion.
When is ulnar collateral flow considered to be adequate?	If blushing of the hand occurs in less than 5 seconds.
Describe the steps involved in radial artery cannulation.	1. Dorsiflex the hand with a roll of gauze and an arm board.

2. Palpate the radial pulse just proximal to head of the radius.
3. Insert a 20-gauge needle-catheter at a 30° angle.
4. Advance the catheter and needle until arterial blood flash.
5. Either (a) slide the catheter over the needle into the artery or (b) pass the needle and catheter together through artery wall, remove the needle, withdraw the catheter until blood spurts, thread the guide wire into the vessel, advance the catheter, and remove the wire.
6. Attach to pressure tubing.

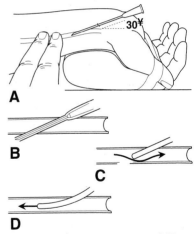

Radial artery catheterization using the Seldinger technique (step 5b of sequence). From Hurford WE, et al. Critical Care Handbook of the Masschusetts General Hospital. 3rd Ed. Baltimore: Lippincott Williams & Wilkins, 2000:15.

What are 8 complications associated with arterial cannulation?

1. Thrombosis
2. Thromboembolism
3. Distal ischemia
4. Hemorrhage

5. Hematoma
6. Infection
7. AV fistula
8. Neurologic injury

What are 5 risk factors associated with ischemic complications?

1. Low cardiac output
2. Vasoconstricting agents
3. Multiple failed attempts to cannulate
4. Peripheral vascular disease
5. Prolonged duration of cannulation

AIRWAY ACCESS

Name 4 ways to access the airway.

1. Orotracheal intubation
2. Nasotracheal intubation
3. Tracheostomy
4. Cricothyroidotomy

What are the indications for endotracheal intubation?

Respiratory rate more than 40 breaths per minute
Inadequate oxygenation ($PO_2 < 60$)
Inadequate ventilation ($PCO_2 > 60$)
Need to control airway
Decreased level of consciousness
Loss of laryngeal reflexes
Anticipated airway obstruction
Anticipated general anesthesia
Need to remove pulmonary secretions

What equipment is required for intubation?

Laryngoscope with blade and functioning light, supplemental O_2, bag-valve mask, suction, ETT with stylet (check balloon with 10-mL syringe), IV access, pulse oximeter, end-tidal CO_2 indicator

What determines the size of the tube to be used?

Age, body habitus, and indication for intubation. Use a 7-mm tube for most women and an 8-mm tube for most men.

What is the appropriate position for intubation?

"Sniffing position"

Pharyngeal-laryngeal axis

Oral axis

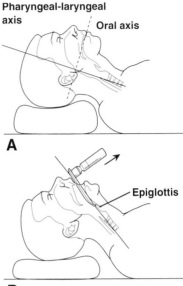

A

Epiglottis

B Straight blade placement

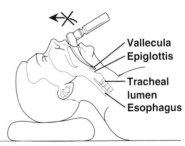

Vallecula
Epiglottis
Tracheal lumen
Esophagus

C Curved blade placement

Adapted from Hurford WE, et al. Critical Care Handbook of the Masschusetts General Hospital. 3rd Ed. Baltimore: Lippincott Williams & Wilkins, 2000:52.

How does trauma complicate intubation?

All multiple-trauma patients are considered to have a cervical spine injury until proven otherwise. Debris or blood may obscure visualization of the airway.

What method can be used to safely intubate a trauma patient?

In-line cervical traction by an assistant

What do you do when you cannot see the vocal cords?

Suction the oropharynx, apply gentle cricothyroid pressure, increase head flexion (in nontrauma patients), remove the laryngoscope, and ventilate with the bag-mask. **Do not permit hypoxemia during prolonged attempts at intubation.**

How do you verify correct tube placement?

Visualize the tube passing through cords, observe chest rise and fall as well as water vapor in the tube on exhalation, auscultate the stomach and both lung fields, and check end-tidal CO_2.

How else can you check for correct tube placement?

Fiberoptic endoscopy, CXR to ensure the tube is above the carina

When would you use nasotracheal intubation?

Oral trauma, intraoral surgery, and awake prehospital intubation

How is nasotracheal intubation accomplished?

Blindly in a spontaneously breathing patient
Over a fiberoptic laryngoscope
Direct laryngoscopy with Magill forceps assistance

What complication is associated with long-term nasotracheal intubation?

Sinusitis

Name 3 contraindications to nasotracheal intubation.

1. Epistaxis
2. Midface trauma
3. Skull base fracture

EMERGENT CRICOTHYROIDOTOMY

What are 3 indications for emergent cricothyroidotomy?

1. Immediate airway after trauma to oropharynx
2. Unsuccessful endotracheal intubation with desaturation
3. Upper airway obstruction

What are the bare necessities for performing emergent cricothyroidotomy?

Knife blade and handle; tracheostomy tube; and pediatric ETT or 14-gauge catheter-over-needle, bag-valve ventilation unit and O_2 source

Where is the cricothyroid membrane?

Between the cricoid cartilage and the thyroid

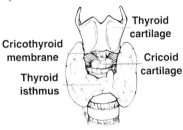

Blackbourne LH. Surgical Recall. 3rd Ed. Baltimore: Lippincott Williams & Williams, 2002:217.

Describe the standard technique of emergent cricothyroidotomy.

1. Vertical skin incision.
2. Horizontal incision in cricothyroid membrane.
3. Insert knife handle, and rotate 90°.
4. Insert ETT or trach tube.
5. Inflate cuff.
6. Hand ventilate.

What 3 complications may be associated with emergent cricothyroidotomy?

1. Hemorrhage
2. Perforation of esophagus
3. Inability to cannulate trachea

TRACHEOSTOMY

Is there a role for emergent tracheostomy?

Probably not. The significant time required and the risk of bleeding often preclude its use.

Are there other options to surgical tracheostomy?

Percutaneous tracheostomy

What is the appropriate time to convert an ETT to a tracheostomy?

Controversial. Elective tracheostomy is usually performed before 3 weeks.

Why are ETTs converted to a tracheostomy?

The incidence of glottic damage is related to the duration of intubation.

What are 6 advantages to tracheostomy?

1. Improved comfort
2. Decreased laryngeal injury
3. Improved oral hygiene
4. Ability to speak
5. Improved mobility
6. Allows gradual ventilator weaning

What are 4 disadvantages of tracheostomy?

1. Tracheal stenosis at stoma site
2. Stomal infection
3. Erosion of neighbor vascular structures
4. Scarring and granulation

Describe the general technique used in percutaneous tracheostomy.

Sterile prep and local anesthetic.
Withdraw the ETT to just below the cords.
Make a transverse incision long enough to accommodate the largest dilator.
Under bronchoscopic guidance, puncture the trachea between the 2nd and 3rd ring with a 16-gauge catheter.
Remove the needle, and advance the guide wire.
Pass serial dilators over a Teflon guiding catheter.
Place the tracheostomy tube over the last dilator.
After proper visualization and confirmation of placement, remove the ETT.

What are 5 complications associated with percutaneous tracheostomy?

1. Bleeding
2. Infection
3. Esophageal perforation
4. Tracheal ring fracture
5. Tracheal stenosis

Is a bronchoscope necessary?

Some authors report success without one; however, most still recommend its use.

How is speech made possible with a trach?	If the cuff is deflated or the tube is fenestrated, the lumen can be occluded with a finger or a speaking valve, thus allowing air to flow proximally and permitting phonation.

INTRACRANIAL PRESSURE MONITORING

Several nonneurosurgical textbooks describe this procedure in great detail, but the author feels this procedure is best performed by a neurosurgeon, particularly in the ICU setting. For this reason, this review does not include detailed "how-to" instructions but does provide some helpful bedside hints.

Name 4 different methods for transducing ICP.	1. Subarachnoid (ICP bolt) 2. Intraventricular 3. Intraparenchymal 4. Epidural

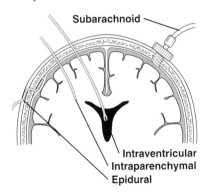

From Hurford WE, et al. Critical Care Handbook of the Masschusetts General Hospital. 3rd Ed. Baltimore: Lippincott Williams & Wilkins, 2000:505.

What are 2 indications for ICP monitoring?	1. Decreasing level of consciousness 2. Risk of undetectable rise in ICP (paralyzed patient, intraoperative)
What is the goal of therapy following traumatic brain injury?	Reducing ICP while maintaining CPP
How should one best follow the effectiveness of therapy?	Serial examinations with a reproducible method

What are 5 modalities one may use to treat elevated ICPs?	1. Elevated head position 2. Deliberate hyperventilation 3. Osmotic diuretics, loop diuretics, corticosteroids, barbiturate coma 4. Ventricular drainage 5. Craniectomy with duroplasty
How important is sterility during insertion and maintenance of a monitoring device?	Extremely important! Infection related to these devices is devastating. Meticulous attention to detail during insertion and maintenance is crucial. Prophylactic antistaphylococcal coverage (Vancomycin) should be used.
On which side is a ventriculostomy normally performed?	The right (or nondominant) side

THORACENTESIS

What are 2 indications for thoracentesis?	1. Obtaining pleural fluid for diagnosis 2. Drainage of restricting pleural effusion
If possible, what should be the position of the patient?	Seated, leaning forward with arms propped up on a bedside table
How is the effusion located?	Percussion (dull over fluid-filled area)
Where should the catheter be placed in relation to the fluid level?	2 interspaces below the fluid level
What is the lowest interspace in which one should place the thoracentesis catheter?	8th intercostal space
In relation to the rib, where should local anesthesia be administered?	Skin, deeper tissue, periosteum of the superior aspect of the rib below the chosen interspace

Should the anesthesia be administered deeper than the rib?	Yes. The pleural cavity should be entered, administering anesthesia to the pleura.
Describe the general technique of thoracentesis.	Sterile prep and local anesthesia. Insert catheter-over-needle in the interspace just over the rib. Remove the needle. Attach a stopcock and large syringe to the catheter. Send fluid for diagnosis. Alternatively, connect tubing to the stopcock, and collect fluid in the chamber.
What 9 laboratory studies should be ordered with the pleural fluid when drawn for diagnosis?	1. Cell count with differential 2. Gram stain and bacterial culture 3. Fungal and mycobacterium cultures 4. Cytology 5. Protein 6. Glucose 7. Amylase 8. LDH 9. pH

CHEST TUBES

What is the purpose of a chest tube?	To remove any unwanted material from the thorax: air, blood, pus, chyle, and pleural fluid
What size tube should one use to drain air, serous effusion, and blood, respectively?	Pneumothorax: 24 French (smaller tube is more comfortable) Pleural effusion: 28 French Hemothorax: 32 French (clotting blood may clog smaller tubes)
Where is the correct anatomical site for chest tube insertion?	4th intercostal space, anterior axillary line

Why not place the tube more inferiorly?

Risk of intra-abdominal injury. The diaphragm can rise to the 4th or 5th interspace during expiration.

Are there alternative sites at which to place a chest tube?

Yes. With loculated pneumothorax or pleural effusions, the chest tube can be directed to a specific location.

How can you predict the depth at which the chest tube is to be inserted?

Measure the chest tube from the site of insertion to the inferior border of the clavicle, and mark the tube with a suture.

List the steps of the general technique of chest tube insertion.

Sterile prep and local anesthesia.
Skin incision.
Create a SQ tunnel to the desired interspace.
Enter the pleural space just superior to the rib.
Spread the pleura by opening the clamp.
Confirm intrathoracic penetration with a gloved finger, and sweep away lung.
Direct the tip of the tube into the pleural space with a Kelly clamp.
Ensure that the last hole in the chest tube is in the chest.
Connect the tube to the collection system.
Secure with a suture, and dress.
Secure all connections to the collecting system

Where should the local anesthetic be injected?

Skin, SQ tissue, periosteum, pleura

Where should the skin incision be relative to the desired interspace?

One interspace below

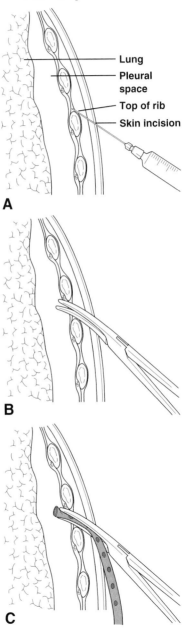

Chest tube insertion. From Hurford WE, et al. Critical Care Handbook of the Masschusetts General Hospital. 3rd Ed. Baltimore: Lippincott Williams & Wilkins, 2000:614.

After entering the chest with a Kelly clamp, what is the one most important step before tube insertion?	Exploring with the index finger to ensure that the lung is free from the chest wall
Where should the chest tube be directed for drainage of hemothorax or hydrothorax?	Posteriorly and superiorly
Where should the chest tube be directed for drainage of pneumothorax?	Anteriorly
What should be done after the chest tube is inserted?	CXR to confirm position and evacuation of air or fluid
What is the significance of the break in the radio-opaque line on the tube?	The break in the line allows you to see the most proximal hole on CXR, to ensure that it is within the chest cavity.
What are 7 complications associated with chest tube insertion?	1. Hemorrhage 2. Laceration of lung 3. Infection 4. Cardiac injury 5. SQ placement 6. Re-expansion pulmonary edema 7. Intraperitoneal placement
What is the role of trocar thoracostomy tubes?	The author feels that these "weapons" have a high complication rate and are not recommended.

Describe the roles of the three chambers (or "three bottles") in the collection apparatus.

The proximal chamber is for pleural drainage. The middle chamber (H₂O seal) prevents air or fluid from being drawn into the pleural space. The distal chamber regulates the level of suction.

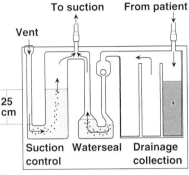

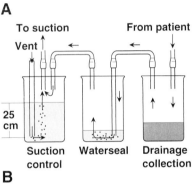

Three chambers in chest tube collection apparatus. From Hurford WE, et al. Critical Care Handbook of the Masschusetts General Hospital. 3rd Ed. Baltimore: Lippincott Williams & Wilkins, 2000:615.

What can cause continuous bubbling in the water seal chamber?

An intrapleural air leak or a leak in one of the connections

How can you differentiate between these two leaks?

Briefly clamp the chest tube near the patient. If the leak continues, the system is flawed and needs to be corrected or replaced. If the leak stops, it is most likely an intrapleural air leak.

A large air leak suddenly develops in an underwater seal draining a chest tube. What event has likely occurred to cause this?

The tube may have slipped partially out of the chest, exposing the proximal drainage hole to room air.

What is the indication from the collection device that the tube is clotted?

Absence of respiratory fluctuation in the water seal column

Should a chest tube be clamped for patient transport?

Never! Clamping a tube in a patient with an air leak may lead to a tension pneumothorax. The tube should be on water seal during transport.

What are the indications for chest tube removal?

When the lung is fully inflated, no air leak is present, and drainage is less than 100 mL over 24 hours

Describe the technique used for chest tube removal.

Remove the securing suture.
Have the patient generate a positive in-trathoracic pressure (deep breath-hold and valsalva).
Hold petroleum gauze and dressings over the tube site.
Rapidly remove the tube.
Dress with occlusive dressings.
CXR to assess for reaccumulation of pneumothorax

PERICARDIOCENTESIS

What are the indications for pericardiocentesis?

Relief of cardiac tamponade and to obtain fluid for diagnostic study

What are the basic instruments required to perform this procedure safely?

A 16-gauge (4-inch) needle with short bevel, a 50-mL syringe, and a sterile alligator connector for ECG lead V.

How can you improve cardiac performance in a patient with tamponade before draining the pericardium?

IV volume infusion

What is the role of ECG lead V attached to the needle?	To indicate when the needle is in contact with the heart
What ECG changes indicate ventricular contact?	ST-segment elevation
What ECG changes indicate atrial contact?	PR-segment elevation
Describe the subxiphoid approach to pericardiocentesis.	Sterile prep and local anesthesia. Insert needle 1 cm to the left of the xiphoid at a 30° angle. Advance the needle while aspirating, and observe ECG.
What should you do if gross blood is obtained?	Assess for coagulation.
Does pericardial blood clot?	No. Pericardial blood has been defibrinated.
What are 7 complications associated with pericardiocentesis?	1. Cardiac dysrhythmias 2. Cardiac puncture 3. Myocardial laceration 4. Coronary artery laceration 5. Air embolism 6. Pneumothorax 7. Bleeding

INTRA-AORTIC BALLOON PUMP

What is an IABP?	A flexible catheter with an elongated balloon that is placed in the descending aorta
How does an IABP work?	It inflates during diastole and quickly deflates at the onset of systole.
What does diastolic augmentation mean?	During diastolic inflation, the balloon displaces 40 mL of blood, thus increasing aortic pressure and diastolic blood flow.

Does IABP affect afterload?

Yes. The rapid deflation leaves a 40-mL "void," decreasing aortic pressure and reducing left ventricular afterload during systole.

What is the overall objective of IABP?

To increase coronary blood flow and decrease myocardial O_2 consumption

What are 7 indications for IABP placement?

1. Postcardiotomy shock: 35% to 40%
2. Medically refractory angina: 15% to 25%
3. Preoperative stabilization after failed PTCI
4. Preoperative stabilization after acute MI
5. Complications of acute MI: acute mitral regurgitation (MR), ventricular septal defect (VSD)
6. Bridge to transplant
7. Prophylaxis for induction of high-risk patients: severe left ventricular dysfunction, long or complex operation

What are 3 contraindications to IABP placement?

1. Significant aortic regurgitation: increase in regurgitant fraction.
2. Aortic dissection: both difficulties in placing the IABP in the true arterial lumen and the reduced afterload increases the force of blood ejection and can extend the aortic dissection.
3. Recently placed (in the last 12 months) thoracic aortic graft: thrombus disruption.

What are the different options for IABP insertion?

1. Percutaneously into femoral artery
2. Open femoral artery cutdown
3. Suprainguinal approach to the iliac artery
4. Transthoracic approach to the ascending thoracic aorta
5. Open axillary artery cutdown

When is surgical placement indicated?

1. Severe ileofemoral atherosclerotic disease (option 2 > 3 > 4 > 5)

2. Aortic occlusion or severe aortoiliac disease (options 4 and 5)
3. Small arteries: small adults or children are more likely to be occluded with sheath (option 2).
4. Heart transplant candidates that are potentially ambulatory (options 3 and 5)

What is the relevance of balloon size and aortic diameter?

The balloon should occlude no more than 85% to 90% of aortic diameter.

Where is the ideal intra-aortic location of the balloon?

The balloon should be above the renal arteries and below the left subclavian artery.

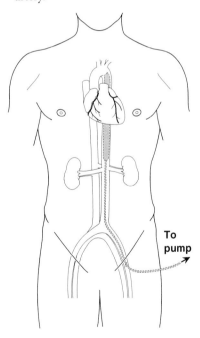

To pump

Intra-aortic balloon pump positioning. From Hurford WE, et al. Critical Care Handbook of the Masschusetts General Hospital. 3rd Ed. Baltimore: Lippincott Williams & Wilkins, 2000:200.

How can you estimate the length of catheter required at the bedside?

Using the catheter, mark the distance from the site of insertion to the angle of Louis with a suture.

Describe the general technique of inserting an IABP.	Sterile prep and local anesthesia. The common femoral artery is cannulated and dilated over wire. The dilator is removed from the introducer. The balloon is deflated, and the catheter is passed over the guide wire to the predetermined length. The guide wire is removed, and the stopcock and pressure tubing are attached for arterial pressure monitoring. Aspirate the catheter lumen before flushing. Attach the balloon tubing. Secure the catheter in place. Perform CXR
How does the tip of the catheter appear on CXR?	As an opaque rectangle
Where should the tip of the catheter be on CXR?	In the 2nd or 3rd intercostal space
What are physiologic "triggers"?	Signals from the patient to initiate inflation and deflation cycles
What are the 2 modes of triggering?	1. ECG 2. Arterial waveform.
Explain the timing of balloon inflation.	Inflation should occur at the onset of diastole (just before the dicrotic notch on the arterial waveform).
Explain the timing of balloon deflation.	Deflation should begin just before systole (coincident with the end-diastolic pressure on the waveform).
What is the complication rate associated with IABPs?	20% to 30%
What are the complications associated with the following steps in this procedure?	
During insertion?	Aortic dissection, ileofemoral injury

During pumping?	Thromboembolism, distal ischemia, infection, balloon rupture
During removal?	Dislodgement of atherosclerotic plaque, balloon entrapment
What is the initial management of most IABP complications?	Balloon removal and vascular surgery consult
What are 2 methods to wean patients from IABP therapy?	1. Changing the ratio of assisted to unassisted beats 2. Reducing the inflation volume of the balloon
What are the 3 goals of balloon removal?	1. To withdraw the balloon intact 2. To minimize bleeding 3. To prevent embolic events
Describe the general steps used to withdraw the balloon.	Deflate the balloon. Withdraw the catheter to the introducer sheath. Apply pressure to the femoral artery below the catheter. Remove the balloon and sheath together, as a unit. Allow bleeding for 1 to 2 seconds to clear embolic material. Apply firm pressure above the insertion site, and release distal pressure to allow back-bleeding for 1 to 2 seconds. Apply firm pressure over insertion site for 30 minutes. Use a handheld Doppler to ensure adequate distal flow during hemostasis.
What should be done if resistance is encountered during removal?	Stop the procedure, and begin surgical removal.

PARACENTESIS

What are 3 indications for paracentesis?	1. Unexplained ascites 2. Suspicion of spontaneous bacterial peritonitis 3. Relief of severe ascites
What are the basic instruments required to perform paracentesis safely?	20-gauge catheter-over-needle, stopcock, 50-mL syringe, extension tubing, and collection chambers
List, in order of preference, 3 insertion sites for paracentesis.	1. Lateral to rectus sheath at umbilical line 2. Periumbilical 3. Adjacent to anterior iliac spine
Describe the general technique for paracentesis.	Sterile prep and local anesthesia. Insert the catheter-over-needle until ascitic fluid is withdrawn. Remove the needle, and attach the stopcock and syringe. Extension tubing may be attached to collection chambers for large volumes.
What 9 laboratory studies should be ordered for the ascitic fluid?	1. Cell count with differential 2. Gram stain and bacterial culture 3. Fungal and mycobacterial cultures 4. Cytology 5. Protein 6. Glucose 7. Amylase 8. LDH 9. pH
What are 6 complications associated with paracentesis?	1. Bleeding 2. Infection 3. Bowel perforation 4. Bladder perforation 5. Persistent ascitic leak 6. Hypotension (secondary to large volume removed)

DIAGNOSTIC PERITONEAL LAVAGE

What is the purpose of DPL?	Evaluation of blunt abdominal trauma and selected cases of penetrating trauma
What are 5 indications for DPL in blunt abdominal trauma?	1. Hypotension with evidence of abdominal injury 2. Unexplained shock 3. Potential abdominal injury in patients with depressed sensorium or altered pain response (head injury, intoxication, paraplegia) 4. Equivocal abdominal exam findings 5. Potential abdominal injury in patients when serial reevaluation is impossible (e.g., anticipated general anesthesia for another injury)
What are the indications with penetrating injury?	Penetration of thoracoabdominal region (between nipples and inferior costal margin), flank wounds, buttocks and perineum wounds
What is an absolute contraindication for DPL?	Obvious indication for exploratory laparotomy (free air, peritonitis, evisceration, gunshot wound, stab wound with hemorrhagic shock)
What must be in place before DPL?	Foley catheter and NG or OG tube
How do these items assist in the procedure?	By decompressing the stomach and the bladder, thus diminishing the chance of perforation
Where must the catheter be placed for DPL with a pelvic fracture?	Supraumbilical position
Why is the supraumbilical position required?	To avoid the high false-positive rate as the hematoma tracks up the medial umbilical ligament

Where should the catheter be placed in pregnant patients?

Supraumbilical position (to avoid injury to the uterus)

What is the DPL blind spot?

The retroperitoneum

If free air is suspected, what should be done before DPL?

Abdominal films (DPL will introduce air into the abdomen)

Describe the general technique used for the open DPL.

Sterile prep to supra- and infraumbilical region.
Local anesthesia.
Vertical midline incision approximately 2 to 4 cm in length down to midline fascia (army-navy retractors are helpful here).
Towel clip both sides of the fascia for traction.
Make a small incision in the fascia.
Use a trochar catheter to pop through the peritoneum.
Direct the catheter alone toward the pelvis.
Aspirate contents with a 12-mL syringe.
If negative aspirate, attach a 1-L bag of lactated Ringer's solution to the catheter, and hang in a pressure bag.
Infuse lactated Ringer's while gently shaking the patient's abdomen.
When only a small amount of fluid remains in the bag, drop the bag to the floor, and collect fluid.

How can you prevent fluid from leaking out of the incision?

By using sponge packs in the incision

How do you avoid incisional blood from entering lavage fluid at the completion of fluid collection?

Clamp the tubing before withdrawing the catheter (this stops the siphoning action).

How do you close the incision after fluid collection?	Heavy figure-of-eight suture to close the fascial defect (optional), and skin staples for the skin.
What should you do if you encounter poor fluid return?	Adjust the catheter position, twist the catheter, place the patient in a reverse Trendelenburg position, apply manual pressure to the abdomen, and instill an additional 500 mL.
What do you do when the system is air-locked?	Check all connections in the tubing. Make sure that all catheter holes are underwater, and re-establish siphon by aspirating on the side port of the drainage tubing.
What are 5 complications associated with DPL?	1. Bowel injury 2. Bladder laceration 3. Vascular injury 4. Hematoma 5. Wound infection
How do you interpret the results of a DPL?	Grossly positive: 5 mL of blood on initial aspirate Microscopic/chemistry criteria: greater than 100,000 RBC/mm^3 ($>$1,000–20,000 RBC/mm^3 for penetrating trauma); greater than 500 WBC/mm^3 ($>$25–100 WBC/mm^3 for penetrating trauma) Presence of particulate (vegetable or fecal) matter Presence of bacteria on Gram stain Elevated amylase, bilirubin

GASTROINTESTINAL INTUBATION

GASTRIC TUBES

What is the purpose of NG intubation?	Gastric decompression and drainage
What is a Levin tube?	A soft tube with a single lumen requiring low, intermittent suction

What is a Salem sump tube?	A dual-lumen tube (suction and vent) that can be placed on continuous suction
How is patency of a sump tube assessed?	The vent tube (blue one) whistles during suction.
How can one minimize patient discomfort before insertion of an NG tube?	Use of viscous lidocaine and Cetacaine spray.
Describe the basic steps for NG tube insertion?	Elevate the head at least 30°degrees, and flex the neck (chin to chest). Lubricate the tube and nostril with lidocaine jelly. Insert the tube into the nostril until it reaches the nasopharynx. Have the patient swallow sips of H_2O. Advance the tube to the stomach, and secure.
What is the quickest test to rule out tracheal intubation?	Ask the patient to speak.
How can you ensure the tube is in the stomach?	Instill 20 to 30 mL of air while listening over the stomach with a stethoscope, and confirm with CXR.
What is an absolute contraindication to NG intubation?	Anterior basilar skull fracture or nasopharyngeal trauma
What is an Ewald tube?	An OG tube used for lavage and evacuation of stomach contents
In patients with diminished mentation and/or loss of gag reflex, what should be done before OG intubation?	Insert a cuffed ETT.

What is a PEG tube?

Percutaneous endoscopic gastrostomy

What are the indications for a PEG?

Long-term gastric access for feeding or decompression

What are 3 contraindications to a PEG?

1. Massive ascites
2. Severe malnutrition (tract formation is impaired, and leaking occurs)
3. Active systemic infection

What sedation and/or analgesia is used for this procedure?

Titrated sequential administration of a narcotic and a benzodiazepine

What is the importance of transillumination with the gastroscope?

This technique indicates close contact of the gastric wall with the abdominal wall and the absence of intervening tissue (e.g., colon or liver).

Describe the general technique used for PEG placement.

Sedation, sterile prep of the abdominal wall.

Gastroscope is introduced into the stomach.

Abdominal wall is observed for transillumination.

Local anesthetic is administered to the abdominal wall at the transillumination site, and a 1-cm incision is made.

Needle-cannula is passed through abdominal wall and into the stomach under direct vision.

A suture or wire is grabbed with biopsy forceps or a snare and then withdrawn with the scope through the mouth.

A suture is then tied to the end of the gastrostomy catheter and pulled down esophagus, or the gastrostomy tube is threaded over a wire and pushed into the stomach and out the abdominal wall

What are 6 complications associated with a PEG?

1. Minor irritation around the site
2. Infection
3. Leak

4. Migration of the tube (SQ or intraperitoneal)
5. Gastrocolic fistula
6. Bleeding

DUODENAL AND SMALL BOWEL TUBES

What is a nasoduodenal feeding tube?	A small, flexible tube that is more comfortable than an NG tube and feeds the duodenum (Entriflex, Dobbhoff, Vivonex)
What are 4 advantages of nasoduodenal feeding tubes?	1. Reduced risk of aspiration. 2. Can feed distal to fistula or obstruction. 3. Can use in patients with gastric atony. 4. Patient comfort
What are 4 disadvantages of nasoduodenal tubes?	1. Low tolerance to high osmolar loads. 2. Cannot bolus feed (requires continuous administration with a pump). 3. Requires frequent irrigation. 4. Must use low-viscosity formula
Where is the ideal location for a small bowel feeding tube?	Distal to the ligament of Treitz
How is this position confirmed?	On a plain radiograph, the tip of the feeding tube is identified distal to the "c-loop" of the duodenum to the left of the vertebral column.

SENGSTAKEN-BLAKEMORE TUBE

What is the indication for the Sengstaken-Blakemore tube (SBT)?	To tamponade endoscopically proven variceal hemorrhage. Usually inserted after failed vasopressin and sclerotherapy.

What should take precedence over all other attempts to treat upper GI bleeding?

Adequate volume resuscitation

Can the SBT be used in conjunction with other therapeutic modalities?

Yes, particularly vasopressin and β-blockade

How many balloons are associated with the SBT?

2

Where are the 2 balloons located?

Esophageal and gastric portions of the tube

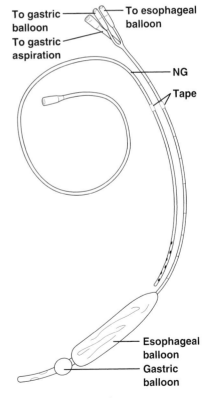

Sengstaken-Blakemore tube.

What are some basic necessities for inserting the SBT?	ECG; supplemental O$_2$; the SBT; suction apparatus; 50-mL syringe; pressure manometer; 10- to 12-French NG tube, Ewald tube; lubrication; supplies for intubation
How should the patient be positioned for placement of the SBT?	In the left lateral decubitus position
Describe the general steps involved with insertion of an SBT.	Empty the stomach with OG or Ewald tube. Test balloons on the SBT, and lubricate. Pass the tube nasally to the 50-cm mark. Fill the gastric balloon with 250 to 500 mL of air or contrast solution, and clamp the tube. Gently withdraw the tube until resistance at the gastroesophageal junction is encountered. Secure to the face with minimal traction. CXR.
What device can be used to anchor the tube?	A football helmet with face mask (the sign of a hard-core surgeon that will certainly earn you style points!)
When should the esophageal tube be inflated?	If bleeding is not controlled by the gastric balloon
How much should you inflate the esophageal balloon?	40 mm Hg (hence the need for the pressure manometer)
How long should the esophageal balloon remain inflated?	The esophageal balloon should be deflated transiently every 4 to 6 hours.
What are 2 complications associated with prolonged esophageal balloon inflation?	1. Mucosal ischemia 2. Perforation

Is an NG tube needed?	Yes
Where should the NG tube be placed?	In the other nostril, proximal to the esophageal balloon
What is the purpose of the NG tube?	To control secretions and prevent regurgitation
What are 3 complications associated with SBTs?	1. Esophageal rupture 2. Aspiration 3. Refractory variceal bleeding
Is there a role for endotracheal intubation?	Yes, in altered consciousness, respiratory compromise, aspiration, shock, or complex medical problems

ENDOSCOPY: BRONCHOSCOPY AND ESOPHAGOSCOPY

What are the 2 basic forms of endoscopy?	1. Rigid 2. Flexible
Is one technique superior to the other?	Both techniques have advantages and disadvantages. Therefore, both should be mastered by all surgeons caring for critically ill patients.
Name 4 advantages of flexible endoscopy.	1. Well-tolerated 2. Requires only local anesthesia 3. Requires minimal sedation 4. Patient acceptability
Name 4 advantages of rigid endoscopy	1. Accepts larger forceps for biopsy and/or debridement 2. Accepts larger suction tubing for high volume 3. Better for evaluation of fixation and/or rigidity 4. Better for dilation and stent placement
What 3 monitoring modalities are required for conscious sedation?	1. ECG 2. Noninvasive blood pressure 3. Pulse oximetry

What other 3 items should be available during conscious sedation?

1. Supplemental O_2
2. IV access
3. An assistant for drug delivery and monitoring

What standard equipment is required for endoscopic examination?

Working scope, light source, suction, biopsy forceps, irrigation solution

What are the 2 general indications for bronchoscopy?

1. Diagnostic
2. Therapeutic

Name 12 diagnostic indications for bronchoscopy.

1. Severe cough or change in cough
2. Abnormal CXR
3. Hemoptysis
4. Unresolved pneumonia
5. Abnormal sputum cytology
6. Bacteriologic sampling
7. Metastatic malignancy
8. Smoke inhalation
9. Airway obstruction
10. Bronchoalveolar lavage
11. Bronchogenic cancer
12. Esophageal cancer

Name 4 therapeutic indications for bronchoscopy.

1. Atelectasis
2. Lung abscess
3. Foreign body
4. Stricture

Where is the optimal place to stand to successfully perform bronchoscopy?

The right side of the patient, facing the head of the bed

How is the bronchoscope held?

The controls of the scope are held with the left hand. The right hand manipulates the scope and passes instruments down the scope as needed.

In which anatomic direction is the apex of the vocal cords?

Anterior. This can help to orient you, because the cords separate posteriorly.

Past the vocal cords, how can you orient yourself in the AP plane?

C-shaped rings are anterior, and the membranous trachea is posterior.

What is the normal length of the trachea before the bifurcation?

Approximately 10 cm

As one enters the right mainstem, what branch is first encountered?

The right upper lobe bronchus. This branch typically occurs within 1 cm from the carina and extends laterally from the right mainstem bronchus.

What is the name for the continuation of the bronchus after the right upper lobe branch?

Bronchus intermedias

Describe the typical course of the bronchus intermedias.

The bronchus intermedias extends approximately 2 cm before dividing into the distal branches.

Describe the location of the right middle lobe bronchus.

Directly anterior and usually opposite the superior segmental bronchus of the lower lobe

Describe the initial course of the left mainstem bronchus.

It typically extends approximately 3 cm from the carina before bifurcating to the upper and lower lobes.

What is the first branch of the left mainstem?

The left upper lobe bronchus. This takes off at a 110° angle from the left mainstem.

Describe the continued path of the left mainstem after the upper lobe take off.

The continuation of the left mainstem immediately becomes the lower lobe orifice.

What is required for bronchoscopy of an intubated patient?

A 2-way adapter for simultaneous bronchoscopy and ventilation

What 2 structures are not visualized during bronchoscopy through an ETT?

1. Larynx
2. Upper trachea

Is visualization of the bronchial anatomy best performed "on the way in" or "on the way out"?

On the way in. This allows observation of any abnormality that is undisturbed by any scope trauma.

Which side of the airway is usually observed first?

The opposite side of the suspected pathology

Describe the position required for successful rigid bronchoscopy.

The patient's head should be placed on blankets in the hyperextended position to straighten the route through the oropharynx to the trachea.

Describe the hand position used to best introduce and manipulate a rigid bronchoscope.

The left hand is used to stabilize the patient's head by placing the middle and ring fingers on the hard palate, leaving the thumb and forefinger to stabilize and advance the scope.

After reaching the carina, how are the right and left mainstem bronchi intubated?

By rotating the patient's head to the side opposite where one wishes to go

What are 6 complications associated with bronchoscopy?

1. Arrhythmias
2. Hypoxemia
3. Bronchospasm
4. Pneumothorax
5. Bleeding
6. Pulmonary infection

Describe the 2 major aspects that differentiate esophagoscopy from bronchoscopy.

1. The esophagus is more friable and prone to full-thickness injury and perforation.
2. A much broader spectrum of pathology affects the esophagus than affects the tracheobronchial tree, and many of these conditions can be

managed with endoscopy, which is not the case with the tracheobronchial tree.

In what position should the patient be placed for successful esophagoscopy?

The left lateral decubitus position, with the endoscopist facing the patient. This position allows oral secretions to drain easily.

Describe the 2 techniques for passing the endoscope into the esophagus.

1. Direct vision: the scope is passed posterior to the corniculate tubercles of the larynx into the upper esophagus.
2. Blind pass: using the fingers, the tongue is pushed anteriorly, and the scope is passed through the upper esophageal sphincter.

What structure is first encountered during esophagoscopy?

The upper esophageal sphincter

What pathologic finding should one inspect for in this region?

Zenker's diverticulum

What technique can be used to help visualize the esophageal mucosa as the scope is being passed?

Intermittent air insufflation

How would an area of fixation or rigidity be identified?

These areas do not insufflate well.

How does one observe the undersurface of the lower esophageal sphincter?

Retroflexing the scope within the stomach allows visualization of the cardia and lower esophageal sphincter.

Should one do most of the evaluation of the esophagus and stomach "on the way in" or "on the way out"?

Typically, the operator should concentrate on navigation of the scope during insertion and evaluate pathologic entities as the instrument is pulled back.

Describe the techniques used for rigid esophagoscopy.	Rigid esophagoscopy is performed in a manner similar to that of rigid bronchoscopy (see above); however, the patient is usually intubated. The scope is held in the same manner as the rigid bronchoscope and is passed under direct vision into the upper esophagus.
What are 3 contraindications for esophagoscopy?	1. Significant arthritis: patients who cannot extend their neck sufficiently 2. Large thoracic aortic aneurysm 3. Zenker's diverticulum
What are 3 complications associated with esophagoscopy?	1. Perforation (0.8% in rigid and 0.3% in flexible) 2. Aspiration 3. Arrhythmia
What is the most common site of esophageal perforation associated with esophagoscopy?	Just above the cricopharyngeous, secondary to problems with esophageal intubation
How does an esophageal perforation manifest?	Pain, fever, SQ emphysema, and/or pleural effusion

COMPARTMENT SYNDROME

Define compartment syndrome.	Increased pressure within a fascial compartment
What are the 2 etiologic mechanisms?	1. Increased volume of compartment contents 2. Decreased compartment size

ABDOMINAL COMPARTMENT SYNDROME

What 3 organ systems are most affected by increased abdominal pressure?	1. Renal 2. Pulmonary 3. Cardiovascular

What are 5 common manifestations of abdominal compartment syndrome (ACS)?

1. Decreased urine output
2. Increased systemic vascular resistance
3. Decreased cardiac output
4. Hypoxemia
5. Elevated peak airway pressures

What is the normal pressure of the abdominal cavity?

0 cm H_2O or subatmospheric

What compartmental pressure is suggestive of ACS?

25 cm H_2O

What compartmental pressure is diagnostic of ACS?

Greater than 30 cm H_2O. A relative increase in pressure over time may also be diagnostic.

What is the most direct and accurate way of measuring intra-abdominal pressure?

An intraperitoneal catheter attached to a water manometer or transducer

Why is this technique not often used clinically?

Because of the potential complications: peritoneal contamination, viscous perforation

Name 3 abdominal compartments in which the intra-abdominal pressure can be indirectly assessed.

1. Bladder: by a Foley catheter
2. Stomach: by an NG tube
3. Rectum: by an esophageal catheter

What instruments are required for assessing abdominal pressure using the bladder technique?

Foley catheter with an aspiration port, large-piston syringe, 20-gauge needle, water manometer or pressure transducer, Kelly clamp, sterile saline

Where is the manometer placed as a "zero" reference point?

At the level of the pubic symphysis

Describe the general technique for measuring abdominal pressure using the bladder technique.

Sterile saline (50 mL) is instilled into the bladder via the aspiration port. The drainage tube is simultaneously clamped with a Kelly.

The Foley is cannulated with a needle attached to the manometer.

Are there other acceptable bladder techniques?

Yes

Describe the "no-clamp technique."

The bladder is instilled with 50 mL of sterile saline.

The "Y" of the Foley is considered to be the zero point and is placed at the level of the pubic symphysis.

The drainage tube is held vertically above this point, and the height of the column is measured from the "Y" or zero point.

Why is only a limited volume of saline infused into the bladder?

To maintain a passive reservoir. When the bladder volume exceeds 100 mL, the intrinsic muscles of the bladder begin to contract and falsely elevate "intra-abdominal" pressures.

EXTREMITY COMPARTMENT SYNDROME

What are 5 specific etiologies of extremity compartment syndrome?

1. Trauma (most common)
2. Revascularization procedures with prolonged ischemia
3. DVT
4. External compression (military anti-shock trousers [MAST] or dressings)
5. Bleeding secondary to anticoagulation

Name the 4 compartments of the lower leg and the nerve within each compartment.

1. Anterior compartment: deep peroneal nerve
2. Lateral compartment: superficial peroneal nerve
3. Superficial posterior compartment: sural nerve
4. Deep posterior compartment: tibial nerve

What is the most commonly affected compartment?

Anterior

What are the 3 clinical "hallmarks" of compartmental hypertension?

1. Increased tissue tension
2. Neurologic and muscular dysfunction
3. Occlusion of venous outflow within the compartment

What is often the first manifestation of compartment syndrome?

Pain out of proportion to findings of the physical exam

What is the normal compartment pressure of the lower extremity?

Less than 10 mm Hg

What is considered to be an abnormal compartment pressure?

Greater than 30 mm Hg

In what position should the limb be placed before assessing compartment pressures?

Flat, or at the level of the heart

Describe the simple percutaneous technique of measuring compartmental pressures.

Sterile prep and local anesthesia.
Insert an IV catheter attached to a pressure transducer into the lower limb (preferably away from any vascular structures).

What is the treatment of lower extremity compartment syndrome?

Fasciotomy of all 4 compartments

What are the 3 tenets of a successful 4-compartment fasciotomy?

1. Complete incision of the skin overlying the compartments
2. Longitudinal incision of entire fascia
3. Aggressive local wound care

What incisions are required to release all 4 compartments of the lower extremity?

Anterolateral and medial skin incisions allow all 4 compartments to be easily released.

What is an alternative approach with a single incision?

A single lateral incision is made starting at the fibular head and extending to the ankle. This incision requires more skill than the 2-incision approach to release the deep posterior compartment.

Section 2

Organ Systems

9   Central Nervous System

CENTRAL NERVOUS SYSTEM ICU EMERGENCIES THAT LEAD TO RAPID DEATH

What 8 issues arise in the CNS that can lead rapidly to neurologic devastation or death?

1. Posterior fossa hematomas or swelling (call Neurosurgery)
2. Hydrocephalus (HCP) (call Neurosurgery)
3. Status epilepticus (call Neurology)
4. Meningitis
5. Anoxia
6. Hypotension
7. Hypoglycemia
8. Stroke (many hospitals now have a "stroke team" for emergent neurological evaluation and treatment of suspected stroke)

PHYSIOLOGY

Why is CNS physiology data important?

Both intracranial and systemic parameters affect blood flow to the brain. A continuous supply of oxygen and glucose is required for survival of neural tissue.

What is CBF?

Cerebral blood flow

How is CBF calculated?

CBF = CPP/cerebrovascular resistance (CVR)

What is a normal CBF?

50 mL of blood per 100 g of brain tissue per minute

What is a pathologic CBF?

Less than 25 mL/100 g results in EEG flatline; less than 10 mL/100 g results in cell death.

How is CPP calculated?	CPP = MAP − ICP
What is a normal CPP?	It is a pressure **gradient**, normally 60 to 70 mm Hg
What is CVR?	Cerebrovascular resistance (net resistance to blood flow into brain)
What is MAP?	Mean arterial pressure
How is MAP calculated?	MAP = diastolic + $\frac{1}{3}$ (systolic - diastolic)
What is a normal MAP?	60 to 80 mm Hg
What is ICP?	Pressure inside the cranial vault ("intracranial pressure")
What is a normal ICP?	2 to 12 mm Hg
What is a pathologic ICP?	Greater than 20 mm Hg
What is cerebral autoregulation?	Automatic dilatation and constriction of midsize cerebral blood vessels to maintain normal CBF in the face of a CPP of 50 to 150 mm Hg; often lost in pathologic states
What 3 components fill the cranial vault?	1. Blood 2. Brain 3. CSF
Why is this relevant?	The cranial vault has **fixed volume** and is entirely occupied by these three components. An increase of the volume of any one or an addition of a fourth element must be compensated by an equal decrease of the volume of the others; otherwise, ICP will rise.
What eponym is applied to this hypothesis?	Munroe-Kellie Hypothesis

What are 4 common causes of increased ICP based on this concept?

1. HCP (excess CSF)
2. Tumor
3. Blood clot
4. Brain edema

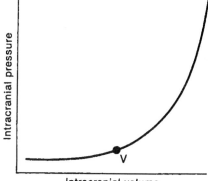

From Jarrell BE, Carabasi III RA, Radomski JS. NMS Surgery. 4th Ed. Philadelphia: Lippincott Williams & Wilkins, 2000:532.

What is the effect of PEEP on ICP?

PEEP elevates ICP by impairing venous drainage from head

What is the effect of barbiturates on the brain?

Decrease of cerebral metabolic rate by 60%

NEUROLOGIC EVALUATION

What do you do when called to see a patient with a neurologic problem?

Get information: ABC (airway, breathing, circulation), history, neurologic exam, imaging, invasive monitors

What must you look for on neurologic exam?

Decreased level of consciousness or focal neurologic deficit

What are the 4 levels of consciousness?

1. Alert
2. Lethargic: awakens, requires continuous stimulation to keep attention

3. Stuporous/obtunded: does not follow commands, responsive to irritating or painful stimuli
4. Comatose: no purposeful response to deep pain

What are 3 clinical indications of intracranial HTN (IC-HTN)?

1. Pupillary dilation or asymmetry to light
2. Decorticate or decerebrate posturing
3. Progressive deterioration of neurologic exam not attributable to extracranial factors

What is Cushing's triad, and what does it represent?

Cushing's triad is a clinical syndrome resulting from IC-HT. It represents:
1. HTN
2. Bradycardia
3. Respiratory irregularity (Cheyne-Stokes respirations)

What fraction of patients with IC-HTN have the full triad?

About one third

What are focal neurological deficits?

Focal neurological deficits may include cranial nerve palsy, asymmetric weakness or numbness, loss of reflexes, and posturing. Deficits are typically associated with a discrete CNS lesion.

What is "posturing"?

An involuntary pathologic motor response to deep pain

What are 2 types of posturing, and what damage does each type signify?

1. Decorticate/flexor posturing: damage **above** the brainstem; elbow flexion, internal rotation of arm
2. Decerebrate/extensor posturing: damage **in** the brainstem; elbow extension, external rotation of arm.

When should you order brain imaging?

Whenever you even consider it. It is particularly important in the face of any new, unexplained change in mental status or focal neurologic deficit.

What is the brain imaging study of choice in a patient with acute neurologic change?

Head CT **without** contrast

What are the advantages of CT?

Fast, available, shows most acute pathology (blood, stroke, HCP, mass lesions, herniation)

What are 5 types of invasive monitors, and what does each assess?

1. **ICP Monitor ("bolt"):** fiberoptic intraparenchymal probe that monitors ICP; this focal reading usually reflects global ICP.
2. **Jugular bulb venous oximetry:** assess cerebral extraction of oxygen from blood.
3. **Brain tissue oxygen probes:** focal assessment of parenchymal oxygen tension to assess delivery of oxygen to brain tissue
4. **Ventriculostomy catheter:** transduce ICP and drain CSF to decrease ICP.
5. **CVP, Swan-Ganz, A-line:** assess systemic problems.

Which patients need ICP monitoring?

Those with known intracranial pathology (bleed, contusion, edema/swelling) who do not have reliable neurologic exams (i.e., depressed mental status, pharmacologic sedation, paralysis). **Remember: a neuro exam is always better than an ICP monitor.**

What are the specific indications for bolting a trauma patient?

1. Severe head injury (GCS < 8) with abnormal head CT (See description of the GCS later in this section.)
2. Severe head injury (GCS < 8) with normal head CT and at least one of

the following risk factors:
a. Age greater than 40 years
b. SBP less than 90 mm Hg
c. Posturing

You have a patient with high ICPs as measured by your bolt. What 10 things can you do?

1. Notify the neurosurgical team who placed the bolt.
2. Elevate HOB to 30°.
3. Ensure no neck constriction (tight C-collar or trach ties).
4. Maintain BP for good CPP (remember, CPP is a gradient).
5. Mild hyperventilation (arterial partial pressure of carbon dioxide [$PaCO_2$] = 33–37 mm Hg).
6. Sedation.
7. Head CT to evaluate for surgical mass lesion.
8. Mannitol, 0.25 to 1.0 g/kg (increased serum osmolality to extract free water from brain).
9. Ventriculostomy to drain CSF.
10. Decompressive hemicraniectomy.

How does hyperventilation drop ICP?

Hyperventilation results in decreased $PaCO_2$, which causes cerebral vasoconstriction.

Why is hyperventilation controversial?

Little long-term benefit has been demonstrated. Cerebral vasoconstriction induced may produce ischemia; $PaCO_2$ levels lower than 30 mm Hg are rarely indicated. Hyperventilation to $PaCO_2$ should only be done with jugular bulb venous oximetry catheter in place and at a neurosurgeon's discretion.

What is GCS?

Glasgow **C**oma **S**cale: a scoring system with good interrater reliability for assessing level of consciousness in trauma patients. Total score ranges from 3 to 15, derived from the addition of

Table 9-1. Glasgow Coma Scale

Category	Points for a Given Response
Motor	**6:** Obeys verbal command to move **5:** Localizes to pain **4:** Withdraws from pain **3:** Stimulus causes flexure posturing **2:** Stimulus causes extensor posturing **1:** No response to stimulus
Verbal	**5:** Fully oriented **4:** Not fully oriented **3:** Intelligible but not organized **2:** Unintelligible sounds **1:** No vocalization
Eye opening	**4:** Spontaneous **3:** Opens to speech **2:** Opens to pain **1:** No eye opening

Motor, Verbal, and Eye scores. (See Table 9-1.)

How can you remember the number of points per category?

A **V-6 motor**, **4-eyes**, and **V**erbal (roman numeral 5)

How is the GCS modified for an intubated patient?

In place of a number value, the verbal score is denoted T for endotracheal/tracheostomy "tube" (i.e., a nonresponsive patient who does not open his eyes is designated 2T). The highest possible intubated GCS is 10T.

What are some causes of altered mental status in the ICU?

Use the mnemonic **VITAMIN D**:
Vascular: anoxic-ischemic encephalopathy, stroke, disseminated intravascular coagulation (DIC), vasculitis, hypertensive encephalopathy

Infectious: bacterial or fungal meningitis, viral encephalitis

Traumatic: diffuse axonal injury, subdural hematoma (SDH)

Affective: depression, pseudocoma

Metabolic: hypoglycemia, hypercalcemia, hypercapnia, metabolic alkalosis, thyroid disorders, adrenal crisis, uremia, hepatic encephalopathy, hypothermia, Wernicke's encephalopathy

Inflammatory: aseptic meningitis, vasculitis

Neoplastic: metastases, primary CNS tumor, paraneoplastic limbic encephalitis

Drugs

What are 4 ways to minimize delirium in ICU patients?	1. Minimize use of neurologically active drugs (narcotics, BDZs). 2. Maintain normal day/night cycles when possible. 3. Make surroundings familiar and calm. 4. Frequently reorient the patient to time, place, and events.
What percentage of patients have an acute, transient change in mental status after a major operation?	~30%
What are 6 risk factors for postoperative delirium?	1. Older age 2. Alcoholism (recent) 3. Preoperative organic brain disease 4. Severe cardiac disease 5. Multiple comorbid illnesses 6. Prolonged cardiopulmonary bypass time ("pumphead")
What are 8 common causes of postoperative delirium?	1. Medications (narcotics, BDZ) 2. Metabolic disorders (uremia) 3. Alcohol withdrawal 4. Low cardiac output

5. Hypoxia
6. Sepsis
7. Recent stroke
8. Perioperative hypoperfusion (anesthesia, bypass, blood loss)

STROKE

What are the 2 major classifications of stroke and their relative incidences?	1. Hemorrhagic (15%) 2. Ischemic (85%)
What are 2 main causes of cerebral ischemia?	1. Global anoxia (often systemic, e.g., hypotension) 2. Vascular occlusive disease (ischemic stroke)
What is the main cause of ischemic stroke?	Almost always an embolic source (cardiac, aortic, carotid, peripheral if patent foramen ovale present).
How is stroke diagnosed?	New focal neurologic deficit on exam; may be confirmed by head CT.
What does the head CT show in stroke?	Initially following ischemic stroke, nothing; subtle density change or sulcal effacement at 12 to 24 hours; hypodensity by 24 to 48 hours
Why perform CT emergently?	To evaluate for bleeding or a surgically amenable lesion
What strokes could cause sudden unresponsiveness?	Left MCA (speech centers) and basilar (brainstem)
What are the 8 initial steps in managing *ischemic* stroke?	1. ICU monitoring. 2. Normal saline at 100 mL/hr (no dextrose). 3. SBP ~160 in a normotensive patient, SBP ~180 in a hypertensive patient (to maintain CPP gradient). 4. HOB flat for CPP. 5. Normal arterial partial pressure of oxygen; no hypercarbia.

6. Aspirin, 325 mg stat and then QD.
7. Intubate for airway protection if patient is not following commands or is hypoventilating.
8. Consult neurologist to assist with ICP management, workup, and possible anticoagulant/lytic therapy.

What are the initial steps in managing *hemorrhagic* stroke?

All of the same steps as for an ischemic stroke, except maintain MAP near the patient's baseline to balance perfusion versus rebleeding risk and consider Dilantin.

In what 3 situations do you consult a neurosurgeon for a stroke patient?

1. Hemorrhagic cerebellar stroke or ischemic cerebellar stroke with worsening mass effect (may cause very rapid sudden death—a **true emergency**)
2. Large right MCA ischemic stroke unresponsive to medical management (may benefit from decompressive hemicraniectomy)
3. Factors favoring surgical clot evacuation in hemorrhagic stroke (young patient, large clot, worsening neuro exam, superficial or frontal location)

What are 9 risk factors for focal neurologic deficits after cardiac surgery?

1. Increased age.
2. Diabetes mellitus.
3. Pre-existing cerebral vascular disease (especially history of a stroke)
4. Perioperative hypotension
5. Known or discovered ascending aortic atherosclerosis and calcification
6. Left ventricular mural thrombus
7. Opening of a cardiac chamber during surgery
8. Postoperative atrial fibrillation
9. Long duration of cardiopulmonary bypass

What is the incidence of stroke immediately after CEA?

3% to 5%

Is there proof that intraoperative shunts decrease stroke rate?

No

What are 2 mechanisms of perioperative neurologic injury?

1. Cerebral hypoperfusion because of cerebrovascular disease or hypotension
2. Particulate embolism because of atherosclerotic debris, thrombus, platelet debris, or air

INTRACRANIAL HEMORRHAGE

What is IPH?

Intraparenchymal hemorrhage (hemorrhagic stroke)

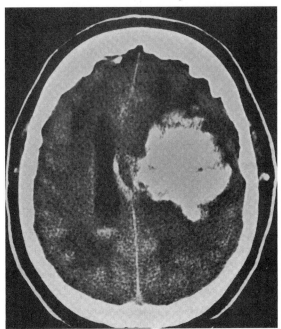

Intraparenchymal hemorrhage. From Miller J, Fountain N. Neurology Recall. 2nd Ed. Philadelphia: Lippincott Williams & Wilkins, 2003:334.

What is the most common cause of IPH?	Rupture of small perforating arteries in deep brain structures in patients with **HTN**
What are 3 less common causes of IPH?	1. Vascular anomalies (AVMs, aneurysm) 2. Arteriopathies 3. Tumors
What are the 4 most common locations of IPH in decreasing order?	1. Basal ganglia (50%) 2. Thalamus (15%) 3. Pons (15%) 4. Cerebellum (10%)
What is the treatment of IPH?	Same as the treatment for ischemic and hemorrhagic stroke. Most basal ganglia, thalamic, and brainstem bleeds are not helped by surgery.

EPIDURAL HEMATOMA

What is the most common mechanism of epidural hematoma (EDH)?	Temporal skull fracture that causes tearing of the middle meningeal artery. This artery is between the bone and dura (i.e., epidural).
What is the classic temporal clinical sequence in EDH?	1. Brief posttraumatic LOC 2. "Lucid interval" of several hours 3. Deterioration: stupor, ipsilateral blown pupil, contralateral hemiparesis
Why does this temporal clinical sequence occur?	The initial LOC caused by immediate concussion effects (seconds to minutes of neuronal dysfunction). This resolves and results in the lucid interval. The subsequent deterioration is caused by the expanding mass lesion (EDH) causing herniation.

In what percentage of EDH patients is this triad seen?

10% to 30% of cases

What is the classic description of an epidural blood clot seen on head CT?

Lentiform, meaning lens-shaped, or biconvex

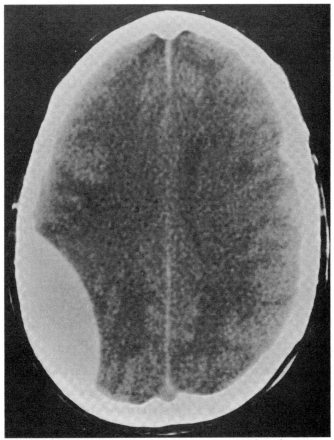

Epidural hematoma. From Miller J, Fountain N. Neurology Recall. 2nd Ed. Philadelphia: Lippincott Williams & Wilkins, 2003:332.

SUBDURAL HEMATOMA

What is the most common cause of SDH?

Head trauma. May also occur in patients taking Coumadin without history of trauma.

What are the 2 main types of SDH?

1. Acute: usually presents immediately after head trauma.
2. Chronic: usually presents in elderly people with history of minor trauma within the last month.

How are the 2 types of SDH different on head CT?

Acute blood is bright white (hyperdense). Chronic blood is dark (hypodense).

Where does the blood come from in SDH?

Tearing of bridging veins that originate in the cortical neural tissue and traverse the subdural space to drain into the dura and the dural sinuses

Which has higher mortality, SDH or EDH?

SDH. The initial impact injury to the brain parenchyma generates a very high force from rapid acceleration or deceleration. Mortality is 20% to 50% for EDH versus 50% to 90% for SDH after closed-head injury.

What is the classic appearance of SDH on head CT?

Lunate or crescent shaped. It never crosses midline, because the falx is in the way.

SUBARACHNOID HEMORRHAGE

Where does the blood come from in SAH?

Most of the major blood vessels supplying the brain rest on top of the pia mater and are covered by the arachnoid mater (in the subarachnoid space). Rupture of any of these vessels causes SAH.

What is the most common mechanism of SAH?

Trauma

What are the 2 most common causes of nontraumatic SAH and their incidences?

1. Ruptured intracerebral aneurysm (80%)
2. Ruptured AVM (5%)

What are the symptoms of nontraumatic SAH?

From mild headache to sudden-onset worst headache of life, nausea/vomiting, confusion, focal neurologic deficit, lethargy, coma, or death

What test does a patient with nontraumatic SAH need?

Four-vessel cerebral angiography within 24 hours to evaluate for surgical lesion (cerebral aneurysm)

What 2 factors are prognostically important in SAH?

1. Extent of brain damage from initial bleed (may be negligible to devastating)
2. Early successful obliteration of aneurysm by surgical clipping to prevent rebleeding

What is the prognosis for unclipped ruptured aneurysm?

50% will rebleed within 6 months (20% within 2 weeks). Rebleeds are much more likely to be fatal.

What is the classic appearance of SAH on head CT?

Five-point star outlining the interhemispheric fissure, sylvian fissures, and brainstem.

Identify the SDH, SAH, and IPH.

A: SAH
B: IPH
C: SDH

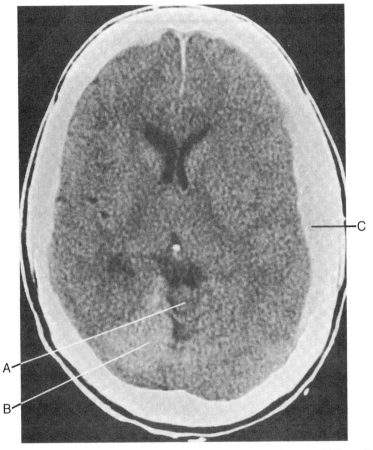

From Miller J, Fountain N. Neurology Recall. 2nd Ed. Philadelphia: Lippincott Williams & Wilkins, 2003:332.

HERNIATION

What is herniation?

A pathologic shift of brain structures

What typically causes herniation?

A mass lesion (hematoma, brain tumor) or brain swelling

Name 4 types of herniation.

1. Uncal herniation (shift of medial temporal lobe to crush the brainstem)
2. Transtentorial herniation (upward or downward movement of the midbrain)
3. Subfalcine (shift of cingulate gyrus under the falx cerebri)
4. Tonsillar herniation (cerebellar tonsils through foramen magnum)

What is the pathologic consequence of herniation events?

Vessel occlusion by compression causing stroke and damage by direct compression (e.g., CN III). Herniation events are emergencies. Mass effect must be removed to have the possibility of survival.

SPINE

What must be checked before placement or removal of a spinal, epidural or LP?

PT, PTT, and platelet count

Why must these be checked?

Risk of spinal EDH

What symptoms would suggest spinal EDH?

Progressive weakness and numbness below the level of the lesion

What specific syndrome could result after LP in a coagulopathic patient?

Cauda equina syndrome

What are the important features of cauda equina syndrome?

1. Urinary retention (>90% sensitivity).
2. "Saddle anesthesia": numbness of anus, perineum, genitals, buttocks, upper posterior thighs (75% sensitivity).
3. May also have decreased anal sphincter tone, fecal incontinence, and urinary overflow incontinence.

How do you confirm your diagnosis of epidural clot?

Urgent spine MRI

What do you do if you find a clot?

Call for a neurosurgery consult to evaluate for urgent decompressive laminectomy. Patients who have decompression delayed for more than 72 hours are very unlikely to recover function.

What major spinal morbidity may result from aortic aneurysm surgery?

Spinal cord infarction and anterior spinal syndrome

What are 4 other causes of cord infarction?

1. Hypotension in an elderly atherosclerotic patient
2. Aortic dissection
3. Spinal epidural abscess (inflammation causes venous thrombosis and, therefore, venous infarct)
4. Emboli to radicular arteries (e.g., during cath lab procedures)

What is the treatment for cord infarction?

Reverse any underlying causes (e.g., restore BP). There are few options and a poor prognosis for recovery.

What medical therapy can improve prognosis for traumatic spinal injury?

Early high-dose steroids

OTHER NEUROLOGIC CONDITIONS

HYDROCEPHALUS

What is HCP?

Increased volume of CSF within the skull, most frequently in the ventricles (water on the brain)

What are the 2 main types of HCP?

Communicating and noncommunicating

Describe each type of HCP.	1. Communicating: blockage of the arachnoid granulations, so no drainage of CSF to venous system. Often a sequela of meningitis or SAH. 2. Noncommunicating: mechanical obstruction of CSF flow. Often seen with tumors of the foramen of Monro, cerebral aqueduct, or fourth ventricle.
What are 5 clinical signs of HCP?	1. Headache 2. Nausea and vomiting 3. Ataxia 4. Papilledema 5. Upward gaze palsy (inability to look up, "Parinaud's syndrome")

MENINGITIS

What are the 6 common symptoms of meningitis?	1. Fevers/chills 2. Severe headache 3. Neck pain, stiffness, rigidity 4. Vomiting 5. Photophobia 6. Altered mental status (**focal** neurologic deficit is rare)
How do you diagnose meningitis?	By performing an LP
What concern would delay performing an LP?	History or exam concerning for intracranial mass (e.g., history of tumor, trauma, focal neurodeficit) or risk of herniation following decompression by LP
So, in that situation, what do you do?	Obtain head CT, and do an LP if no mass lesion is depicted.
What LP findings make you suspect meningitis?	Elevated WBC, pressure, protein; organisms on Gram's stain; depressed CSF glucose:serum glucose ratio (<6)

What are the 3 most common meningitis organisms found in patients aged 3 months to 7 years?	1. *Haemophilus influenzae* 2. *Streptococcus pneumoniae* 3. *Neisseria meningiditis*
What are the 3 most common organisms in patients older than 7 years?	1. *Streptococcus pneumoniae* 2. *Neisseria meningiditis* 3. *Listeria monocytogenes*

SEIZURES

What is a seizure?	An uncontrolled neuronal electrical activity

What are the 2 main types of adult seizures?	1. Generalized: bilaterally symmetric activity, immediate LOC
	2. Partial (also called focal): asymmetric activity
	  a. Simple partial: normal consciousness
	  b. Complex partial: depressed consciousness

What are 7 common etiologies of seizures?	1. Head trauma (20%–30% posttrauma) 2. Intracranial blood 3. Intracranial infection 4. Metabolic abnormalities (low sodium or glucose) 5. Alcohol withdrawal 6. Stimulant drugs 7. Fever
What decreases the incidence of posttraumatic seizure?	Phenytoin (Dilantin)
What is status epilepticus?	1. Seizure lasting more than 30 minutes 2. Multiple seizures without full recovery of consciousness in between
What are the 3 initial steps in managing a seizure?	1. Give Ativan, 2 mg IV push, if seizure lasts more than 2 minutes.

Repeat every 5 minutes up to 10 mg total.
2. Simultaneous Dilantin load, 20 mg/kg IV, at 50 mg/min. (May cause hypotension!)
3. If seizure persists, discuss phenobarbital, intubation, and pentobarbital coma with EEG monitoring with neurology.

By what iatrogenic mechanism can seizure remain occult?

Seizure or continuing status can be missed in the paralyzed patient.

GUILLAIN-BARRÉ SYNDROME

What is Guillain-Barré syndrome (GBS)?

Acute-onset, progressive muscle weakness (usually ascending) because of peripheral motor nerve demyelination

What is a main concern in severe cases of GBS?

Respiratory and oropharyngeal muscle paralysis requiring intubation and ventilation

What causes GBS?

Likely an autoantibody against peripheral nerve myelin sheaths

What are 4 classic findings in a patient's history for GBS?

1. Viral infection
2. Surgery
3. Immunization
4. Mycoplasmal infection

What is the treatment for GBS?

1. Plasmapheresis
2. Supportive care (e.g., ventilation)
3. DVT prophylaxis and physical therapy

MYASTHENIA GRAVIS

What is the key clinical feature of myasthenia gravis (MG)?

Fatigable weakness: strength **decreases** on repeated use of a muscle group.

What 3 muscle groups are most commonly weakened by MG?	1. Ocular (ptosis, diplopia) 2. Bulbar (dysphagia, dysarthria) 3. Limbs (very rarely occurs without ocular or bulbar symptoms)
What is the etiology of MG?	Autoantibodies to nicotinic Ach-receptors at the neuromuscular junction
What is the main treatment of MG?	1. Immunosuppression (azathioprine, cyclosporine, mycophenylate, corticosteroids) 2. Anticholinesterases (neostigmine; increased concentration of acetylcholine) 3. Thymectomy (addresses underlying immune disorder) 4. Plasmapheresis (short-term intervention for crisis or prethymectomy) 5. Supportive care (intubation) for crisis episodes
What is a key differential diagnosis of MG?	Eaton-Lambert syndrome (also known as Lambert-Eaton syndrome)
What distinguishes Eaton-Lambert syndrome from MG?	Strength initially **increases** on repeated use of a muscle group (eventually fatigues).
What is the etiology of Eaton-Lambert syndrome?	Antibodies to presynaptic calcium channels in the neuromuscular junction
What does Eaton-Lambert syndrome make you consider?	Malignancy (present in 66%)
What is the malignancy most commonly associated with Eaton-Lambert syndrome?	Oat-cell carcinoma of the lung (associated with thymoma)

10   Head and Neck

AIRWAY MANAGEMENT

What is a tracheotomy?

A surgical procedure to create an airway. "Tracheotomy" and "tracheostomy" are used interchangeably because the hole may be temporary or permanent.

What is a tracheostoma?

A permanent opening created by suturing the cut edges of the trachea circumferentially to the skin. It is not synonymous with a tracheostomy.

What are 10 possible complications from long-term endotracheal intubation?

1. ETT obstruction (could result in death)
2. Tube displacement (tube should lie midway between the glottis and carina)
3. Intubation granuloma
4. Interarytenoid adhesion
5. Posterior glottic stenosis
6. Vocal cord paralysis
7. Arytenoid cartilage dislocation
8. Subglottic stenosis
9. Failure to wean
10. Difficulty managing secretions and increased risk of aspiration

What are 4 advantages of a tracheotomy compared to endotracheal intubation?

1. Significantly decreased work of breathing
2. Improved control of secretions
3. Decreased risk of aspiration
4. Decreased risk of laryngeal complications

List the possible complications associated with a tracheotomy.

Intraoperative?

Bleeding
Pneumothorax
Pneumomediastinum
Tracheoesophageal fistula
Recurrent laryngeal nerve injury
Airway fire

Early postoperative?

Incisional bleeding
Mucous plugging
Tube displacement
Respiratory arrest (loss of hypoxic
    drive)
Postobstructive pulmonary edema
Severe wound infection

Late postoperative?

Tracheal stenosis
Tracheo-innominate fistula
Tracheal granulation tissue
Persistent tracheocutaneous fistula

How is each type of tracheotomy complication managed in the ICU?

Early bleeding (within 48 hours)?

Mild bleeding is common. Suture, cautery, or coagulant materials may be used. Watch for hematomas causing airway compression or intratracheal bleeding. Never fully close the skin.

Mucous plugging?

Meticulous trach care with frequent suctioning and humidification. Change inner cannula often.

Tube displacement?

Use stay sutures, particularly with pediatric patients. Tape obturators to head of bed, and have additional tracheostomy tubes and ETTs immediately available.

Respiratory arrest?

Be aware of potential loss of hypoxic drive. Have a backup rate on ventilator if necessary.

Postoperative pulmonary edema?

Look for frothy sputum, particularly during the first 30 minutes after operation. Be vigilant in patients with a long history of upper airway obstruction.

Wound infections?

Do not make tracheotomies too low in the neck, particularly after recent sternal incisions. Perform meticulous trach care. Aggressively control glucose levels in diabetic patients.

Tracheal stenosis?

Minimize cuff pressure on tracheostomy tube.

How are late tracheal complications avoided?

By downsizing tracheostomy tubes and decannulating as expeditiously as possible

What is a tracheo-innominate fistula?

A devastating complication resulting when a tracheostomy tube erodes through the tunica intima of the innominate artery

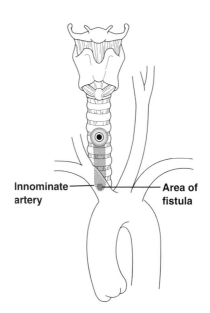

Tracheo-innominate arterial fistula. Adapted from Bailey BJ. Head and Neck Surgery—Otolaryngology. 3rd Ed, Vol 1. Baltimore: Lippincott Williams & Wilkins, 2001:684.

How does a tracheo-innominate fistula present?

Massive hemorrhage inside the tracheal tube

What clinical finding may warn you of an impending fistula?

A **sentinel bleed** may occur hours to days before erosion of the artery. This bleeding comes from the vaso-vasorum.

How is a tracheo-innominate fistula managed?

Hyperinflate the tracheostomy tube cuff. If unsuccessful, perform the Utley maneuver. Definitive repair is performed by ligating innominate artery.

What is the Utley maneuver?

Place an ETT with the cuff inflated below the level of bleeding. Then, insert a finger into trachea, and apply anterior pressure on bleeding artery.

What is the mortality rate of tracheo-innominate fistula?

Greater than 70%

When should someone with an ETT be converted to a tracheostomy?

This is controversial. Current literature suggests after the patient has failed extubation once or if the patient is expected to require mechanical ventilation for more than 2 weeks.

How are tracheostomy tubes sized?

The number of the tube corresponds to the diameter of the cannula. The larger the number, the larger the cannula.

How are tracheostomy tubes secured?

Initially, four sutures typically secure the tracheostomy flange to the skin. A trach tie is also secured around the patient's neck. These ties are typically changed to softer ties during the first trach change or on POD 5 to 7.

Which tube should be initially placed?

Men typically receive a Shiley 8.0 cuffed tube; women receive a Shiley 6.0 cuffed tube. The tracheostomy tube should be approximately 2/3 to 3/4 the size of the trachea.

When do you need a cuffed tube?

Cuffs (balloons on the end of the tracheostomy tubes) prevent air leaks during positive-pressure mechanical ventilation. Also, a cuff can minimize pneumonia in a patient who is grossly aspirating. Cuffs do not prevent microaspiration of oropharyngeal secretions.

How do you minimize cuff pressures?

Aspirate as much air from the inflated cuff as possible until a very minimal leak occurs at peak inspiratory pressures.

When should you use an uncuffed tube?

When mechanical ventilation is not needed or anticipated in the near future. Pediatric patients should avoid cuffed tubes because of an increased risk of subglottic stenosis.

What is an inner cannula?

A disposable tube that fits and locks inside the body of a tracheostomy tube.

What are the advantages of an inner cannula?

They are typically disposable, are regularly changed (every 8 hours and as needed), and can be removed in the event of a mucous plug.

What are the disadvantages of an inner cannula?

Most only fit tracheostomy tubes of standard sizes. Patients with obese necks may need special tubes that may, or may not, have inner cannulas.

What is an obturator?

A plastic rod that fits into a tracheostomy tube and aids insertion. The beveled head allows the tracheostomy tube to more easily pass through the skin and prevents damage to the trachea.

What are stay sutures?

Unknotted sutures that are placed into the trachea during surgery. The free ends of the suture are taped to the patient's chest. They allow the physician to pull the trachea anteriorly, which aids in placement of a dislodged tube.

What is a Bjork flap?

An inferiorly based flap consisting of the anterior portion of one tracheal ring sutured to the inferior skin margin. This greatly reduces the incidence of accidental decannulation and eases reinsertion if necessary

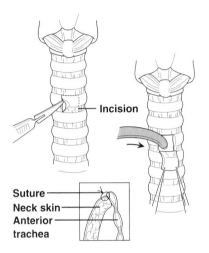

Bjork flap. Adapted from Bailey BJ. Head and Neck—Otolaryngology. 3rd Ed, Vol 1. Baltimore: Lippincott Williams & Wilkins, 2001:684.

What are routine trach care orders?

First trach change to be performed by house officer
Humidified trach collar
Suction tracheostomy with normal saline bullets every 4 hours and as needed (more frequently if necessary)
Change inner cannula every 8 hours and as needed
Do not remove trach ties
Continuous pulse oximetry for the first 24 hours after tracheostomy
Tape obturator to head of the bed
Extra tracheostomy tube and ETT at the bedside

When should a tracheostomy tube be downsized?

The first tracheostomy tube change occurs on nonventilated patients on **POD 5 to 7** to allow a tract to form (may take longer if wound healing is delayed). Tubes are **serially downsized every 2 to 3 days afterward** until they are capped and then decannulated.

What is a Passy-Muir speaking valve?

A one-way valve placed on the tracheostomy tube that opens during inspiration but closes during expiration, thus forcing air through the larynx and allowing a patient to speak.

When should a tracheostomy be decannulated?

After a patient can ventilate independently with the tracheostomy tube capped, has no evidence for upper airway obstruction, has minimal suction requirements, and can cough on demand

How do you dress a decannulated tracheostomy site?

With an occlusive dressing. Place petroleum gauze over the stoma, then place two folded 4 × 4 gauze, then tape to provide an air-tight seal. Change the dressing daily until the stoma closes.

What is a percutaneous dilatational tracheotomy?

Tracheotomy at the bedside using a modified Seldinger technique with or without bronchoscopic visualization. In addition, various amounts of sharp and blunt dissection are performed.

What are the advantages of the percutaneous method?

Decreased costs associated with transport and OR time.

What are the disadvantages of the percutaneous method?

Paratracheal intubation
Possible pneumothorax, pneumomedi-astinum, hemorrhage, or death
Inability to pass dilators into calcified trachea
Difficulty in addressing intraoperative complications
Increased expense of disposable percuta-neous tracheostomy kits

HEAD AND NECK POSTOPERATIVE CARE

LARYNGECTOMY AND NECK DISSECTION

What structures are removed with a laryngectomy?

They range from having the entire larynx removed, including the thyroid cartilage, cricoid cartilage, and hyoid bone, to partial laryngectomies that allow for voice preservation.

What is a radical neck dissection?

The en bloc removal of lymph node–bearing tissues on one side of the neck. Included in the specimen are the spinal accessory nerve, internal jugular vein, and sternocleidomastoid muscle.

What is a modified radical neck dissection?

Preservation of one or more of the following structures:
1. Spinal accessory nerve
2. Internal jugular vein
3. Sternocleidomastoid muscle

What is a selective neck dissection?

Removal of only the lymph node groups with the highest risk of metastasis. The spinal accessory nerve, internal jugular vein, and sternocleidomastoid muscles are spared.

What is a TEP?

A tracheoesophageal puncture. A small, white tube (known as a TEP prosthesis), is placed in this puncture site.

What is a TEP used for?

Patients digitally occlude their tracheostoma, which forces air through the prosthesis into the esophagus and out their mouth. This allows the patient to have esophageal speech.

How do you care for a stoma of a laryngectomy patient?

Regularly remove crusts, and frequently suction to prevent airway occlusion.

What mistake should be avoided with laryngectomy patients in respiratory distress?

Do not attempt oral bag masking and/or oral intubation! Laryngectomy patients must be ventilated through their stoma, because there is no connection of their airway to their mouth (except, in most cases, the small TEP)

What follow-up study is typically obtained for laryngectomy patients?

A leak study (cervical contrasted swallow study) to look for a pharyngeal leak that may progress to a pharyngocutaneous fistula.

What are the risk factors for pharyngocutaneous fistula formation?

Previous irradiation
Diabetes
Advanced head and neck cancer
Age
Poor preoperative nutritional status

Which aspects are particularly important in the postoperative physical exams?

Thorough cranial nerve exam: Patients are at risk for damage to marginal mandibular branch of facial nerve, hypoglossal nerve, vagus nerve, and spinal accessory nerve.
Thorough neck exam: Close attention to neck swelling, drain output, stoma patency, incision breakdown, or necrosis. Drain output should be checked for consistency and volume; it may indicate bleeding, a spit fistula, or chylous leak.
Thorough chest exam: Laryngectomy patients are at risk for aspiration pneumonia and postoperative myocardial infarction.

HEAD AND NECK RECONSTRUCTION

What are the reconstruction options for head and neck defects?

Primary closure/secondary intention
Split-thickness skin grafts
Local flaps
Regional myocutaneous flaps/osteomyocutaneous flaps
Microvascular free flaps

What complications can lead to graft failure for microvascular free flaps?

Venous thrombosis
Arterial thrombosis
Hematoma

How should free flaps be followed postoperatively?

Examined, at minimum, every 4 hours for 48 to 72 hours (jejunal free flaps need to be examined every 2 hours). Doppler signals should be checked to follow arterial flow. Venous sufficiency should be followed by direct visualization and/or pinpricks of the flap.

How does a flap appear when thrombosis occurs?

Venous?

Flap appears swollen, purple, and warm. Pinprick shows copious return of dark blood.

Arterial?

Flap appears cool and very pale. Pinprick shows very minimal blood return.

How is venous thrombosis managed?

Initially, with leeches to temporize the flap. Surgical exploration with thrombectomy is the definitive treatment.

How do leeches work?

They secrete hirudin to anticoagulate the flap and suck out blood to decrease vascular engorgement.

What else does the patient need with leech therapy?

Antibiotics to prevent bacterial suprainfection (particularly with *Aeromonas hydrophilic*). Fluoroquinolones are typically used.

SINUS SURGERY

What are symptoms of a CSF leak?

Clear rhinorrhea
Salty-tasting drainage
Headache

How are CSF leaks repaired?

Lumbar drain
Endoscopic versus open surgical repair

What is invasive fungal sinusitis?	A grave sinus infection in which fungi invade the bloodstream and the underlying infected sinus mucosa
What does invasive fungal sinusitis cause?	Avascular necrosis of underlying tissues secondary to microthromboses
How is invasive fungal sinusitis diagnosed?	Positive biopsy results Decreased uptake of gadolinium on T_1-weighted MRI Failure of nasal mucosa to bleed on pinprick
Who is at risk for invasive fungal sinusitis?	Diabetic patients and immunosuppressed patients
How is fungal sinusitis treated?	Extensive surgical debridement of infected tissue and reversal of immunosuppression
What are the two most critical aspects of treatment?	Reversal of immunosuppression and aggressive control of glucose levels
What is the mortality of invasive fungal sinusitis?	50%

COMMON ICU ISSUES

EPISTAXIS

What are 3 common causes of epistaxis in the ICU?	1. Nonhumidified oxygen via nasal cannula 2. Underlying coagulopathy 3. Hypertension
How are these common causes of epistaxis treated?	Humidified oxygen Reverse coagulopathy Blood pressure control Direct pressure Nasal packing Surgical ligation or embolization

HOARSENESS

What is hoarseness?	Laryngeal dysfunction caused by abnormal vocal cord function
Is stridor a form of hoarseness?	No! Stridor is a medical emergency with noise during breathing caused by airway obstruction. It may coexist with hoarseness, with glottic sources of obstruction.
What are common causes of ICU hoarseness?	Postintubation hoarseness Reflux-induced laryngitis Mucosal drying Postnasal drip from sinusitis Stroke
How can intubation cause hoarseness?	Vocal cord edema Intubation granuloma Interarytenoid adhesion Posterior glottic stenosis Vocal cord paralysis Arytenoid cartilage dislocation
What nerve innervates voice production?	The vagus nerve via the superior laryngeal nerves and recurrent laryngeal nerves
What does the superior laryngeal nerve innervate?	The external branch innervates the cricothyroid muscle. The internal branch provides sensation to the larynx.
What does the recurrent laryngeal nerve innervate?	Motor innervation to the intrinsic muscles of the larynx and sensation to the subglottis
What is meant by a "high vagal" lesion?	Injury to the vagus nerve above the branchpoint of the superior laryngeal and recurrent laryngeal nerves
Do patients with a "high vagal" lesion carry a worse prognosis?	Yes, because sensory innervation to the larynx provided by the superior laryngeal nerve is lost. These patients are more prone to aspirate.

What is the danger of a single paralyzed vocal cord?

Vocal cords adduct and meet at the midline during swallowing to prevent aspiration. A paralyzed vocal cord typically remains fixed laterally, thus allowing aspiration and causing hoarseness.

How is a unilateral vocal cord paralysis treated?

Gelfoam, alloderm, or other type of medialization procedure if one cord is paralyzed

Isshiki and other forms of thyroplasty on awake patients with safe airways

Other advanced forms of laryngeal surgery

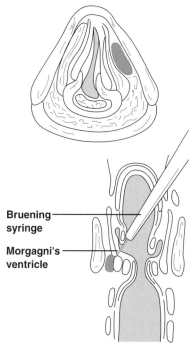

Bruening syringe

Morgagni's ventricle

Gelfoam injection for vocal cord medialization. Adapted from Bailey BJ. Head and Neck—Otolaryngology. 3rd Ed, Vol 1. Baltimore: Lippincott Williams & Wilkins, 2001:633.

11

Respiratory System

ANATOMY AND PHYSIOLOGY

What is TV?

Tidal volume; the volume of air inspired during a single, regular breath

What is TLC?

Total lung capacity; the volume of gas contained within the lung at maximal inspiration

What is VC?

Vital capacity; the greatest volume that can be exhaled after maximal inspiration

What is residual volume (RV)?

The gas remaining in the lung after maximal exhalation (VC + RV = TLC)

What is FRC?

Functional residual capacity; the volume of air that remains in the lung after a *normal* exhalation. Therefore, it is greater than the RV. The difference between the FRC and the RV is known as the expiratory reserve volume.

What 5 types of cells line the peripheral respiratory tree?

1. Type I pneumocyte (predominant): a squamous cell involved in gas exchange.
2. Type II pneumocyte: a stem cell capable of producing new alveolar epithelial cells; it produces surfactant.
3. Clara cell: nonciliated epithelial cells in the terminal bronchioles; their function is unknown.
4. Alveolar macrophage: scavengers that remove debris from the air spaces; this is the most common type of cell recovered in bronchoalveolar lavage.

5. Mast cells: participate in immunologic processes.

What is surfactant?

A phospholipid secreted by type II pneumocytes that lowers surface tension and improves compliance

What is bronchial constriction?

A reflexive bronchial smooth muscle constriction mediated by vagal afferents

List 9 causes of bronchial constriction.

1. Instrumentation
2. Foreign body
3. Cold air
4. Chemicals
5. Gastric acid
6. Cigarette smoke
7. Histamine
8. Some prostaglandins
9. Leukotrienes

How many circulations does the lung possess?

2 circulations:
1. Pulmonary: brings in deoxygenated blood
2. Bronchial: brings in oxygenated blood supplying the bronchial arteries

What is ventilation to areas of the lung with no perfusion called?

Dead space

What is perfusion of an area of lung with no ventilation called?

A shunt

What is HPV?

Hypoxic pulmonary vasoconstriction; the response of the pulmonary vasculature to alveolar hypoxia. Oxygenation is maintained by diverting blood flow to well-ventilated areas of the lung.

What is V/Q mismatch?

Blood flow (Q) is "matched" to ventilation (V) through HPV.

Significant regional abnormalities in blood flow or ventilation may overwhelm local autoregulation, causing a V/Q mismatch and resultant hypoxemia.

Which 3 common drugs can cause a V/Q mismatch?

1. Nitroprusside
2. Nitroglycerin
3. Dihydropyridines

All 3 can interrupt the ability of the lung arterioles to constrict in response to hypoxia.

ARTERIAL BLOOD GASES

What are the basic measurements reported with an ABG?

In order:
1. pH
2. $PaCO_2$: arterial carbon dioxide
3. PaO_2: arterial oxygen
4. HCO_3: serum bicarbonate

How do acute changes in $PaCO_2$ affect pH?

For each rise of 10 mm Hg, pH decreases by 0.08.

How fast does $PaCO_2$ rise in an apneic patient?

6 mm Hg in the first minute, then 3 mm Hg/min

What 3 clinical scenarios might cause respiratory acidosis?

1. Inadequate respiratory drive: oversedation, head injury
2. Inability to maintain work of breathing
3. Airway obstruction: foreign body, blood, mucous plug, bronchospasm

What clinical scenarios might cause respiratory alkalosis?

Hyperventilation from pain, fear, head injury, or certain brain tumors; psychogenic causes

What is the most common cause of respiratory alkalosis in the ICU?

Iatrogenic hyperventilation

What underlying conditions would cause metabolic acidosis?

Mnemonic **SLUMPEDD**:
Salicylate toxicity (aspirin overdose)
Lactic acidosis
Uremia
Methanol intoxication
Paraldehyde intoxication
Ethylene glycol poisoning
Diabetic ketoacidosis
Diarrhea

How do you determine when a patient has respiratory compensation for a metabolic acidosis?

Use the Winter's equation:
$1.5(HCO_3) + 8 \pm 2 = P_{CO_2}$

When one compensates for an acidosis or alkalosis, can a completely normal pH be achieved?

No

List 3 causes of metabolic alkalosis?

1. Excessive loss of gastric acid: vomiting, NG suction
2. Severe dehydration: contraction alkalosis
3. Ingestion of alkaline substances: milk-alkali syndrome

For each of the following blood gases, identify the appropriate physiologic state:

pH = 7.24, P_{O_2} = 80, P_{CO_2} = 61, HCO_3 = 25

Respiratory acidosis

pH = 7.56, P_{O_2} = 100, P_{CO_2} = 20, HCO_3 = 24

Respiratory alkalosis

pH = 7.32, P_{O_2} = 120, P_{CO_2} = 30, HCO_3 = 15

Metabolic acidosis (with respiratory compensation)

pH = 7.58, P_{O_2} = 130, P_{CO_2} = 40, HCO_3 = 35

Metabolic alkalosis

VENTILATION

What are 4 indications for intubation and mechanical ventilation?	1. Inability to maintain a patent airway 2. Inability to prevent aspiration of secretions 3. Inadequate alveolar ventilation: rising P_{CO_2} 4. Inadequate alveolar oxygenation: falling P_{O_2} or O_2 saturation
How is proper intubation confirmed?	1. Bilateral auscultation over chest 2. Bilateral chest movement 3. End-tidal CO_2 4. CXR verification
What is the greatest danger of ET intubation?	Unrecognized esophageal intubation
How is pulmonary compliance calculated?	Compliance = $\Delta V/\Delta P$ where V = lung volume and P = pulmonary pressure (cm H_2O)

BASIC VENTILATOR MODES

What is pressure-cycled ventilation?	Delivery of set airway pressure to the patient. The volume delivered depends on lung compliance.
What is volume-cycled ventilation?	Delivery of set TV to the patient. The pressure attained depends on lung compliance.
What is the IMV mode?	Intermittent mandatory ventilation; a volume-cycled mode in which the TV and mechanically delivered respiratory rate are set. Each breath is delivered at a constant flow rate with variable peak pressures. The patient may take additional breaths above the set rate, but *without* help from the ventilator.
What are 2 weaknesses of the IMV mode?	1. Breathing over the ventilator may be difficult for the patient because of high resistance in the tubing.

2. The patient's own breathing pattern is interrupted.

What is the SIMV mode?

Synchronized intermittent mandatory ventilation. SIMV is similar to IMV, except that the ventilator senses the patient's spontaneous breathing pattern and attempts to time the machine-delivered breaths with the patient's breathing cycle.

What is the theoretical advantage of SIMV over IMV?

SIMV prevents "breath stacking" (i.e., superimposing a mechanical inhalation or exhalation on spontaneous breathing, with resulting increased airway pressures).

What is the AC mode?

Assist control mode; a volume-cycled mode. The physician inputs the TV and respiratory rate, as with IMV and SIMV. In the AC mode, however, the machine senses any patient-generated respiratory effort and immediately follows with a full, machine-powered breath. Thus, the patient does no work even to carry out his own spontaneous breaths.

What are 2 weaknesses of the AC mode?

1. Patient does little work of breathing.
2. One must watch for respiratory alkalosis.

What is PSV?

Pressure support ventilation. PSV senses initiation of the patient's spontaneous breath and delivers a specified amount of pressure support during that breath.

What is the danger of using PSV alone?

An apneic patient would receive no breaths at all if PSV only is used.

For what is PSV used?

As an adjunct to the SIMV mode to decrease the work of spontaneous breaths. PSV can also be used alone when weaning the chronic ventilator patient.

What is the primary difference between the AC mode and the SIMV with PSV mode?

In AC, patient-initiated breaths over the set rate each have a set volume. In SIMV with PSV, patient-initiated breaths over the set rate have a volume that is dependent on patient effort with the aid of the pressure support.

What is the difference between the AC mode and the SIMV with PSV mode when the patient is not breathing over the set rate?

Nothing!

What is the PC mode?

Pressure control; a pressure-cycled mode in which the peak airway pressure and respiratory rate are set. The effective TV varies depending on the lung compliance.

What measurement varies throughout an inspired breath during the PC mode to maintain constant peak airway pressures?

Flow rate

What is a benefit of the PC mode over the volume-controlled modes?

In the PC mode, high peak airway pressures are avoided in patients with low compliance.

What are 2 weaknesses of the PC mode?

1. Abrupt decrease in pulmonary compliance can decrease the minute ventilation and cause a rapid rise in P_{CO_2}.
2. Agitated patients who fight the ventilator get minimal TVs.

What is the PRVC mode?

Pressure-regulated volume control. TV and respiratory rate are again set; however, the flow rate varies to prevent exceeding a set peak airway pressure.

Which is the best ventilation mode for each of the following clinical scenarios?

    A trauma patient who is totally apneic

AC (although when not breathing over the ventilator, SIMV is identical)

    A patient with ARDS and very low lung compliance

PC (PRVC would also be a good choice)

    A patient 24 hours out from a large GI surgery who is beginning to take spontaneous breaths

SIMV with pressure support

    A trauma patient 40 days out, weaning from the vent, and awake with a tracheostomy

PSV

CONCEPTS OF MECHANICAL VENTILATION

What 5 important components determine the PIP obtained during mechanical ventilation?

1. Lung–thorax compliance
2. Airway resistance
3. Delivered TV
4. Inspiratory flow rate
5. End-expiratory pressure

What effect does positive-pressure ventilation have on hemodynamics?

Positive-pressure ventilation causes a rise in intrathoracic pressure, which may decrease venous return, causing a subsequent fall in CO and blood pressure.

What are 2 potential complications of high airway pressures?

1. Barotrauma
2. Decreased CO

How can high airway pressures lead to decreased CO and hypotension?

The high positive pressure is referred to all intrathoracic structures, thus reducing the venous return of blood to the heart.

At what PIP does barotrauma become a significant risk?

At less than 50 cm H_2O, barotrauma rarely occurs. At 50 to 70 cm H_2O, there is an 8% incidence of barotrauma. The incidence increases to 43% at a PIP greater than 70 cm H_2O.

What is the difference between ventilation and oxygenation?

Ventilation: removal of CO_2 from the alveoli (Pa_{CO_2})
Oxygenation: delivery of oxygen to red blood cells (Pa_{O_2})

What blood gas parameter primarily reflects alveolar ventilation?

Pa_{CO_2}

What is an acceptable range for Pa_{CO_2} in a patient without chronic obstructive pulmonary disease (COPD)?

30 to 40 mm Hg

Name 2 methods of increasing the alveolar ventilation of a patient on a volume respirator.

1. Increase the rate of ventilation.
2. Increase the TV.

Your patient acutely develops inadequate alveolar ventilation despite correct ventilator settings. What causes must you rapidly rule out?

Mnemonic **LIFE**:
Lung: mucous plugging of bronchus, pneumothorax
Internal tubing: dislodgment of ETT, right mainstem intubation, plugging of tube
Fight: agitated patient fighting ventilator
External tubing: disconnection of ventilator from patient, kinking of tubing, patient biting ETT

How does one determine the appropriate TV for a specific patient?

10 to 12 mL/kg of patient's ideal body weight

What is minute ventilation?

TV × rate of ventilation

What 2 blood parameters reflect the patient's oxygenation status?

1. PaO_2
2. Oxygen saturation

How do you estimate the PaO_2 based on the oxygen saturation?

The 40,50,60–70,80,90 rule! A PaO_2 of 40 correlates with a saturation of 70, 50 with 80, and 60 with 90.

What is FIO_2?

The fraction of the inspired gas mixture comprised of oxygen

What is PEEP?

Positive end-expiratory pressure

What does PEEP do?

Holds alveolar sacs open, and recruits more alveoli. Oxygenation may be enhanced as PEEP increases.

How much PEEP is usually required?

Most intubated patients require at least 5 mm Hg; however, increasing amounts may be required achieve adequate oxygenation.

What 2 problems are associated with high PEEP?

1. Barotrauma: SQ emphysema, bleb formation, pneumothorax
2. Decreased venous return, causing decreased CO and hypotension

At what FIO_2 levels will oxygen toxicity occur?

50% to 60% for more than 24 hours (100% oxygen for short periods of time is usually well tolerated)

How accurate are the FIO_2 designations of the various face masks?

It is impossible to deliver reliably more than 50% oxygen except by ETT. (Thus, oxygen toxicity is not a risk unless the patient is intubated.)

What are the 2 most common causes of hypoxia in the ICU?

1. Atelectasis
2. Pulmonary edema

What is the lowest acceptable PaO_2?

60 to 70 mm Hg

What 6 steps can you take to improve oxygenation?

1. Increase PEEP.
2. Increase F_{IO_2}.
3. Diurese and optimize CO if in pulmonary edema.
4. Decrease oxygen consumption: sedation, treat fevers with Tylenol, treat infections.
5. Increase inspiratory to expiratory (I:E) ratio on ventilator
6. Transfuse if severely anemic

What 3 factors influence DO_2 to tissues?

1. Oxygen saturation (SpO_2)
2. Hemoglobin content of blood
3. CO

where $DO_2 = 13.4 \times SpO_2 \times Hgb \times CO$

What is dead space ventilation (Vd/Vt)?

The ratio of physiologic dead space (volume of inspired air not participating in gas exchange) to TV. This ratio (usually <0.4) is often associated with failure to wean from ventilatory support when greater than 0.6.

How can Vd/Vt be calculated?

$Vd/Vt = (PaCO_2 - PeCO_2)/PaCO_2$
where $PeCO_2$ = exhaled PCO_2.

What are 3 common modes of weaning patients from a ventilator?

1. SIMV supplemented by pressure support
2. Intermittent periods of T-piece ventilation
3. PSV

What is the Tobin Index?

Respiratory rate/spontaneous TV. If less than 100 breaths/min/L, then success with extubation is more likely.

What are 8 useful weaning parameters?

1. Resolution of the original problem
2. Patient awake and following commands
3. Negative inspiratory pressure greater than 20 cm H_2O
4. Resting minute ventilation less than 10 L/min

5. Respiratory rate less than 30 breaths/min
6. pH 7.33 to 7.48
7. Po_2 greater than 70 mm Hg on Fio_2 of 40%
8. Tobin Index less than 100 breaths/min/L

Why is early weaning from mechanical ventilation preferred?

To prevent atrophy of the respiratory muscles and to minimize complications of mechanical ventilation

List 7 complications associated with mechanical ventilation?

1. Barotrauma
2. Oxygen toxicity
3. Secretion accumulation
4. Nosocomial infections: pneumonia
5. Laryngotracheal stenosis
6. Atrophy of respiratory musculature
7. Tracheo-innominate fistula

What are 7 causes of weaning failure?

1. Premature attempt to wean
2. Oversedation
3. Bronchospasm
4. Excessive secretions
5. Acid-base imbalances
6. Hypothyroidism
7. Electrolyte imbalances

What is a RQ?

Respiratory quotient; the ratio of the rate of CO_2 production to the rate of O_2 consumption (normally 0.8 in a healthy person)

Why measure RQ when patients are difficult to wean from ventilatory support?

Large carbohydrate loads in the nutritionally supported patient lead to increased CO_2 production. This may increase RQ to 1.0 or greater and prevent weaning from ventilatory support.

How could you modify nutrition to reduce RQ?

Increasing the percentage of calories provided as fats can reduce the production of CO_2.

NONINVASIVE MECHANICAL VENTILATION

What is CPAP?

Continuous positive airway pressure. It is PEEP applied during spontaneous inspiration and expiration and may be administered with a face mask.

What is the benefit of CPAP?

Increased expiratory transpulmonary pressure and lung volume (increased functional reserve capacity). This pressure is intended to keep alveoli open and lung compliance optimal.

What is NPPV?

Noninvasive positive-pressure ventilation. Both inspiratory pressure and expiratory pressure are set and delivered via face mask.

What are 3 indications for NPPV?

1. Decreased ventilation
2. Increased work of breathing
3. Post extubation for some COPD patients

What are 5 contraindications to NPPV?

1. Facial deformity or fracture
2. Inability to protect airway
3. Excessive secretions
4. Decreased mental status
5. Hemodynamic instability

LUNG PATHOLOGY

Name 6 ways to improve pulmonary toilet.

1. Frequent suctioning of the airways
2. Chest percussion
3. Turning the patient frequently
4. Encouraging cough
5. Using inhaled bronchodilators
6. Using incentive spirometry if patient is not intubated

What are 5 indications for CXR in the ICU?

1. Central line or pulmonary artery catheter placement
2. Chest tube insertion
3. Thoracentesis

4. Any significant change in patient status
5. Recent intubation

What 6 conditions may cause wheezing?

1. Bronchospasm
2. Aspiration
3. Pulmonary edema
4. Pulmonary embolus
5. Pneumothorax
6. Endobronchial intubation

What are 7 respiratory health maintenance issues for patients in the ICU?

1. Avoid aspiration by elevating the head of the bed and frequently checking for gastric residuals.
2. Encourage aggressive pulmonary toilet.
3. Keep FIO_2 less than 50%.
4. Ensure a favorable RQ.
5. Check daily CXR in patients with ETTs, chest tubes, and pulmonary artery catheters.
6. Avoid fluid overload.
7. Implement DVT prophylaxis.

HEMOPTYSIS

What is hemoptysis?

Blood in the sputum

What defines massive hemoptysis?

More than 600 mL of blood produced in 24 hours

Name 5 causes of hemoptysis?

1. Infection: pneumonia, tuberculosis, bronchiectasis
2. Malignancy
3. Instrumentation: bronchoscopic biopsy
4. Trauma
5. Vasculitis: Goodpasture's or Wegener's diseases

What is the best position for a patient with massive hemoptysis?

On the side with the bleeding lung down to prevent spillage of blood into the contralateral lung

What are 4 treatment priorities in massive hemoptysis?	1. Intubate (people die of asphyxiation, not from exsanguination).
	2. Correct coagulopathies.
	3. Localize the site of bleeding.
	4. Use 1 of 3 treatment options:
	   a. Selected bronchial balloon tamponade.
	   b. Bronchial artery embolization.
	   c. Surgical resection of the source of bleeding.

ASPIRATION

What are 6 factors in the ICU that predispose a patient to aspiration?	1. Altered sensorium 2. Impaired swallowing or cough 3. Slowed gastric emptying 4. Ileus 5. Poorly functioning NG tube 6. Premature extubation
List 2 ways to lessen the likelihood of aspiration.	1. Check gastric residuals and mental status frequently. 2. Keep the head of the bed elevated.
What is the treatment of aspiration pneumonitis?	1. Eliminate the cause. 2. Pulmonary toilet. 3. Consider intubation for deterioration. 4. Monitor oxygen saturation. 5. Culture sputum. 6. Consider prophylactic antibiotics.
What are 6 complications associated with aspiration?	1. Upper airway colonization 2. Bronchospasm 3. Tracheobronchitis 4. Pneumonia 5. ARDS 6. Death

PULMONARY EDEMA

What is pulmonary edema?	Accumulation of fluid in the interstitial and air spaces of the lung

What are the 2 general categories of pulmonary edema?

1. Cardiogenic: increased hydrostatic pulmonary capillary pressure as in fluid overload or left heart failure
2. Noncardiogenic: either altered permeability of the capillary membrane (sepsis, ARDS) or decreased plasma oncotic pressure (nephrotic syndrome)

What is the initial treatment of pulmonary edema?

Oxygen and diuresis should supplement treatment of underlying cause.

ACUTE RESPIRATORY DISTRESS SYNDROME

What causes ARDS?

Injured alveolocapillary membrane allows both inflammatory cells and protein-rich fluid to enter the interstitium and alveoli. The capillary–endothelial barrier is further damaged by inflammatory cells and their mediators, contributing to the large V/Q mismatch.

What are the 3 primary features of ARDS?

1. Severe hypoxemia refractory to increased inspired oxygen concentration
2. Diffuse pulmonary infiltrates: interstitial and alveolar
3. Low lung compliance

What are the 3 criteria for the diagnosis of ARDS?

1. Ratio of PaO_2 to FIO_2 less than 200
2. Pulmonary capillary wedge pressure less than 18 mm Hg
3. Diffuse pulmonary infiltrates

Name 9 conditions that can precipitate ARDS.

1. Sepsis
2. Multiple trauma
3. Shock
4. Aspiration
5. Multiple blood transfusions
6. Disseminated intravascular coagulopathy

7. Pancreatitis
8. Fat embolism syndrome
9. Cardiopulmonary bypass

Describe the radiographic finding of ARDS.

1. Initially, diffuse or patchy bilateral infiltrates sparing the costophrenic angles.
2. Later, patchy or nodular infiltrates.
3. If the condition progresses, a pattern of diffuse interstitial fibrosis may occur.

How can you differentiate between cardiogenic pulmonary edema and ARDS on CXR?

Generally, with ARDS you will not see pulmonary vascular redistribution, pleural effusion, or cardiomegaly.

How can the impact of ARDS on the patient be lessened?

Treat the underlying condition! Maximize DO_2. Maintain the lowest possible pulmonary capillary wedge pressure compatible with adequate CO.

How should patients with ARDS be mechanically ventilated?

The significant decrease in pulmonary compliance increases the risk for barotrauma. Ventilate with TVs of 5 mL/kg and plateau pressures less than 30 cm H_2O.

What is the mortality rate of ARDS?

Greater than 50%. When accompanied by sepsis, mortality approaches 90%!

What is the most common cause of death in patients with ARDS?

Nonpulmonary multiple organ system failure

PNEUMOTHORAX

What is a pneumothorax?

Air or gas in the pleural space

What is the pleural space?

The area between the visceral and parietal pleura

What are 4 common causes of pneumothorax in the ICU patient?

1. Barotrauma
2. Central line insertion or thoracentesis
3. Air spaces left in the chest after cardiothoracic surgery
4. Tracheostomy placement

How is a pneumothorax diagnosed?

CXR or physical exam (decreased breath sounds and hyperresonance to percussion on the ipsilateral side)

What is a tension pneumothorax?

Air in the pleural space with a pressure greater than atmospheric pressure. The increased intrathoracic pressure can lead to hemodynamic changes, cardiovascular compromise, and death.

What is the treatment of a tension pneumothorax?

Decompression of the chest with a large-bore needle in the second intercostal space in the midclavicular line, unless a chest tube can be placed immediately

Why are patients on ventilators at greater risk for a tension pneumothorax?

Air can be forced into the pleural space with positive-pressure ventilation and trapped there because of a ball valve–like effect.

Why does tension pneumothorax cause hemodynamic compromise?

Tension pneumothorax causes impairment of venous return to the heart secondary to increased pressure in the thoracic cavity.

What is the implication of an air leak after a chest tube is placed?

The lung or bronchus has an opening that allows air to escape into the pleural space and out through the chest tube. One must rule out an improperly positioned tube or a faulty connection.

What characteristics are seen in a chest tube suction apparatus when a patient has a parenchymal air leak versus a bronchial leak?

Parenchymal leaks: typically smaller and less voluminous
Bronchial leaks: more often continuous and higher volume

Can a patient with a chest tube in the pleural space develop a pneumothorax?	Yes. The chest tube may be in a loculated space, or the tube may be clogged.
What is SQ emphysema?	The bubbly sensation on palpation that can occur when a pneumothorax decompresses itself into the soft tissues
Is SQ emphysema dangerous?	No. It should, however, alert the clinician to the possibility of a pneumothorax or proximal airway injury. It can also occur in the setting of a chest tube or tracheostomy when air dissects into SQ tissue planes around the tubes.
What is the treatment of SQ emphysema?	Better evacuation of air from the chest

PLEURAL EFFUSION

What is a pleural effusion?	A collection of fluid in the pleural space
Name 7 causes for development of pleural fluid in an ICU patient.	1. Heart failure 2. Fluid overload 3. Pancreatitis 4. Nephrotic syndrome 5. Pneumonia 6. Cirrhosis 7. Central line infusing fluid into the pleural space
How are pleural effusions categorized?	As exudates and transudates
What are the Light's criteria?	1. Pleural/serum LDH ratio greater than 0.6 2. Pleural LDH greater than $2/3$ upper limit for normal serum LDH 3. Pleural/serum protein ratio greater than 0.5
What is the significance of the Light's criteria?	If any criterion is met, a transudative effusion is excluded.

What test can be used with the Light's criteria to improve its specificity?	Serum albumin - plural albumin < 1.2 g/dL suggests an exudative effusion.
Why categorize pleural effusions into these two categories?	Exudates often require aggressive treatment of the pleural space, such as chest tubes or even decortication. Transudates usually respond to thoracentesis and treatment of the underlying problem.
What is the name of a pleural effusion associated with pneumonia?	Parapneumonic effusion. These sometimes are sterile, but when they contain bacteria, they often progress to an empyema.
What pleural fluid pH suggests an empyema that will require chest tube drainage?	Less than 7.0
How is a pleural effusion drained in an ICU patient?	By insertion of a catheter (chest tube or pigtail) or by thoracentesis
What are 3 indications for drainage of pleural fluid?	1. To make a diagnosis 2. To allow more efficient ventilation 3. To prevent "trapped lung" in the case of hemothorax or empyema
What should one suspect when a large pleural effusion is present in the hours after central line insertion?	Hemothorax (vascular injury) or IV fluids (catheter in the pleural space)
What is the treatment of this type of pleural effusion?	Insertion of a chest tube for drainage of blood or fluid from the pleural space

PULMONARY EMBOLISM

What is a PE?	A thrombus formed in the peripheral venous circulation that breaks free and travels to the lung, where it lodges in

the pulmonary vascular tree and causes an inflammatory reaction

Where do most clinically important thrombi form?

The large veins of the pelvis and thigh

What 5 factors in the ICU predispose a patient to a PE?

1. Immobility
2. Surgery (particularly orthopedic)
3. Malignancy
4. Pregnancy
5. History of smoking or using oral estrogens

Name 4 ways to prevent a PE.

1. Mobility
2. Sequential compression devices
3. Low-dose heparin
4. LMW heparin

What 8 symptoms might a patient report?

1. Commonly asymptomatic
2. Pleuritic chest pain
3. Difficulty breathing
4. Easy fatigability
5. Cough
6. Hemoptysis
7. Low-grade fever
8. Pain or swelling in a leg

What 4 physical findings are associated with a PE?

1. Sinus tachycardia
2. Mild to severe respiratory distress
3. Cyanosis
4. Hypotension

What are the usual findings on lung exam?

The lung exam is usually normal, although there may be focal wheezing, a pleural friction rub, or rales.

What is the most common ECG finding?

Sinus tachycardia

What are the 4 "classic" ECG findings?

1. A deep S wave in lead I
2. A prominent Q wave in lead III
3. An inverted T wave in lead III
4. Right-axis deviation

These 4 findings are associated with moderate to severe PE.

How is the diagnosis of a PE confirmed?

1. ABG studies show hypoxia with a large A-a gradient.
2. V/Q scan or spiral CT of the chest.
3. An echocardiogram may show right ventricular strain.
3. Pulmonary arteriogram is the gold standard.

What happens to the central pressures during massive acute PE?

The central venous pressure and pulmonary artery systolic pressure should increase acutely and markedly, especially if there is cardiovascular compromise.

What are the most common radiographic findings on CXR?

Normal or unchanged

Does everyone suspected of having a PE need a pulmonary angiogram?

No. If clinical suspicion is low with a normal physical exam, "low probability" V/Q lung scan, or negative spiral CT of the chest, a pulmonary angiogram is not mandatory.

What are 5 treatment modalities for acute PE?

1. IV heparin: acute treatment
2. Thrombolytic therapy
3. Coumadin: long-term prophylaxis
4. Vena cava filter: for recurrent emboli during anticoagulation therapy or when a patient has a contraindication to anticoagulation
5. Pulmonary embolectomy: last option for massive PE

What treatment do most patients with a PE require?

IV heparin only

What are 3 indications for emergency surgical pulmonary embolectomy?

1. Refractory hemodynamic compromise
2. Severe hypoxia despite mechanical intubation and ventilation

3. Continued deterioration despite anticoagulation with heparin or thrombolytic therapy

LIFE-THREATENING SITUATIONS

What are the 2 most common respiratory disasters in an ICU?

1. Loss of an airway
2. Aspiration

What are the 5 components in treatment of acute bronchospasm?

1. Oxygen administration
2. Steroids
3. Inhaled bronchodilators
4. β-Agonists (SQ epinephrine may be considered in an emergent setting)
5. Mechanical ventilation

A patient with known severe COPD, if treated with supplemental oxygen, may experience impaired breathing and increasing CO_2 retention. What physiologic impairment explains this phenomenon?

The patient's respiratory center in the brain no longer responds to rising CO_2, because CO_2 is chronically elevated. The patient's breathing is driven by hypoxia, and excessive supplemental oxygen eliminates that drive.

A patient who was just intubated and placed on a ventilator has no breath sounds on the left side. What is the most likely explanation?

An ETT extending into the right mainstem bronchus and occluding the left mainstem bronchus

What 6 respiratory issues could arise in the next 24 hours that could kill the patient in the previous question?

1. Loss of airway
2. Pulmonary edema
3. Virulent pneumonia
4. PE
5. Aspiration
6. Pneumothorax

Name 4 ways to lessen the likelihood of airway loss.

1. Intubate the patient sooner rather than later.
2. Be sure the tubes are secure.

3. Make sure the patient cannot bite the tube.
4. Ensure optimal large airway toilet.

Name 3 ways to lessen the likelihood of pulmonary edema.

1. Maximize cardiac status.
2. Use diuretics and manage fluid status to keep lungs dry.
3. Intubate if necessary.

Name 3 ways to lessen the likelihood of virulent pneumonia.

1. Monitor cultures.
2. Treat virulent organisms aggressively.
3. Wash your hands and stethoscope between patients.

Name 3 ways to lessen the likelihood of a PE.

1. DVT prophylaxis
2. Prompt diagnostic workup if PE is suspected.
3. Inferior vena cava filter if PE is suspected in a patient already on anticoagulation or if a high-risk patient has a contraindication to anticoagulation

Name 3 ways to lessen the likelihood of aspiration.

1. Keep the GI tract decompressed.
2. Do not rely on cuffed tubes for protection.
3. Keep the patient's head raised at approximately 30°.

Name 3 ways to lessen the likelihood of a pneumothorax.

1. Ensure chest tubes are working properly.
2. Avoid excessive needle sticks during difficult procedures.
3. Try to avoid PIPs greater than 45 cm H_2O.

12   Cardiac Arrhythmias

MONITORING

How are disturbances in cardiac rhythm usually detected in the ICU?

ICU patients are usually monitored by a continuous cardiac rhythm monitor to detect aberrant rhythms and to monitor response to treatment.

What lead should be chosen for the cardiac rhythm monitor?

Any lead that best shows the P wave and the QRS complex (typically, leads II and V_1).

When should a rhythm strip be recorded?

At admission, the start of each shift, the time of any arrhythmia, and during treatment

Is a rhythm strip by itself adequate for the correct diagnosis of an arrhythmia?

No. A 12-lead ECG should be obtained to adequately interpret the rhythm.

What is the most important ECG that you should obtain?

The previous ECG for comparison and/or the admit ECG for the patient's baseline

If you cannot establish a diagnosis with the 12-lead ECG, what 3 other diagnostic options do you have?

1. Lewis lead
2. Intra-atrial ECG: invasive and requires fluoroscopy
3. Esophageal ECG: pill electrode or catheter

What is the Lewis lead?

A maneuver performed to optimize visualization of the P wave. This involves moving the right-arm lead to the 2nd right parasternal space (base of the heart) and the left-arm lead to the 4th or 5th left parasternal space.

The P wave is typically upright in which 4 leads?	1. I 2. II 3. aVF 4. V_4 through V_6
Can the rate of the arrhythmia give any clue regarding the type of arrhythmia?	Yes. Certain rhythms will have a characteristic rate: 100 to 180 bpm: sinus tachycardia 140 to 220 bpm: atrial tachycardia/ re-entrant 260 to 320 bpm: Aflutter 150 to 200 bpm: Vtach 150 to 300 bpm: ventricular flutter
What is the normal QRS duration?	Less than 0.12 milliseconds. This is consistent with a supraventricular impulse conducted normally through the AV conduction pathway.
If a patient presents with a wide QRS complex, what 4 items should be in your differential diagnosis?	1. Vtach 2. SVT with bundle branch block 3. Aberrant ventricular conduction 4. Accessory AV conduction

BASIC SCIENCE OF ARRHYTHMIAS

What are the 3 pacemaker cells of the heart, and what are their intrinsic rates?	1. SA node: 60 to 100 bpm 2. AV node: 40 to 60 bpm 3. His-Purkinje system: 20 to 40 bpm
From where do the impulses for the normal heart rate originate?	SA node
Describe the impulse propagation from the SA node to depolarization of the ventricle.	SA node → AV node → His bundle → right and left bundle branches → Purkinje network → ventricular depolarization
Describe the role of the subsidiary pacemakers.	If the impulse of the SA node is blocked, fails to conduct, or falls below the rate of the subsidiary pacemaker,

the subsidiary pacemaker determines the rate of ventricular depolarization.

What 5 pharmacologic agents work at the AV node?

1. Atropine
2. Adenosine
3. Calcium-channel blockers
4. Digoxin
5. β-blockers

What is the activation time of the ventricle?

80 to 100 milliseconds. This correlates with the QRS complex width on ECG.

What are the 3 mechanisms of arrhythmia formation?

1. Abnormal automaticity: spontaneous depolarizations
2. Re-entry
3. Triggered activity: caused by oscillations in the membrane potential

What 4 factors can decrease automaticity?

1. Increased parasympathetic activity
2. Hyperkalemia
3. Moderate hypothermia
4. Antiarrhythmics

Conversely, what 6 factors can increase automaticity?

1. Increased sympathetic activity
2. Hypokalemia
3. Severe hypothermia
4. Myocardial ischemia
5. Cardiac stretching
6. Digoxin can increase sinus node automaticity

Describe the 4 steps in the pathogenesis of re-entry.

1. A conducted impulse encounters two divergent, functional pathways, which converge into a more distal pathway.
2. There is a unidirectional block in one limb.
3. The unblocked impulse conducts retrograde up the blocked limb, but a gap must remain between the re-entrant impulse and the refractory tail to maintain the re-entrant pathway.

4. The re-entrant pathway can generate depolarizing impulses as it cycles.

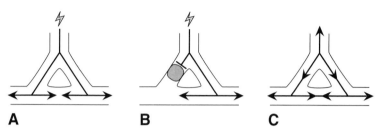

A   **B**   **C**

Lightning bolts indicate sites of impulse formation, arrows indicate the directions of impulse conduction, perpendicular lines indicate the block of impulse conduction, and shaded areas indicate those areas that have not completed the repolarization process.

BRADYCARDIA AND HEART BLOCK

What 6 items are in the workup for patients with bradyarrhythmias?

1. 12-lead ECG
2. Rhythm strip
3. Atrial tracings from epicardial wires (if present)
4. CXR
5. CBC
6. Electrolytes

What is the priority in assessing a patient with bradycardia?

Determine if the bradycardia is symptomatic by monitoring BP, peripheral perfusion, urine output, and mentation.

If the patient is hypotensive and bradycardic, what interventions should be initiated?

ACLS should be instituted immediately. Then, after the airway and breathing are secured (remember your ABCs), begin the following:

1. Atropine: 1 mg IV every 3 to 5 minutes
2. Defibrillator: to assist in monitoring and for transcutaneous pacing if necessary
3. Either of the following:
   a. Dopamine: 5 to 20 μg/kg/min
   b. Epinephrine: 2 to 10 μg/kg/min
4. Diagnostic workup

5. Establish central access, preferably right IJ, for possible transvenous pacing wire or pacing swan.

What are the indications for permanent pacemaker placement?

Severe sinus node dysfunction and complete heart block that is symptomatic and persistent (7–14 days). It is important to document the patient's underlying rhythm while he or she is being temporarily paced, because up to 70% with sinus node dysfunction and up to 35% with AV block will recover their normal intrinsic rhythm.

What is sinus bradycardia?

A sinus rhythm with a rate lower than 60 bpm

What are 6 causes of sinus bradycardia?

1. Drugs: β-blockers; calcium-channel blockers; digoxin; class Ia, Ic, and III antiarrhythmics; lithium.
2. Hypothyroidism.
3. Profound hypoxia.
4. Moderate hypothermia.
5. Sick sinus syndrome.
6. Athletes: sinus bradycardia is a normal variant in athletes.

What is the management for sinus bradycardia?

1. Treat only if symptomatic.
2. Treat the underlying cause.
3. Atropine, theophylline, or temporary transvenous pacing if necessary.

Describe respiratory sinus arrhythmia.

Heart rate is elevated with inspiration and decreased with exhalation.

Is respiratory sinus arrhythmia normal?

Yes

Describe 1st-degree AV block.

PR interval greater than 0.2 seconds with a conducted QRS after each P wave

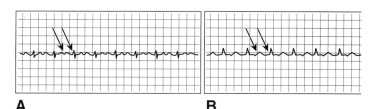

A   **B**

Arrows indicate PR intervals of 0.25 (**A**) and 0.35 second (**B**).

What are 4 causes of 1st-degree AV block?

1. Normal variant in healthy people
2. Ischemia
3. High vagal tone
4. Drugs: β-blockers, calcium-channel blockers, digitalis, amiodarone

What is the management for 1st-degree AV block?

Treatment typically is not needed, but if symptomatic, drug dosage may need to be adjusted.

Describe Mobitz type I or Wenckebach's 2nd-degree AV block.

Results from a conduction block in the AV node, which manifests as *progressive* PR prolongation and failure to conduct a P wave.

What condition predisposes patients to Mobitz type I?

Acute MI. Consequently, these patients don't need management for the conduction defect as much as they need evaluation for coronary artery disease.

How is Mobitz type I described?

As a ratio of P waves to QRS complexes. For instance, 4:3 block indicates that the 4th P wave is not conducted.

Describe Mobitz type II 2nd-degree AV block.

A conduction defect that manifests with a *consistent* PR interval but sudden failure to conduct one or more P waves.

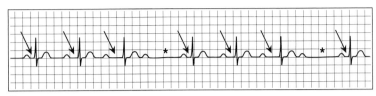

A

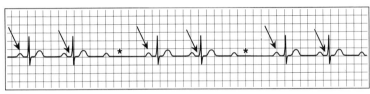

B

Mobitz type I (**A**) and type II (**B**) 2nd-degree AV block. Arrows indicate conducted beats, and asterisks indicate second-degree AV block.

What is the management for Mobitz type II?

Transvenous pacing typically is necessary, because Mobitz type II frequently is progressive to complete block.

Describe 3rd-degree AV block.

Complete heart block with AV dissociation. The ventricular escape rate is determined by the subsidiary pacemaker in the His-Purkinje system. The atrial rate remains regular, and P waves can be superimposed on T waves or hidden in QRS complexes. (see opposite)

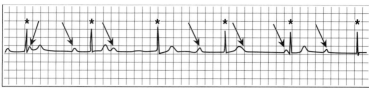

A

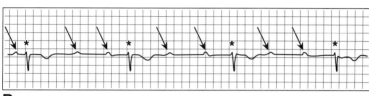

B

Arrows indicate the varying PR-interval relationships, and asterisks indicate the regular junctional (**A**) and ventricular (**B**) escape rates.

What are 6 common causes of 3rd-degree AV block?	1. Medications: digitalis, calcium-channel blockers, β-blockers, etc. 2. Lev's disease and Lenegre's disease: degenerative diseases of the conduction system 3. Cardiomyopathies 4. Acute MI 5. Valvular disorders: endocarditis, mitral valve replacement, etc. 6. Lyme disease
What is the management of 3rd-degree block?	Transcutaneous pacing until transvenous pacing can be established
What are 6 risk factors for postcardiac surgery bradyarrhythmias?	1. Valvular surgery 2. Age 3. Perivalvular calcifications 4. History of left bundle branch block 5. Left main disease and extensive coronary artery disease 6. Prolonged bypass time
What percentage of sinus node dysfunction in cardiac transplant patients will require permanent pacing?	As high as 21% (average, 8%)

What is the likely cause of sinus node dysfunction in postoperative (PO) noncardiac patients?	Increased vagal tone (from spinal or epidural, laryngoscopy, surgical intervention)
What is the most likely cause of transient AV block in PO noncardiac patients?	Acute MI
What is the management for transient AV block?	1. Manage and correct the underlying coronary artery disease. 2. Temporary pacing if needed, with electrophysiology service evaluation. 3. Permanent pacemaker if symptomatic and high-grade 2nd- or 3rd-degree AV block.
What are the 2 preferred sites of placement for temporary pacing wires?	1. Right IJ vein 2. Left subclavian vein

SUPRAVENTRICULAR TACHYARRHYTHMIAS

How do you work up a patient with a tachy-arrhythmia?	1. Determine if the patient is hemodynamically stable. If unstable, ABCs and ACLS. 2. 12-lead ECG, rhythm strip, previous ECG, CXR, ABG, CBC, and electrolytes
What is the rate for sinus tachycardia?	The lower limit is usually 100 bpm; the upper limit is 220 minus age (in years).
What are 7 causes of sinus tachycardia?	1. Fever 2. Pain 3. Infection 4. Volume depletion 5. Heart failure 6. Thyrotoxicosis 7. Drugs
What is the management of sinus tachycardia?	Treat the underlying cause. If the diagnosis is in doubt, adenosine or

vagal maneuvers may aid in elucidating the rhythm.

What are premature atrial contractions?

Premature beats arising in the atrium and occurring before the expected sinus beat. The P-wave morphology is different from the sinus beat.

Which patient population needs to be treated for premature atrial contractions?

Patients who are at risk for Afib or who cannot tolerate Afib (i.e., chronic obstructive pulmonary disease, postthoracic surgery, hypertrophic cardiomyopathy, severe mitral stenosis) may require prophylaxis.

What 5 types of SVTs comprise paroxysmal SVTs?

1. AVNRT: 50%
2. Concealed AV bypass tract: 15% to 50%
3. Intra-atrial re-entry: 6%
4. Sinus node re-entry: 3%
5. Automatic atrial tachycardia: 3%

Describe the ECG findings for AVNRT.

1. Abrupt-onset tachyarrhythmia with regular QRS interval (150–200 bpm).
2. P waves buried in the QRS complex.
3. QRS morphology is normal as long as there is no bundle branch block or ventricular conduction delay.

What maneuver can be performed to help differentiate AVNRT with aberrant conduction from Vtach?

Carotid massage. The rate in Vtach will be unaffected, but a supraventricular rhythm will be slowed.

What are the management options for AVNRT?

If symptomatic and progressive:
1. Adenosine
2. Vagal maneuvers
3. Cardioversion (20–50 J) with hemodynamic compromise or symptoms of heart failure
4. Verapamil and diltiazem for acute and chronic management

5. β-Blockers, class Ia and Ic antiarrhythmics, amiodarone, and digitalis for chronic management
6. Radiofrequency ablation (RFA) for persistent arrhythmia

How do pharmacologic agents and surgical intervention terminate sustained re-entrant tachyarrhythmias?

1. Drugs can either prolong the recovery period or accelerate an impulse so that it encounters a refractory period, thus terminating the circuit.
2. Artificial pacemakers can depolarize or capture part of the reentrant circuit, thus making it refractory to the re-entrant impulse.
3. Cardioversion can capture all receptive parts of the re-entrant circuit, thus making it refractory to any re-entrant impulse.
4. Ablation of an accessory pathway surgically or by catheters will remove a component of the re-entrant circuit.

Describe the pathophysiology of a concealed AV bypass tract tachycardia.

This arrhythmia is dependent on a retrograde AV tract that bypasses the AV node and activates the atria ectopically.

What are the ECG findings?

A P wave may be seen more than 70 milliseconds after the QRS complex, and bundle branch block ipsilateral to the re-entrant circuit will prolong the tachycardic cycle by approximately 35 milliseconds.

What is the treatment?

Similar to AVNRT. Treat if symptomatic.

What is WPW syndrome?

A form of re-entrant tachyarrhythmia associated with early ventricular depolarization via an accessory AV tract

What are 3 characteristic ECG findings of WPW syndrome?

1. Short PR interval
2. Wide QRS
3. Delta wave: a slur in the upswing of the QRS, which represents early depolarization.

What is the difference between orthodromic reciprocating tachycardia and antidromic reciprocating tachycardia?

Orthodromic reciprocating tachycardia: involves antegrade conduction through the AV node with retrograde conduction via the accessory pathway.

Antidromic reciprocating tachycardia: involves antegrade conduction via the accessory pathway with retrograde conduction via the AV node.

What is the greatest threat to the patient with WPW syndrome?

Development of Afib with degeneration into Vfib

What drugs should be avoided in Afib with rapid antegrade conduction down the accessory pathway?

Drugs that block the AV node should be avoided, because they may permit unopposed conduction down the accessory pathway and precipitate Vfib. These drugs include adenosine, digoxin, and verapamil.

What is the management for WPW syndrome?

1. Emergent cardioversion for hemodynamically significant Afib
2. Procainamide for stable Afib
3. RFA of the accessory pathway for any patient with WPW and rapid Afib

What are 3 ECG findings with multifocal atrial tachycardia (MAT)?

MATs result from increased automaticity. Consequently, the ECG will show the following:
1. Atrial rate greater than 100 bpm
2. At least 3 different P-wave morphologies and PR intervals
3. Irregular RR intervals

What chronic condition typically is associated with MAT?

Chronic obstructive pulmonary disease

What is the management for MAT?

Treat the underlying cause:
1. Hypoxemia
2. Hypercapnia
3. MI
4. Congestive heart failure
5. Electrolyte derangements
Calcium-channel blockers or β-blockers may have to be used to control the rate. Amiodarone can be used in refractory cases.

What drug do you want to avoid in managing MAT?

Digitalis, which may worsen the arrhythmia

ATRIAL FIBRILLATION AND ATRIAL FLUTTER

Describe the pathophysiology of Afib.

Afib results from random depolarization of the atrium with the possible generation of re-entry loops and random conduction through the AV node.

In addition to re-entrant pathways, what other mechanism promotes Afib?

Aberrant foci, most commonly from the pulmonary veins

What are 3 typical ECG findings of Afib?

1. Rapid, irregular undulation of baseline ECG corresponding to rapid multiple depolarizations of the atrium (rate, 400–600 bpm)
2. Narrow QRS (unless aberrant conduction occurs)
3. Irregular, usually rapid ventricular response (rate, 100–160 bpm)

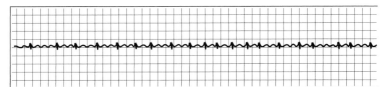

A Flutter

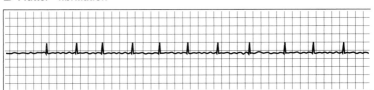

B Flutter - fibrillation

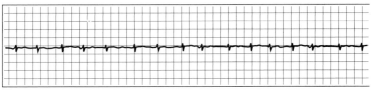

C Coarse fibrillation

D Fine fibrillation

Flutter (**A**), flutter–fibrillation (**B**), coarse fibrillation (**C**), and fine fibrillation (**D**).

What is the Ashman's phenomenon?	Aberrant conduction in Afib, which results in a widened QRS. This can be seen when a shorter RR interval following a longer RR interval is delayed by the partially refractory period of the right bundle.
What are 3 symptoms of Afib?	1. Heart failure 2. Hypotension 3. Angina

Symptoms typically result from the rapid rate, shorter diastolic filling time, and loss of atrial kick to the ventricle.

What are 8 causes of Afib in nonsurgical patients?

1. Systemic hypertension (most common)
2. Coronary artery disease
3. Valvular heart disease
4. Cardiomyopathies
5. Hyperthyroidism
6. Pulmonary disease
7. Hypoxia
8. Drugs: aminophylline, alcohol, caffeine

What are the indications for immediate synchronized, electrical cardioversion of a patient in Afib?

Hemodynamically unstable patient with hypotension, heart failure, and/or ischemia.

How much energy should be used for cardioversion in this patient?

100 J should be the initial dose.

Which is more effective: anteroposterior patches or right parasternal–left paraspinal patches?

Anteroposterior patches provide a better vector for defibrillation.

How is cardioversion for Aflutter different than for Afib?

The initial dose typically is 25–50 J for Aflutter. If the patient has pacing wires, atrial overdrive pacing can be attempted for flutter.

How do you overdrive pace for Aflutter?

Gradually increase the pacing rate until the impulse captures (usually 20%–30% greater than the flutter rate), and abruptly discontinue pacing.

If the patient is hemodynamically stable, what is the next concern?

Controlling the ventricular rate

How is the ventricular rate best controlled?

β-Blockers, calcium-channel blockers, and digoxin are most often used to attain a goal rate of 70 to 100 bpm.

Once rate control is attained, what is the next step?

If the arrhythmia persists for longer than 24 hours, attempt cardioversion.

What are 3 pharmacologic drugs used for cardioversion?

1. Amiodarone
2. Procainamide
3. Ibutilide

What are 2 indications for anticoagulation in patients with Afib?

1. Afib for more than 48 hours
2. Recurring Afib that may require cardioversion

Why is anticoagulation indicated?

To decrease the risk of thromboembolic stroke and transient ischemic attack

Describe the pathogenesis of Aflutter.

Macro re-entry phenomenon within the atria

What are 3 typical ECG findings in Aflutter?

1. Saw-toothed flutter waves in the inferior leads.
2. Flutter waves at a regular frequency (220–350 bpm)
3. Ventricular rate is dependent on the conduction limitation. For instance, a patient with 2:1 conduction will have a rate of 150 bpm, and a patient with 3:1 conduction will have a rate of 100 bpm.

What is the management for Aflutter?

1. Cardioversion (25–50 J) for hemodynamically significant arrhythmia: this may precipitate Afib and will simply require repeat cardioversion at higher voltage.
2. Atrial pacing to terminate the rhythm.
3. β-Blockers, verapamil, quinidine, and amiodarone.
4. Anticoagulation

When should patients be anticoagulated for Aflutter?	Patients are at risk for thrombus formation (like patients with Afib), but no consensus on the timing of anti-coagulation is available. Rarely, a patient will have hemodynamically stable Aflutter for 24 to 48 hours and may be prophylactically anticoagulated, or an echocardiogram may be performed before treatment.

VENTRICULAR TACHYARRHYTHMIAS

What cardiac disorder is most commonly associated with ventricular arrhythmias?	Coronary artery disease and history of MI. The structurally normal heart does not typically develop ventricular arrhythmias.
Describe the pathogenesis of PVCs.	Increased automaticity or re-entry in the ventricle initiates development of a premature QRS complex more than 0.12 milliseconds in duration. The PP interval typically is uninterrupted.
What are 5 typical causes of PVCs?	1. Atherosclerotic heart disease and left ventricular dysfunction 2. Cardiomyopathy 3. Drugs: caffeine, theophylline, alcohol, antiarrhythmics 4. Infiltrative diseases: tumors, infection, sarcoidosis 5. Electrolyte derangements: magnesium, potassium
What is Vtach?	Ventricular tachycardia; the occurrence of 3 or more PVCs in succession with a ventricular rate of more than 100 bpm

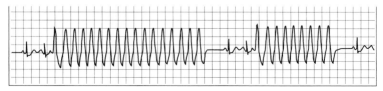

Nonsustained Vtach.

What strategy should be used for prevention of malignant ventricular arrhythmias in patients with hemodynamically tolerable Vtach?

1. Post-MI patients with ejection fraction (EF) of 40% or less benefit from ICD placement.
2. If the EF is 40% or greater and there is no history of MI, patients with frequent Vtach episodes require either RFA or chronic drug therapy (amiodarone).

What is torsades de pointes?

Polymorphic Vtach with QT prolongation. It typically manifests on ECG as Vtach undulating on the QRS axis.

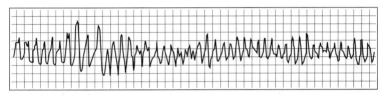

Torsades de pointes.

What are 5 causes of acquired QT prolongation and torsades?

1. Medications: type IA and type III antiarrhythmics, tricyclic antidepressants, nonsedating antihistamines, azole antifungals, erythromycin, pentamidine
2. Electrolyte derangements: especially hypomagnesemia and hypokalemia
3. Hypothyroidism
4. Cerebrovascular accident
5. Organophosphorous insecticide poisoning, liquid protein diets, and alcoholism

What is the management for torsades de pointes?

1. Correct the underlying causes.
2. Give IV magnesium immediately, even if normal.
3. Isoproterenol infusion.
4. Temporary pacing.

Significant ventricular arrhythmias in noncardiac patients typically occur in what setting?

Postoperative infarction/ischemia or structural heart disease. These patients may have initiating stressors, such as hypoxia, medications, hypokalemia, and hypomagnesemia. They should all be evaluated for treatable coronary artery disease.

What is ventricular flutter?

Vtach with a rate of more than 300 bpm

What is the management for ventricular flutter?

Unsynchronized, emergent cardioversion

What is Vfib?

Ventricular fibrillation; disorganized rhythm with multiple areas of depolarization in the ventricle. The electrical activity eventually ceases.

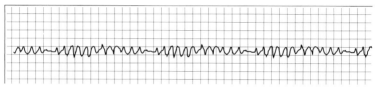

Vfib.

What is the appropriate management algorithm for pulseless Vtach and Vfib?

Initiate ACLS:
1. Establish a secure airway and breathing (remember your ABCs).
2. Assess circulatory status, and perform immediate, unsynchronized external defibrillation if unstable. Defibrillate up to 3 times (200–360 J).
3. If refractory to electrical cardioversion, use either a single dose of 40 U of IV vasopressin or 1 mg of epinephrine every 3 to 4 minutes.
4. Defibrillate once with 360 J.
5. Amiodarone loading (150 mg IV loading dose over 10 minutes, followed by 360 mg over 6 hours).
6. Remember to always go back to the airway and breathing as you cycle down your algorithm.
7. Defibrillate.
8. Other drugs that can be used include lidocaine and procainamide.

What is the strategy for primary prevention of malignant ventricular tachyarrhythmias in patients with previous MI?

1. ICD placement for patients with EF of 40% or less carries carry a survival benefit.
2. β-Blockers reduce mortality and decrease the risk of sudden death.
3. Angiotensin-converting enzyme inhibitors also reduce mortality.
4. Prophylactic antiarrhythmics have not unequivocally demonstrated a survival benefit.

How do you manage patients with hemodynamically intolerable Vtach?

They should all be evaluated for ICD placement, but amiodarone can be used in those with a short life expectancy or who refuse the procedure.

What is the prognosis for patients with sustained ventricular arrhythmias?

In-hospital mortality can be as high as 50%, with a 40% chance of recurrence for initial survivors. Consequently, these patients should be aggressively managed with electrophysiology service and, possibly, an implantable cardioverter-defibrillator (ICD) placement with or without antiarrhythmic medications.

Which group of patients benefits the most from the above interventions?

Those with EF of 40% or less and a history of MI

What is the acute management for hemodynamically stable PVCs and short runs of Vtach?

Correct any reversible causes.

What is the acute management for hemodynamically stable sustained Vtach?

1. Lidocaine
2. Procainamide
3. Amiodarone
4. Overdrive ventricular pacing if ventricular epicardial wires are in place

In patients with sustained ventricular arrhythmias, what is considered to be first-line therapy?	ICD placement because of the high risk of recurrence and mortality.

PHARMACOTHERAPY

What are 6 different types of antiarrhythmic drugs, and how are they classified?	1. Class Ia: sodium-channel blockers (quinidine, procainamide, disopyramide) 2. Class Ib: sodium-channel blockers (lidocaine) 3. Class Ic: sodium-channel blockers (flecainide, propafenone, moricizine) 4. Class II: β-blockers 5. Class III: potassium-channel blockers (sotalol, amiodarone, bretylium, ibutilide) 6. Class IV: calcium-channel blockers
What are 6 medications for ACLS?	1. Epinephrine 2. Vasopressin 3. Amiodarone 4. Lidocaine 5. Atropine 6. Adenosine
What is the mechanism of action for adenosine?	Adenosine is a naturally occurring nucleoside that slows AV node conduction and inhibits re-entry. The half-life is less than 10 seconds.
What is the indication for adenosine?	Paroxysmal SVT
What is the dosage for adenosine?	6 mg IV rapid bolus (over 1–2 seconds), followed by 12 mg IV rapid bolus after 1 to 2 minutes for up to 2 doses.
What are 3 contra-indications for adenosine?	1. 2nd-degree block 2. 3rd-degree block 3. Sick sinus syndrome

What happens if adenosine is given to a patient in Afib or Aflutter?

A brief, transient decrease in the ventricular rate

What are 4 side effects of adenosine?

1. Apprehension, light-headedness, tingling
2. Chest pain, facial flushing, headache, palpitations
3. Metallic taste
4. Shortness of breath

What is the mechanism of action for amiodarone?

Amiodarone is a class III potassium-channel blocker that increases the action potential duration and effective refractory period. It also has β-blocker activity with minimal negative inotropic effect.

What is the dosage for amiodarone?

150 mg IV for 10 min, followed by 1 mg/min IV over 6 hours. This is followed by a maintenance infusion at 0.5 mg/min for 18 hours.

What are 3 advantages of amiodarone?

1. Anti-ischemic effects
2. Low proarrhythmic profile
3. No depression of left ventricular function

What are 3 indications for amiodarone?

1. Vfib and unstable Vtach
2. Supraventricular arrhythmias (Afib)
3. Hypertrophic cardiomyopathy

What are 2 contraindications for amiodarone?

1. 2nd-degree block
2. 3rd-degree block

What are 7 side effects of amiodarone?

1. Bradycardia, arrhythmias, heart block, sinus arrest
2. Nausea, vomiting, constipation
3. Hyper- and hypothyroidism
4. Hepatic dysfunction
5. Pulmonary fibrosis, alveolar and interstitial pneumonitis

6. Peripheral neuropathy
7. Blue-gray skin pigmentation

What is the mechanism of action for atropine?

Atropine is an anticholinergic that blocks the effects of Ach at the SA and AV nodes, thus increasing the discharge rate and conduction velocity and decreasing the refractory period.

What is the indication for atropine?

Symptomatic bradycardia

What is the dosage of atropine?

0.5 to 1.0 mg IV push every 3 to 5 minutes to a maximum dose of 0.04 mg/kg. Paradoxically, a dose less than 0.5 mg may cause bradycardia.

What are 5 contraindications for atropine?

1. Acute-angle glaucoma
2. Obstructive uropathy
3. Obstructive disease of the GI tract
4. Asthma
5. Myasthenia gravis

What are 3 side effects of atropine?

1. Headache, insomnia, agitation, dry mouth
2. Palpitations, bradycardia, tachycardia
3. Photophobia, increased intraocular pressure, blurred vision

What is the mechanism of action for lidocaine?

Lidocaine is a class Ib sodium-channel blocker with low proarrhythmic potential.

What is the indication for lidocaine?

Ventricular arrhythmia

What is the dosage of lidocaine?

1 to 1.5 mg/kg IV bolus at 25 to 50 mg/min, with repeat boluses of 0.5 mg/kg given every 3 to 5 minutes until a total dose of 3 mg/kg is given. An infusion of 1 to 4 mg/min is begun once a perfusing rhythm is obtained.

Decrease the infusion rate by half after the first 24 hours.

What are 6 contraindications for lidocaine?

1. Stokes-Adams syndrome
2. WPW syndrome
3. Severe heart block
4. Hypotension
5. Myocardial depression
6. Neurologic disorders.

Lidocaine should be used cautiously in which groups of patients?

1. Elderly patients
2. Those with hepatic or renal dysfunction

What are 3 side effects of lidocaine?

1. Seizures, lethargy, slurred speech, tinnitus, blurred vision
2. Bradycardia, cardiac arrest, arrhythmia
3. Respiratory depression and status asthmaticus

What is the mechanism of action for procainamide?

Procainamide is a class Ia sodium-channel blocker that depresses phase 0 of the action potential. It effectively reduces conduction velocity and effective refractory period in the atria, ventricle, and His-Purkinje system. It is also a moderate potassium-channel blocker with anticholinergic activity.

What are 3 indications for procainamide?

1. Vtach
2. Afib and Aflutter
3. Paroxysmal atrial tachycardia

What is the dosage for procainamide?

50 to 100 mg slow IV push every 5 minutes up to a total of 1.5 g. Give until arrhythmia disappears, hypotension occurs, QRS widens by 50%, or maximum dose is reached. Once arrhythmia disappears, start an infusion at 1 to 6 mg/min.

What are 5 contraindications for procainamide?

1. 2nd-degree block
2. 3rd-degree block
3. Myasthenia gravis
4. Systemic lupus erythematous
5. Torsades de pointes

What are 4 side effects of procainamide?

1. Seizures
2. Asystole, bradycardia, Vfib
3. Thrombocytopenia, neutropenia, agranulocytosis, hemolytic anemia
4. Lupus-like syndrome, positive antinuclear antibody (ANA), positive Coombs' test

What is the mechanism of action for Sotalol?

Sotalol is a class III potassium-channel blocker with high nonselective β-blocker activity. Unlike amiodarone, it decreases left ventricular function and can be very proarrhythmic.

What are 2 indications for sotalol?

1. Life-threatening ventricular arrhythmias
2. Prophylaxis for Afib in high-risk patients

What is the dosage for sotalol?

Start at 80 mg PO BID and increase every 2 to 3 days to a daily dose of 160 to 320 mg. Adjust dose for renal impairment.

What are 5 contraindications for sotalol?

1. 2nd-degree block
2. 3rd-degree block
3. Long QT syndrome
4. Heart failure
5. Asthma

What are 3 side effects of sotalol?

1. Bradycardia, heart failure, ventricular arrhythmia
2. Bronchospasms
3. Elevated LFTs

13

Cardiovascular Pump Problems

BASIC CONCEPTS

What are the 2 functions of the cardiovascular pump?

1. Delivery of oxygen to all vascular beds in the body
2. Removal of waste products of metabolism

What is the formula for oxygen delivery?

$DO_2 = CI \times 13.4 \times Hgb \times SaO_2$

What is a normal DO_2?

520 to 570 mL/min/m²

List 3 ways to maximize DO_2.

1. Maximize CI (normal = 2.4 – 4.0 L/min/m²)
2. [Hgb] of 10 mg/dL or greater (optimal DO_2/work at 11 mg/dL)
3. SaO_2 greater than 95%

What can we learn from mixed venous oxygenation?

SvO_2 measures the amount of oxygen left in the blood returning to the heart. This will depend directly on both the oxygen delivery and the oxygen extraction. This is the theory behind the Fick principle to determine CO.

What is a normal SvO_2, and what level would be worrisome?

Normal is greater than 70%. Less than 65% warrants investigation for inadequate oxygen delivery.

How is the mixed oxygen level sampled?

A slow withdrawal of blood from the PA via a PAC.

What is the formula for oxygen consumption?

$VO_2 = CI \times 13.4 \times Hgb \times (SaO_2 - SvO_2)$

What is a normal V_{O_2}?	110 to 160 mL/min/m²
What is the formula for CI?	CI = CO/BSA where CO = heart rate (HR) × stroke volume (SV) BSA = (ht [in cm] + wt [in kg] − 60)/100
What is a normal CI?	2.4 to 4.0 L/min/m²
Below what level is the CI significant and requiring aggressive intervention?	Less than 2.0 L/min/m²
What are the 5 factors that influence CO?	1. HR 2. Preload 3. Compliance (distensibility) 4. Contractility 5. Afterload
How do these factors fit into the equation for CO?	CO = HR × SV or CO = HR × (EDV − ESV) where EDV is end-diastolic volume (determined by both preload and distensibility) and ESV is end-systolic volume (determined by both afterload and contractility).

MANIPULATING CARDIAC OUTPUT

HEART RATE

What would be optimal HR in ICU patients?	Less than 100 bpm
What are the 2 main reasons to avoid higher HRs?	1. Time for diastolic filling decreases. 2. Less time for coronary perfusion. As above, tachycardia is usually a marker for some underlying problem.

At what point in the cardiac cycle does flow occur in the coronary arteries?

During diastole. The force involved in contraction must be greater than the aortic pressure to eject the blood; therefore, blood flow through the coronary arteries and perfusion of the myocardium does not occur until ventricular relaxation in diastole.

What drugs are used to manipulate the HR?

Increase: β-agonist (i.e., isoproterenol, epinephrine, dobutamine, dopamine) or antimuscarinics (i.e., atropine, glycopyrolate).
Decrease: β-blockers are commonly used to slow rates in sinus rhythm, and diltiazem and digoxin are used to reduce SVT rates (e.g., Afib and AV-node re-entrant tachycardia).

Is cardiac rhythm a consideration for ICU patients?

Yes. In addition to the rate of ventricular response, atrial dysrhythmias can lead to lower filling pressures because of inadequate atrial kick.

How much can the restoration of sinus rhythm improve CO?

Conversion to NSR can increase CO by 25% to 30% in some patients. The average is closer to 10%, but patients with stiff ventricles (i.e., diastolic dysfunction) may improve by 30%.

PRELOAD

Who were the first 3 people to describe fundamental causes of variation in SV?

1. William Howell in 1884
2. Otto Frank in 1894
3. E. H. Starling in 1918

What is the Starling principle?

Heart muscle contracts more forcefully during systole the more the ventricle is filled during diastole.

Draw a Starling curve

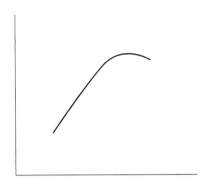

What is the *x*-axis of the Starling curve?

SV

What is the *y*-axis of the Starling curve?

Some estimation of preload: myocyte length or stretch; LVEDV, LVEDP, left atrial pressure, PA pressure, CVP

What is preload?

LVEDV

What is the best indicator of volume status?

LVEDP

List 2 ways in which LVEDP can be determined.

1. Left heart catheterization to measure the LVEDP directly
2. A PAC to measure the PCWP

What is PCWP?

Pulmonary capillary wedge pressure, or PA occlusion pressure. Because the pulmonary arterial and venous system do not have valves, inflation of the balloon at the tip of a PAC allows the transducer to "look" downstream to the left atrial pressure. This is the closest approximation of LVEDP without catheterization of the left heart.

If the catheter cannot be wedged, what is the next best correlate of the LVEDP?

PAD pressure. This is usually 5 mm Hg higher than the PCWP.

What 3 assumptions are made when equating PCWP to cardiac preload (LVEDV)?

1. LVEDP correlates to LVEDV, unless compliance is decreased.
2. Left atrial pressure equals LVEDP, unless the mitral valve is diseased (remember, the mitral valve is open at the end of diastole).
3. PCWP approximates left atrial pressure in the absence of pulmonary venous hypertension and/or high PEEP.

Why is PCWP not a good predictor of volume status in the first few hours after a coronary artery bypass graft?

The ventricle tends to be poorly compliant in the early postoperative period secondary to cold-induced injury, ischemia, or reperfusion injury.

What is a normal PCWP?

4 to 12 mm Hg

How high would you push PCWP in an ICU patient before considering other therapy?

Generally 18 to 20 mm Hg, but it also depends on the PEEP and other factors.

Would a person with a normal CO need to the PCWP raised to this level?

No. The best volume status is the lowest filling pressure that leads to an adequate CO.

Who *may* need a higher PCWP?

Some patients with CHF because of previous MI or other causes
Some patients with recent MI and consequent diastolic abnormality
Some patients with diastolic abnormalities, such as pericardial constriction or restrictive heart disease
Some patients with chronic valvular disease (generally aortic insufficiency or mitral regurgitation)
Patients who have had difficult or long open heart procedures

What are 3 problems with excess preload?

1. Law of Laplace: wall tension is proportional to pressure and diameter (i.e., may worsen ischemia).

2. Pulmonary venous pressure greater than 20 mm Hg can cause pulmonary edema.
3. Overdistension of myocytes may decrease their ability to contract by a shift to a lower Starling relationship.

What are 3 major determinants of myocardial oxygen demand?

1. Myocardial wall tension
2. Contractility
3. HR

What are 2 determinants of myocardial oxygen supply?

1. Arterial oxygen content
2. Coronary blood flow

What is the definition of coronary blood flow?

Coronary blood flow = coronary perfusion pressure/coronary vascular resistance
Coronary vascular resistance is affected by coronary artery stenosis in addition to metabolic, hormonal, and autonomic nervous system parameters.

What percentage of CO is used for normal coronary artery blood flow?

3% to 5% (80 mL/100 g/min)

What are 2 implications of increased wall tension on myocyte function?

1. Increased myocardial oxygen demand as the ventricular work increases
2. Decreased myocardial oxygen supply as the coronary artery perfusion decreases

DISTENSIBILITY

What 3 factors determine distensibility?

1. Valvular disease
2. Chronic hypertension
3. Ventricular scarring

Can this distensibility be addressed acutely?

No. It may improve over weeks to months if the cause is treated.

CONTRACTILITY

What would indicate that contractility is inadequate?	Poor CO with normal or high filling pressures
How would you treat poor contractility?	Inotropic support

List 6 items that should be in the differential diagnosis for an unexpected need for inotropic support in any patient, but especially in those following chest surgery.

1. Pericardial tamponade
2. Tension pneumothorax
3. MI
4. Valvular prosthetic malfunction
5. Acidosis
6. Electrolyte imbalance

Knowing that the above 6 factors can affect contractility, what 5 tests must be checked directly following open heart surgery?

1. Electrolytes
   a. K^+: keep at high-normal levels required for normal electrical conduction.
   b. Ca^{2+}: keep at high-normal levels for both conduction and contractility.
   c. Mg^{2+}: allows calcium to function adequately.
   d. Na^+: hyponatremia is one of more common causes of Afib
2. CBC for adequate Hgb and platelets
3. CXR for ETT placement, atelectasis, and fluid accumulation
4. Coagulation parameters to evaluate for adequate reversal of heparin or clotting factor deficiencies
5. ABG for assessment of oxygenation

AFTERLOAD

What hemodynamic measurement represents afterload?	Systemic vascular resistance (SVR)
Why is BP not a good determinant?	BP is dependent on the cardiac pump in addition to the vascular resistance.

What is the equation for SVR?

$SVR = (MAP - CVP)/CO \times 80$

What is the normal range of SVR?

900 to 1,400 dyne sec cm^{-5}

How does afterload manipulation affect CO?

Afterload is the pressure the ventricle must overcome to eject blood, so decreasing this pressure will allow the heart to eject more blood with less work.

What must be avoided with afterload reduction?

Dropping the systemic pressure below the end-organ perfusion pressure

Who is particularly susceptible to significant afterload reduction?

Patients with fixed stenosis, most commonly in the heart, brain, kidneys, or intestines

Where should the BP be maintained?

100 to 140 mm Hg systolic(chronic hypertensives or cerebrovascular patients may need higher pressures). An MAP of greater than 60 mm Hg is needed to maintain perfusion to the brain.

What 4 pathologies benefit most from afterload reduction?

1. Aortic regurgitation: decreases backflow across the incompetent valve.
2. Mitral regurgitation: decreases ventricular peak pressure, thereby decreasing the fraction of blood flowing back through the diseased valve.
3. Ventricular septal defect: similar to MR; decreases the fraction passing from left to right.
4. Heart failure of any cause: decreases the pressure, allowing further increase in CO.

What would be used for afterload reduction?

Vasodilators: nitroglycerin, sodium nitroprusside, Fenoldopam, Nesiritide (b-type natriuretic peptide), α-blockers

DIAGNOSIS

What common feature explains dyspnea in all types of cardiomyopathy?

Elevated left atrial pressure, leading to increased pulmonary venous pressure that results in pulmonary edema and decreased oxygenation

What are 11 potentially reversible causes of dilated cardiomyopathy?

1. Alcoholic cardiomyopathy
2. Hypocalcemia, hypokalemia, hypophosphatemia
3. Hemochromatosis
4. Pheochromocytoma
5. Myocarditis
6. Sarcoid heart disease
7. Lead poisoning
8. Selenium deficiency
9. Uremic cardiomyopathy
10. Ischemic cardiomyopathy
11. Peripartum

What are 7 classic physical signs of ventricular dysfunction?

1. Distended neck veins
2. Lateral point of maximal impulse
3. S_3 gallop
4. Mitral or tricuspid regurgitation murmurs
5. Moist crackles
6. Distended or pulsatile liver
7. Peripheral or sacral edema

What is the significance of a narrow pulse pressure in patients with cardiomyopathies?

Associated with a CI of less than 2 L/min/m^2

What 3 hemodynamic values would you expect in right heart failure?

1. Low CI
2. High RAP
3. High PVRI

What 3 hemodynamic values would you expect in left heart failure?

1. Low CI
2. High PCWP
3. High SVRI
Left heart failure may also lead to elevated right sided pressures.

What is the definition of shock?

Inadequate oxygen delivery to meet the metabolic demands of the peripheral tissue

What 4 hemodynamic values would you expect to see with hypovolemia?

1. Low CI
2. Low CVP
3. Low PCWP
4. High SVRI

What 3 hemodynamic values would you expect in vasogenic (neurogenic) shock?

1. High CI
2. Low CVP
3. Low SVRI
   Similar to sepsis, but this responds to volume and/or vasoconstriction

What 2 hemodynamic values would you expect in hyperdynamic and hypodynamic sepsis?

Hyperdynamic:
1. High CI
2. Low SVR
Hypodynamic:
1. Low CI
2. High SVR

What 5 hemodynamic values would you expect in cardiogenic shock?

1. Low CI
2. High CVP
3. High PCWP
4. High SVRI
5. Low Vo_2

What distinguishes left heart failure from cardiogenic shock?

Vo_2 is maintained in left heart failure.

What 5 hemodynamic values would you expect in massive pulmonary embolus?

1. Low CI
2. High CVP
3. High PAS
4. High PAD
5. Normal to low PCWP

What 4 hemodynamic values would you expect in pericardial tamponade?

1. Elevated equilibration of CVP
2. Elevated equilibration of PAD
3. Elevated equilibration of PCWP
4. Low CI

What hemodynamic values would you expect in tension pneumothorax?	Similar to tamponade plus respiratory symptoms, decreased oxygenation

PUMP OPTIMIZATION

Give a general algorithm to optimize the pump function of the heart.	1. Optimize fluid status. 2. Maximize inotropy and afterload pharmacologically. 3. Add mechanical facility.

VOLUME

What would be the most important feature of volume status to control?	Control of bleeding (especially in postoperative patients)
Why could pericardial tamponade be considered a volume problem?	Pericardial tamponade prevents the heart from being able to fill with blood.
What should be done when a low PCWP is found but the patient has a normal CI?	No intervention is necessary with adequate CO at any given PCWP.
Can the PCWP be pushed higher than 20 mm Hg?	Yes, especially in patients with stiff ventricles and those with high PCWP preoperatively.
What are the 2 major risks of increasing preload above 20 mm Hg?	1. Overdistension of the ventricle, leading to worsening CO 2. Pulmonary edema

PHARMACOLOGY

When should inotropes be used in ICU patients?	Only when CI is low and adequate volume status has been attained (optimal PCWP)

What 3 drugs would you consider in patients with low CI and low SVR?

You want to increase inotropy and increase vascular tone.
1. Dopamine (5–10 μg/kg/min): provides some β stimulation, and α stimulation occurs above 10 mg/kg/min.
2. Norepinephrine: β stimulation occurs at low levels, but α-receptors are stimulated at low doses; increases in potency quickly
3. Epinephrine: β stimulation at most levels, and with increasing doses, α stimulation occurs.

What 4 drugs would be considered in patients with adequate PCWP, low CI, and normal SVR?

You want to increase contractility/inotropy. Inotropes can be used alone or together.
1. Dobutamine (5–40 μg/kg/min): inotrope of choice for acute systolic dysfunction.
2. Milrinone (bolus of 50 μg/kg over 10 min, then 0.375–0.75 μg/kg/min): phosphodiesterase inhibitor that is both a positive inotrope and vasodilator by increasing cAMP levels.
3. Epinephrine (1–10 μg/min): at low doses, looks very much like dobutamine.
4. Norepinephrine(1–12 μg/min): significant vasoconstriction may overcome positive inotropic effects.

What 3 drugs would you consider in a patient with adequate PCWP, low CI, and high SVR?

You want to reduce afterload.
1. Nitroprusside (start with 0.2 μg/kg/min, then titrate up to 5 μg/kg/min): beware of cyanide accumulation at rates above 10 μg/min.
2. Nitroglycerin: viable alternative at rates above 50 μg/min (predominantly venous vasodilator

at <40 µg/min and arterial dilator at >200 µg/min); be wary of methemoglobin accumulation.

3. Fenoldapam (0.25–1.6 µg/kg/min): an alternative to nitroprusside in patients with reduced renal function.

What should you worry about when a patient has high PCWP and low CI with normal or low SVRI?

Suspect diastolic failure.

What would be the treatment for a patient with high PCWP and low CI with normal or low SVRI?

1. Low CO: dobutamine or milrinone, isoproterenol if low HR as well.
2. Low to normal CO: diuresis with furosemide, or try nitroglycerin.

MECHANICAL ADJUNCTS

INTRA-AORTIC BALLOON PUMP

What does an IABP do physiologically?

1. Increases CO: decreases VO_2 by 15% to 20%, increases coronary perfusion.
2. Decreases afterload: decreases myocardial oxygen consumption.

How does an IABP work?

The balloon deflates during systole, decreasing the afterload by lowering the SVR. The balloon inflates during diastole, increasing the SVR and, therefore, the BP. This increase in BP also improves coronary artery perfusion. More succinctly, the IABP causes systolic unloading and diastolic augmentation.

What events on the arterial waveform or the ECG should trigger balloon inflation?

The dicrotic notch of the a-line or the peak of the T wave on the ECG (aortic valve closure)

What events on the arterial waveform or the ECG should trigger the balloon deflation?

The upswing of the arterial pulse (before ventricular contraction) or after the peak of the P wave on the ECG

What are the maximal and minimal support settings?

Maximal support: 1:1
Minimal support: Generally 1:4, because a lower ratio (1:8) increases risk of thrombosis and/or embolism

What are 7 indications for IABP placement?

1. Postcardiotomy shock: 35% to 40%
2. Medically refractory angina: 15% to 25%
3. Preoperative stabilization after failed PTCI
4. Preoperative stabilization after acute MI
5. Complications of acute MI: acute MR, ventricular septal defect
6. Bridge to transplant
7. Prophylaxis for induction of high-risk patients: severe left ventricular dysfunction, long or complex operation

What are the 3 contraindications to IABP placement?

1. Significant aortic regurgitation: increases the regurgitant fraction.
2. Aortic dissection: both difficulties in placing the IABP in the true arterial lumen and the reduced afterload increase the force of blood ejection and can extend the aortic dissection.
3. Recently placed thoracic aortic graft (in the last 12 months): thrombus disruption.

Can an IABP be used in children?

Small catheters are available and are effective in children. (One of the first reported uses was in a child in 1967.)

What are the consequences of early inflation?

Early aortic valve closure, causing impaired SV

What are the consequences of late inflation?	Poor augmentation of coronary perfusion
What are the consequences of early deflation?	Poor reduction of afterload
What are the consequences of late deflation?	Increased afterload, causing increased myocardial O_2 consumption
What are the 3 criteria for weaning the IABP?	1. Normal platelets 2. Normal coagulation parameters 3. Hemodynamically stable on minimal inotropes
What is the algorithm for weaning?	1. Stop heparin for 4 to 6 hours. 2. Change the synchronization ratio to 1:2, or decrease the balloon volume to 30 mL. 3. Wait 4 hours. 4. If stable, decrease the ratio to 1:4, or decrease the balloon volume to 20 mL. 5. If stable, remove.
What are the 3 most catastrophic complications associated with an IABP?	1. Aortic dissection/rupture 2. Iliofemoral dissection/rupture 3. CNS embolization
What is the cause of the dissection?	A catheter tip that erodes though ulcerated plaque
What is the most common complication?	Distal limb ischemia (to some degree in 5%–15%); 5% will require operative repair: patch angioplasty or femoral–femoral bypass.
What are other possible complications associated with an IABP?	1. Local infection 2. Hemorrhage at insertion site 3. AV fistula 4. Pseudoaneurysm formation
Is visceral ischemia a problem?	Renal emboli are not uncommon, but mesenteric complications are rare.

What is the differential diagnosis of diminished distal pulses in patients with an IABP?	1. Hypothermia 2. Inadequate CO 3. Pharmacologic vasoconstriction: usually a side effect of pressors 4. Acute ischemia: secondary to arterial thrombosis or embolism
How is acute peripheral ischemia treated?	1. Remove the introducer sheath. 2. If hemodynamically stable, remove the catheter. 3. If unstable, replace in the contralateral limb. Use smaller sheath if possible. 3. If unstable, perform a femoral–femoral bypass.

ASSIST DEVICES

What are ventricular assist devices (VADs)?	Mechanical pumps that work in parallel with the failing ventricular circuit
What are the 4 indications for an using a VAD?	1. When inotropes and balloon pump are inadequate 2. Postpericardiotomy shock: 4% 3. Cardiogenic shock: MI greater than 40% of left ventricular loss 4. When heart transplantation is the outcome and the patient appears to be failing on inotropic support
What are the 4 different types of pumps in VADs?	1. Roller pumps 2. Centrifugal pumps 3. Accessory ventricles 4. Hemopump
Where can the VAD be placed?	Placed parallel to: 1. Right ventricle: right atrium to PA = RVAD 2. Left ventricle: left atrium to aorta = LVAD 3. Both = BiVAD
What would be the goal CO of the VAD?	To provide greater than 2.5 L/min/m^2

When and how should the patient be weaned from the VAD?

Usually begin to attempt to wean after 24 hours in place (unless placed specifically as a bridge to transplant). Decrease the pump flow rate until the atrial pressure increases to 20 to 25 mm Hg or the BP and CO (patient's) falls.

What is the course of weaning from VAD?

Can range from few hours to months or years. Many patients cannot be weaned, but success can occur in $^1/_3$ of patients

What is ECMO?

Extracorporeal membrane oxygenation

What is the primary difference between ECMO and a VAD?

A membrane oxygenator

Can ECMO be used to bridge patients to transplantation like a VAD?

Less likely. The general time that a patient can be on ECMO is 7 to 10 days, and a heart is unlikely to become available for transplant in that short a time period.

Can patients be weaned from ECMO?

Yes. They either wean, die, or get transitioned to a VAD.

HEART TRANSPLANTATION

What is the limiting factor in cardiac transplantation?

Donor supply. There are approximately 2,000 potential donors for 20,000 potential recipients annually in the United States.

Who needs a heart transplant?

Patients with end-stage heart disease not amenable to optimal medical therapy or surgical procedure (includes revascularization, PTCI, and catheter ablation techniques)
Patients who are unable to wean from inotropes, IABP, or VAD

Who are candidates for heart transplant?

Generally 0 to 60 years (physiologic age)

New York Heart Association class III+ or IV heart failure

Normal or reversible renal, hepatic, and cerebral function system

No malignancy, recent pulmonary infarct, severe PVD, or significant cerebrovascular disease

What are 6 contraindications for heart transplant?

1. Malignancy (nonskin)
2. Ongoing infection
3. Recent pulmonary infarction
4. Severe PVD, cerebrovascular disease (relative)
5. End-organ failure
6. IDDM with end-organ dysfunction

What are the survival outcomes?

1 year: 80% to 90%
5 years: 60% to 70%
10 years: Greater than 50%

Why are brady-, tachy-, and dysrhythmias treated differently in heart transplant patients?

The heart is denervated; therefore, vagolytic (atropine) and vagotonic (digoxin) agents are ineffective.

Does reinnervation occur?

Yes. Of heart patients, 75% show some sympathetic reinnervation at 1 year.

Does reinnervation have any effects on the patient?

Yes. Reinnervation can improve exercise performance because of the ability to increase HR more rapidly. It also can help in the diagnosis of coronary artery disease in recipients, because reinnervation allows patients to feel angina.

Can heart transplant patients have an MI?

Yes. Coronary artery disease can be a manifestation of chronic rejection; 50% of patients have some evidence of coronary artery disease at 5 years, 5% of which is significant.

How long can a heart be preserved before transplantation?	Approximately 4 hours in cold preservation solution
When are infections most common after any transplant?	The first 3 to 6 months
What 5 types of infections are most common after transplantation?	1. Bacterial 2. Atypical bacteria 3. Viral 4. Fungal 5. Protozoal
What 3 organs systems are most commonly involved with cytomegalovirus?	1. GI: stomach, colon 2. Lung: pneumonitis 3. Other, including heart Cytomegalovirus can also stimulate the immune system, so it can be associated with rejection.
When is rejection most common?	During first 2 months after transplantation
What 3 factors are important for successful heart, lung, and heart–lung transplantation?	1. ABO compatibility 2. Size match 3. Short ischemic time
In a heart–lung transplant recipient, is it possible to reject a lung without concomitant heart rejection?	Yes. Either lung may show evidence of rejection without involvement of the contralateral lung or heart.

14   Coronary Syndromes and Cardiac Arrest

OVERVIEW OF CORONARY AND INTENSIVE CARE

What are the top 10 elements of cardiovascular health maintenance in the ICU?

1. Keep a close eye on fluid status. Most patients are relatively fluid overloaded unless they have had recent losses (bleeding, bowel obstruction, sepsis, pancreatitis).
2. Review the rhythm, and try to work toward the closest approximation of sinus rhythm at a rate of 90 bpm that you can attain.
3. Review medications, and eliminate as many cardiac depressants as feasible (i.e., antiarrhythmics, anticonvulsants, benzodiazepines).
4. Be sure that potassium and magnesium are on the high side of the normal range. If they are not, replace them until they are.
5. Consider gentle enhancing of cardiac function with low-dose dobutamine or dopamine (5 μmg/kg/min).
6. Review ECG and rhythm strips daily to keep up with electrical state of the heart.
7. Remember that ICU patients, by definition, are not very stable. Thus, conditions that were appropriate for the heart yesterday may not be appropriate today.

8. Be sure you have instant access to the venous circulation at all times in case some cardiac event occurs suddenly.
9. Consider keeping defibrillator pads on the patient if you have seen some Vtach or if the patient has required defibrillation.
10. Be sure that blood pressure is controlled with a proper regimen.

What cardiovascular issues could arise that would kill your patient in the next 24 hours, and what can you do to lessen the likelihood of these issues arising?

Arrhythmias	Keep the patient monitored. Attach the patient to defibrillator pads if at risk. Keep potassium and magnesium on the high side of normal. Do not let central lines or pulmonary catheters sit in the RV. Consider antiarrhythmics if arrhythmias are prevalent. Prevent and treat alkalosis.
Tamponade	Be sure bleeding is controlled. Ensure that mediastinal tubes are working if present. Obtain echocardiogram if effusion is suspected. Consider possibility of tamponade after heart surgery, uremia, cancer.
Cardiac ischemia	Anti-ischemic agents (β-blockers, calcium-channel blockers, nitrates) Anticoagulants (aspirin; heparin if unstable) Adequate oxygen delivery
Declining cardiac function	Monitor with cardiac output, mixed venous O_2. Have low threshold for inotropes.

Consider IABP.
Intervene if CI is less than 2.0.

Aortic stenosis   No vasodilators
No hypovolemia

CORONARY DISEASE

EPIDEMIOLOGY

**What is the leading cause
of death in North America?**

Since 1900, cardiac disease has been the leading cause of death in the United States for every year except 1918. Currently, cardiovascular disease is responsible for approximately 40% of all deaths, with an average of 1 fatality every 33 seconds.

**In 1918, what was the
leading cause of death?**

The Spanish flu epidemic (675,000 Americans died)

**What percentage of patients
admitted to the hospital
with ischemic-like chest
pain are subsequently diagnosed with an acute MI?**

Less than 25%

**What is acute coronary
syndrome?**

A spectrum of conditions compatible with myocardial ischemia, typically caused by disruption of an atherosclerotic plaque with subsequent limitation of coronary blood flow. These conditions include ST-elevation MI, non-ST-elevation MI, and unstable angina.

CORONARY BLOOD FLOW AND MYOCARDIAL
OXYGEN CONSUMPTION

**What are the 3 major
determinants of myocardial
oxygen demand?**

1. Myocardial wall tension (30% of total)
2. Contractility
3. Heart rate

What are the 2 major determinants of myocardial oxygen supply?

1. Arterial oxygen content
2. Coronary blood flow

Define coronary blood flow.

Coronary blood flow = coronary perfusion pressure/coronary vascular resistance

where coronary vascular resistance is determined by the degree of coronary artery stenosis as well as by metabolic, hormonal, and autonomic nervous system parameters.

Most coronary blood flow occurs during which phase of the cardiac cycle?

Diastole

What is the normal resting coronary arterial blood flow?

80 mL/100 g/min, or 3% to 5% of cardiac output

When is myocardial wall tension highest?

During isovolumic systole

ELECTROCARDIOGRAM

Name 9 causes of ST elevation.

1. Acute MI
2. Ventricular aneurysm
3. Pericarditis: diffuse ST elevations
4. Myocardial contusion
5. Prinzmetal's angina
6. Early repolarization
7. Hypothermia: Osbourne J wave
8. Hyperkalemia
9. Artifact: occasionally seen with LBBB, left ventricular hypertrophy, myocardial neoplasms, hypertrophic myopathies

Name 5 causes of ST depression.

1. Acute posterior MI
2. Ischemia
3. Digoxin
4. Left ventricular hypertrophy
5. Bundle branch blocks

Name 7 important causes of T-wave inversion.	1. Ischemia 2. Electrolyte abnormalities 3. Medications: digoxin 4. Bundle branch blocks 5. Myocarditis 6. Seen with subarachnoid hemorrhages 7. After a ventricular premature beat and some tachycardias
Name 7 causes of ectopy (atrial and ventricular).	1. Ischemia 2. Reperfusion after thrombolytic therapy: the classic example is accelerated idioventricular rhythm. 3. Electrolyte abnormalities: K^+, Mg^{2+}, Ca^{2+} 4. Hypoxia 5. Monitoring lines: Swan-Ganz catheters, CVP lines 6. Medications: β-agonists, antiarrhythmics 7. Endogenous catechols: pain, anxiety

CARDIAC ENZYMES

Name three cardiac isoenzymes.	1. Creatine kinase (CK): myocardial band (MB) fraction 2. LDH 3. Aspartate aminotransferase
Name another marker of myocardial ischemic injury.	Troponin I
What is the timing of detection of troponin I in serum?	6 hour to 7 days after infarct
What is the benefit of troponin I?	Detects minor cardiac injury not detected by other traditional techniques.
Name 7 causes of CK elevation.	1. Acute MI 2. Myocarditis

3. Trauma/status epilepticus/surgery
4. Severe, prolonged exercise
5. Polymyositis/muscular dystrophy
6. Devastating brain injury
7. Familial elevation

Name 3 causes of CK-MB elevation.

1. Acute MI
2. Cardiac surgery
3. Muscular dystrophy

Name 4 causes of CK-BB (brain fraction) elevation.

1. Brain injury/Reye's syndrome
2. Uremia
3. Malignant hyperthermia
4. Small intestinal necrosis

Name 7 causes of LDH elevation.

1. Acute MI
2. Pernicious anemia/sickle cell crisis
3. Large PE
4. Renal infarction
5. Prosthetic heart valves
6. Hemolytic anemia
7. Liver injury

ACUTE MYOCARDIAL INFARCTION

DIAGNOSIS AND TREATMENT

What are the indications for the diagnosis of acute MI and initiating primary reperfusion therapy?

ST elevation greater than 1 mm in 2 or more contiguous leads
or
New bundle branch block with history suggesting acute MI
or
Posterior infarction with RV involvement
and
With any of the above, time to therapy less than 12 hours from onset of symptoms

Can an ST-elevation infarction be diagnosed in the setting of a pre-existing LBBB?

Yes, but it remains somewhat controversial. Criteria include:

1. ST elevation greater than 1 mm in a direction concordant with the QRS complex
2. ST depression greater than 1 mm in leads V_1, V_2, or V_3
3. ST elevation greater than 5 mm discordant with QRS complex

Does right bundle branch block obscure the diagnosis of acute infarction?

No

Among patients with ST-elevation MI, who benefits most from primary reperfusion therapy?

Patients with anterior infarctions who are treated *early*. Although benefit may be seen up to 12 hours following symptom onset, the greatest benefit is appreciated when time to therapy is < 3 hours. Remember, time is muscle.

What are the 4 most important predictors of mortality following MI?

1. Age
2. Ejection fraction
3. Extent of coronary artery disease
4. Burden of residual ischemia

What are the common thrombolytic agents?

1. Tissue plasminogen activator
2. Streptokinase
3. Anosylated plasminogen streptokinase activator complex
4. Urokinase

What are 5 contraindications to thrombolysis?

1. Recent trauma/surgery: active bleeding
2. Recent stroke
3. Significant hypertension
4. Recent history of chest compressions
5. Intracranial bleed

What are 5 other important medications used in the treatment of MI?

1. Aspirin
2. β-Blockers
3. Nitrates
4. Narcotics
5. Heparin

What dose of aspirin should be administered in acute MI?	160 to 325 mg. Consider rectal administration if oral administration is not possible.
What if the patient has a true aspirin allergy?	Ticlid or Plavix may be substituted if a true allergy exists.
What are 5 absolute contraindications to thrombolysis?	1. Previous hemorrhagic stroke 2. Any stroke within 1 year 3. Known intracranial neoplasm 4. Suspected aortic dissection 5. Active internal bleeding
Is menses an absolute contraindication to thrombolysis?	No
What is the incidence of intracranial hemorrhage with thrombolysis, and who is at highest risk for this complication?	Less than 1%, but the outcomes are often catastrophic. Older age, low body weight, and hypertension are risk factors. Certain thrombolytic agents also carry somewhat higher risk but may be more efficacious.
What are 3 signs of successful reperfusion after administration of thrombolytics?	1. Resolution of symptoms 2. Normalization of ECG, or decrease in ST elevation greater than 50% 3. Accelerated idioventricular rhythm
What percentage of patients who receive thrombolytics will have angiographically successful reperfusion?	Approximately 70%
What are 6 potential advantages of primary percutaneous coronary intervention (PCI) over fibrinolysis?	1. Lower rates of intracerebral hemorrhage 2. Improved reperfusion and flow rates (>90%) 3. Allows assessment of both left ventricular function and burden of coronary disease

4. Rapid identification of high-risk coronary anatomy and/or mechanical complications
5. Vascular access for placement of emergent balloon pump (IABP) or temporary pacing wire
6. Fewer contraindications than thrombolysis

Which 4 cardiac drugs should routinely be avoided in acute MIs, and why?

1. *Intravenous* angiotensin-converting enzyme (ACE) inhibitors → hypotension: some studies suggest they may increase mortality.
2. Short-acting calcium-channel blockers → hypotension and tachycardia: increased adverse outcomes
3. Inotropic agents in patients with adequate perfusion → increased myocardial O_2 demand and ischemia
4. Routine antiarrythmics offer no survival benefit. Some have even been shown to increase mortality.

What medication should generally be avoided in patients with MI and suspected cocaine intoxication?

β-Blockers

When is it appropriate to administer nondihydropyridine calcium-channel blockers to patients having a MI?

1. Supraventricular tachyarrythmias not controlled by β-blockade
2. Cocaine-induced MI
3. Evidence for ongoing ischemia when β-blockers are contraindicated or ineffective (only in the absence of significant left ventricular dysfunction)

What is the 1st therapy for hypotension/shock associated with an acute MI?

Vasopressors/inotropes
Invasive hemodynamic monitoring:
  CVP monitor, Swan-Ganz catheter

RV Infarction

When should RV infarction be suspected?	In the presence of any acute inferior infarction. The classic triad of elevated neck veins, hypotension, and clear lung fields is specific but relatively insensitive (~25%).
What is the single most predictive ECG finding in patients with RV infarction?	ST elevation in the right precordial lead (V_4R)
What are the 3 cornerstones of therapy for RV infarction?	1. Maintain preload with volume and avoidance of drugs reducing preload: nitrates/diuretics 2. Inotropic support 3. Reperfusion

COMPLICATIONS

List 5 causes of chest pain after an acute MI.	1. Reinfarction 2. Infarct extension 3. Recurrent ischemia 4. Pericarditis: Dressler's syndrome 5. Noncardiac: GI
True or False: Echocardiography is the diagnostic test of choice for suspected postinfarct pericarditis.	False. Pericarditis is a clinical diagnosis. The absence of pericardial fluid does not rule out the diagnosis.
Which 2 medications should not be used in the treatment of early post-infarct pericarditis?	1. Nonsteroidal anti-inflammatory drugs 2. Corticosteroids Both may interfere with healing and increase the risk of infarct expansion and rupture.
What are 5 possible causes of hypotension in patients with inferior MI?	1. RV infarction 2. Bradyarrhythmia 3. Acute mitral regurgitation (MR) 4. Ventricular septal defect (VSD) 5. Bezold-Jarisch reflex

What is the Bezold-Jarisch reflex?	Parasympathetic discharge secondary to stimulation of receptors in the ventricle. This leads to bradycardia and dilation of peripheral blood vessels.
Of what did Albert von Bezold die?	Tragically, he died of mitral stenosis at the age of 32 years.

Arrhythmias

What percentage of patients with acute MI will experience Vfib?	3% to 5%, with the highest incidence during the first 4 hours.
What is the prognostic significance of Vfib early (hours to days) after an acute MI?	None
What is the prognostic significance of Vfib late (days) after an acute MI?	Significant increase in mortality. This requires evaluation and treatment. This event suggests persistent ischemia.
What are 4 indications for placing a temporary pacing wire in acute infarctions?	1. Asystole. 2. Symptomatic bradycardia 3. Bifascicular block with 1st-degree AV block 4. Mobitz type II 2nd-degree AV block
When else should a pacing wire be considered?	1. Right bundle branch block with 1st-degree AV block. 2. LBBB: new or indeterminate 3. Incessant VT: for atrial or ventricular overdrive pacing. 4. Recurrent sinus pauses (>3 seconds) not responsive to atropine

Mechanical Complications

List 6 mechanical complications after an acute MI.	1. Left ventricular aneurysm
	2. Left ventricular rupture
	  a. Free wall contained = pseudoaneurysm
	  b. Noncontained = death
	  c. Septal = VSD

3. Papillary muscle rupture: acute MR
4. Thromboembolus
5. Reinfarction/extension
6. Pericardial effusion/tamponade

What 3 clinical scenarios should prompt investigation for a mechanical complication of MI?

1. New murmur
2. Hemodynamic deterioration
3. Pulmonary edema

List 2 causes of a new murmur after an acute MI.

1. MR
2. VSD

Name 3 ways to differentiate between MR and VSD?

1. Auscultation: frequently not helpful, because both are holosystolic murmurs. A VSD, however, usually is heard best over the sternum. The MR murmur can be heard at the apex but frequently radiates superiorly in posterior leaflet/papillary muscle ruptures and posteriorly in anterior leaflet/papillary muscle ruptures.
2. Doppler echo.
3. Right heart catheterization with measurement of the oxygen saturation in the various chambers. An increase in oxygen saturation of more than 5% between chambers is consistent with a shunt.

Can the amount of left-to-right shunting be estimated in a VSD (or atrial septal defect)?

Yes. Variables needed include SaO_2, RA O_2 (venous saturation), and SvO_2. The equation itself is
Shunt ratio $(Qp/Qs) = (SaO_2 - RA\ O_2)/(SaO_2 - SvO_2)$
For example:
Arterial saturation = 95%
RA saturation = 61%
PA saturation = 78%
Qp/Qs = 2:1
That is, there is twice as much pulmonary blood flow compared with systemic blood flow with the shunt at the RV level.

In patients with acute MR secondary to papillary muscle rupture, which papillary muscle is more commonly involved, and why?	In more than 90% of cases, the posteromedial ruptures, because it is supplied only by the posterior descending artery whereas the anterolateral has dual blood supply.
What percentage of patients will develop a VSD following MI?	0.5% to 2%
Which groups of patients are at highest risk for VSD?	1. Those with large infarcts 2. Those with single-vessel disease and poor collaterals Location of infarct is *not* a risk factor.
Do all patients with an infarct-related VSD have a murmur?	No. Patients with very large defects and/or shock may not have an audible murmur.
What is the definitive therapy of both VSD and papillary muscle rupture?	Surgical repair
What percentage of patients with a transmural MI will experience free wall rupture?	Only 3%. Rupture, however, accounts for more than 10% of mortality in acute MI.
What is the time course of cardiac rupture after infarction?	50% will occur within 5 days and 90% within 2 weeks.
What is a cardiac pseudoaneurysm?	A contained rupture

UNSTABLE ANGINA AND NON-ST-ELEVATION INFARCTIONS

Provide an algorithm for the management of acute cardiac chest pain.	Mnemonic **HOMEBASE**: **H**eparin **O**xygen **M**orphine **E**CG **B**eta-blocker **A**spirin **S**ublingual nitroglycerin **e**X-ray

What percentage of patients who present with chest pain and have a completely normal ECG will ultimately be diagnosed with a MI by enzymes?

1% to 6%

True or False: ACE inhibitors are only beneficial among those with acute MI with left ventricular dysfunction.

False. Although ACE inhibitors are particularly useful in this subset of patients, all patients with MI benefit from these drugs.

Compared to unfractionated heparin, what are 5 advantages of enoxaparin?

1. Ease of administration
2. No need for monitoring levels
3. Decreased incidence of heparin-induced thrombocytopenia
4. Lower cost
5. Reduction in the rate of death, MI, or urgent revascularization

How do platelet glycoprotein IIb/IIIa inhibitors work?

By blocking the IIb/IIIa receptor on the platelet surface, the drug prevents binding of the platelet to fibrinogen, a final common pathway in the process of platelet aggregation.

According to current guidelines, when should glycoprotein IIb/IIIa inhibitors be administered to patients with unstable non-ST-elevation MI?

1. When catheterization and percutaneous intervention is planned
2. When patients have ongoing ischemia, elevated troponin, or other high-risk features

True or False: Thrombolytics are harmful if administered to patients having a non-ST-elevation MI.

True. Several studies (TIMI IIIb, ISIS-2, and GISSI-1) have shown that these drugs *increase* the rate of adverse outcomes in these patients. The exception is patients with posterior wall infarction having RV involvement.

According to guidelines, in which patients with unstable angina and non-ST-elevation MI should an early invasive approach(cardiac catheterization) be used?

Those with:
1. Evidence for recurrent ischemia despite medical therapy
2. Elevated troponins
3. ST-segment depression
4. Clinical features suggestive of CHF
5. High-risk stress test
6. Depressed ejection fraction
7. Sustained Vtach
8. Percutaneous intervention within the past 6 months
9. Previous coronary artery bypass grafting

What are the 7 components of the TIMI risk score?

1. Age greater than 65 years
2. 3 coronary risk factors
3. Known angiographic coronary obstruction
4. ST-segment changes
5. Greater than 2 anginal events within 24 hours
6. Use of aspirin within the last 7 days
7. Elevated cardiac enzymes

What is the clinical significance of the TIMI risk score?

The scoring system is a well-validated tool for stratifying the risk of patients with acute coronary syndromes, and it may help to select patients who will benefit the most from the more aggressive therapies. Studies have demonstrated an increase in adverse outcomes (mortality, MI, and need for urgent revascularization) with higher TIMI risk scores.

CARDIAC ARREST

How should you prepare to handle cardiac arrests?

1. Read about resuscitation.
2. Take advanced cardiac life support classes.

What are 3 common causes of "near" cardiac arrest?

1. Relatively rapid drop in resistance: bolus of vasodilator, rapid warming.
2. Relatively rapid fluid loss: bleeding is most common.

3. Change in heart rhythm: atrial fibrillation is common.

What should your first moves be when confronted with a patient whose BP seems to be approximately 60 mm Hg?

1. Confirm that BP is low (palpate pulse: must be at least 60 mm Hg to feel carotid, 70 mm Hg to feel femoral, and 80 mm Hg to feel radial; flush A-line; check cuff pressure).
2. Evaluate heart rate and rhythm, and treat accordingly.
3. Consider giving calcium chloride via a central line (which buys time for further evaluation).

What are 3 steps you should follow to diagnose arrhythmias?

1. Think about the patient and history.
2. Rhythm strips are not as helpful as you might hope.
3. ECGs are good for evaluation of P waves, width of QRS, and rate.

MANAGEMENT OF CARDIAC ARREST IN THE ICU

What is the top priority in a cardiac arrest situation?

Mnemonic: **ABCs**
Airway
Breathing
Circulation
Ventilation can be with a mask; it does not have to be via endotracheal tube at first. Circulation includes adequate IV access.

What is a priority of almost equal importance in a cardiac arrest situation?

Chest compression if there is no palpable pulse at any location

Once the ABCs are secured, what should you do next?

Think. You now have time to gather your wits, along with information about the patient, and begin treatment.

Next?

Assess cardiac rhythm.

Treatment for Vfib/pulseless Vtach?

Defibrillation at 200/300/360 J

If there is no response after defibrillation, what next?

Epinephrine (1 mg IV; 10 mL of a 1:10,000 solution) or vasopressin (40 U IV for one dose)

What would be the amiodarone dose?

300 mg IV push. Consider repeating 150 mg IV push in 3 to 5 minutes (maximum dose, 2.2 g IV over 24 hours).

What would be the lidocaine dose?

1 to 1.5 mg/kg bolus, followed by 0.5 to 0.75 mg/kg boluses every 5 minutes until a total dose of 3 mg/kg, then an infusion at 2 to 4 mg/min.

When should you use procainamide?

For ventricular ectopy or sustained Vtach if lidocaine is not successful. Start with 20 to 30 mg/min until rhythm is suppressed, blood pressure drops, or QRS widens 50%, and then run 1 to 4 mg/min.

What is the treatment of asystole?

1. Transcutaneous pacing
2. Epinephrine bolus: 1 mg every 3 to 5 minutes
3. Atropine: 1 mg IV

What is PEA?

Pulseless electrical activity; absence of detectable blood pressure in the presence of organized rhythm on ECG (formerly called electromechanical dissociation)

Most are the frequent causes of PEA?

Mnemonic: **5 H's, 5 T's**
Hypovolemia
Hypoxia
Hydrogen ion (acidosis)
Hyper-/**H**ypokalemia
Hypothermia
Thrombosis (coronary)
Tablets
Tamponade
Tension pneumothorax
Thrombosis (pulmonary)

15 Management of the Postcardiac Surgery Patient

NEW POSTOPERATIVE PATIENT

What 5 studies must be checked ASAP in the new postoperative patient?

1. Cardiac indices
2. ECG
3. CXR
4. chest tube drainage
5. urine output

What 4 things should you check on the CXR?

1. Endotracheal tube placement: it should be at about the level of clavicles.
2. Air or fluid in the pleural space.
3. PA catheter position: this should be within the mediastinal shadow.
4. Check for pneumothorax and chest tube position.

What should you do first when a "fresh" cardiac surgery patient arrives in the ICU?

Feel the femoral pulse, and visually ensure that the chest is moving with ventilation.

What questions should be asked about such a patient?

What procedure was done; any reactions to protamine or drips; heart rate; last hemoglobin; any problems in the OR?

SUPRAVENTRICULAR ARRHYTHMIAS

What is the most common arrhythmia in the cardiac surgery population?

Afib; as high as 40% in CABG surgery and as high as 60% in valve replacement. **When asked on the wards, 30% is typically given as the mean.**

What is the most consistent predictor of postoperative Afib?

Age greater than 70 years

What are 7 other associated risk factors for Afib?

1. History of Afib
2. Use of β-blockers
3. Chronic obstructive pulmonary disease
4. Cardiomegaly
5. Left atrial enlargement
6. Right coronary artery stenosis
7. Sinus node or atrioventricular node disease

Why do cardiac surgery patients have a higher incidence of postoperative Afib?

They tend to have structural changes, such as atrial enlargement and elevated atrial pressures, that can support multiple re-entrant circuits. Factors associated with cardiac surgery itself may also predispose these patients to Afib.

What are 8 of these predisposing factors?

1. Acute atrial enlargement
2. Ischemia
3. Bypass and cross-clamp time
4. Hypertension
5. Cannulation
6. Electrolyte derangements (hypomagnesemia)
7. Inflammation (pericarditis)
8. Pulmonary vein venting

When is the peak incidence for Afib?

Postoperative days 2 and 3

What are some prophylactic measures currently used to decrease the incidence of Afib in cardiac surgery patients who are at risk?

Preoperative β-blockers, sotalol, and amiodarone (as long as the drugs are not contraindicated). The loading doses and side effects (i.e., hypotension) may be prohibitive for some patients.

Why is digoxin rarely used in the postoperative patient?

Because of the high sympathetic tone seen in postoperative patients, digoxin is rarely successful.

VENTRICULAR ARRHYTHMIAS

What is the significance of PVCs?

Simple PVCs are not rare after cardiac surgery and are not associated with an increased risk of developing malignant ventricular arrhythmias.

What about patients with frequent PVCs (>30/hr) and nonsustained Vtach?

There is no impact on short-term outcome, but numerous studies have shown reduced long-term outcome in patients with an LVEF of less than 40%.

What are 6 reversible causes of ventricular arrhythmias after cardiac surgery?

1. Electrolyte abnormality
2. Hypoxia
3. Hypovolemia
4. Ischemia
5. Graft closure
6. Inotropic and antiarrhythmic drugs.

Is there any benefit from prophylactic amiodarone to prevent postoperative ventricular arrhythmias?

No. Studies have shown no decrease in mortality with prophylactic amiodarone.

PERFUSION

What is the purpose of hemodynamic monitoring in the postoperative cardiac patient?

To assess volume status and cardiac output

What is cardiac output?

Heart rate × stroke volume. The normal range is 4 to 6 L/min.

What is cardiac index (CI)

Cardiac output/body surface area. The normal range is 2.5 to 4.0 L/min/m².

For a postoperative cardiac patient, what CI indicates a severe reduction in cardiac output?

Less than 2.0 L/min/m²

What is the role of dopamine in most coronary artery bypass graft (CABG) patients?

Some patients come into the unit on 5 μg/kg/min of dopamine, then are rapidly weaned to the renal dose (3 μg/kg/min) and stopped the morning of postoperative day 1.

What is the most common inotrope used for low CI and high SVRI after cardiac surgery?

Dobutamine

What is the ultimate indicator of volume status?

LVEDP

What is the best means to estimate LVEDP in an ICU patient?

Via a Swan-Ganz catheter that measures left-sided pressures by right heart catheterization

What is pulmonary capillary wedge pressure (PCWP)?

When the balloon catheter tip of the Swan-Ganz catheter wedges at a branched PA, it measures the transmitted left atrial pressure, which most closely approximates the LVEDP.

What is the normal value for the PCWP?

12 to 15 mm Hg in resting adult patients at sea level

Is the PCWP representative of the LVEDP during the first few hours after a CABG?

There may be a poor correlation between PCWP and LVEDP during this period because of a change in compliance of the left ventricle. The ventricle may be stiffer.

If the Swan-Ganz catheter does not wedge, what can be used to approximate LVEDP?

PAD pressure

When does PAD pressure not correlate with the wedge pressure?

In severe lung disease with pulmonary vascular changes (pulmonary hypertension)

What is the most common complication during placement of Swan-Ganz catheters?

Arrhythmias

What is the most dreaded complication of Swan-Ganz catheters?

Pulmonary arterial perforation from overwedging

What is the characteristic Swan-Ganz tracing in acute mitral regurgitation?

A V-shaped wave in the wedge tracing, representing regurgitant flow into the left atrium

What is the characteristic finding in acute ventricular septal rupture?

An oxygen saturation step-up in the PA as compared to the right atrium

What Swan-Ganz tracings are suggestive of a hemodynamically significant pulmonary embolus?

Elevated right heart pressures (CVP, PAS, and PAD) with a normal wedge pressure

Can a postoperative patient with a mediastinal tube develop pericardial tamponade?

Yes. Chest tubes can clot, and even with actively draining tubes, blood can collect in loculations, compressing specific parts of the heart.

What does one see in cardiac tamponade?

Equilibrium of all pressures (CVP, PAD, and PCWP) at a high value

Your patient has a Swan-Ganz PA catheter. You want to check the PCWP, but when you inflate the balloon, the pressure tracing rapidly increases until it is off the scale. What is happening?

The PA catheter is "overwedging." The balloon is too far into the PA. When you inflate the balloon, it squeezes longitudinally, until it covers over the pressure monitoring hole at the catheter tip. This causes the monitor trace to rise off the scale.

Is overwedging dangerous?

Yes! It greatly increases the likelihood of PA rupture by the balloon.

How can overwedging be avoided?

Always inflate the balloon slowly while watching the monitor trace. If it begins to overwedge, STOP, deflate the balloon, and pull back the PA catheter before trying again.

Suppose someone who has not read this book overwedges the PA catheter and ruptures the PA?

The first thing you will notice is hemoptysis. The balloon should be carefully reinflated after pulling the catheter back a bit in an attempt to tamponade the bleeding site. If the patient is not intubated, he or she should be positioned with the injured side down and immediately intubated, preferably with a double-lumen endotracheal tube to prevent aspiration of blood into the noninvolved side. Selective intubation of the opposite mainstem bronchus can also serve the same function. Stop all anticoagulation, and make sure blood is available for transfusion. In severe cases, emergency surgery will be necessary.

What causes a low mixed venous oxygen (SvO$_2$) in postoperative cardiac patients?

Low cardiac output, poor arterial oxygenation, and anemia are common causes of decreased oxygen delivery. Fever and agitation are common causes of increased oxygen demand.

What are 2 causes of a high SvO$_2$?

1. Any septal defect or shunt causing left-to-right flow within the heart.
2. Sepsis.

BLEEDING

What are 6 causes of excess bleeding after heart surgery?

1. Technical problems (e.g., bleeding): from a suture line or a side branch of a vein or mammary graft.
2. Excess of heparin: a common problem when underperfused vascular beds open up postoperatively.

3. Hypothermia: cold blood will not clot; rewarm your patient. This is a big deal.
4. Platelet dysfunction: caused by platelet contact with the cardiopulmonary bypass machine or postoperative aspirin.
5. Clotting factor deficiency: caused by excessive transfusion with packed RBCs or retransfusion of large volumes of washed blood.
6. Fibrinolysis: caused by many factors, including excessive bleeding, blood contact with the bypass machine, retransfusion of shed blood.

How can excess heparin be diagnosed and treated?

Prolonged PTT or activated clotting time. Treatment is with protamine.

How can platelet dysfunction be diagnosed and treated?

Prolonged bleeding time with or without low platelet count. Treatment is to administer DDAVP(deamino-D-arginine vasopressin), transfuse platelets, or both.

How can clotting factor deficiency be diagnosed and treated?

Prolonged PT. Treatment is to administer FFP.

How can fibrinolysis be diagnosed and treated?

Decreased fibrinogen level, increased fibrin split products and/or D-dimer. Treatment is with aminocaproic acid (Amicar).

Which pump cases are at greater risk for factor deficiencies/platelet dysfunction?

The ones that last more than 3 hours, patients in renal failure, or large volume of blood filtered through cell-saver.

How much chest tube output after cardiopulmonary bypass is too much?

It varies for each surgeon. In general, output should not be greater than 250 mL/hr during the first 4 hours; after 4 hours, you want it to be less than 100 mL/hr. Once the output is less than 100 mL/hr, the bleeding will almost always stop.

What cause of increased tube drainage may not require therapy?

Some patients may dump a significant amount of blood/fluid from a pocket when they are repositioned. This increase will not be sustained.

Your patient has been experiencing excessive chest tube drainage over the past several hours because of a coagulopathy. The drainage suddenly ceases. What should you do?

Obtain a CXR. The concern is that the chest tubes have clotted and the blood is now accumulating in the chest, a situation that can lead to cardiac tamponade. Look for a widened mediastinum or a pleural accumulation on the chest film. The CXR is not a good way to establish the diagnosis of tamponade, but it can provide clues regarding whether blood is accumulating.

Is hetastarch an anticoagulant?

Yes. Hetastarch should be avoided in the early care of postoperative patients.

OTHER MANAGEMENT

How should the chest of an arrest patient who has just had cardiac surgery be managed?

Usually, it should be opened. Do not perform closed-chest massage on a patient with a prosthetic mitral valve, because it may be pushed out the back of the heart.

What are 6 indications for mediastinal re-exploration?

1. Tamponade physiology (tachycardia, high filling pressures)
2. Hypotension
3. Decreased urine output
4. Large chest output that stops suddenly
5. Massive mediastinal hemorrhage (e.g., 1,000 mL in 5 min)
6. Refractory asystole/Vtach without a pulse

No postoperative cardiac patient should be coded without opening the chest!

List 6 ways in which hypothermic patients can be warmed.

1. Warm fluids.
2. Heat the ventilator humidifier to 40°C.
3. Warm the room.
4. Heating lamps on bare torso.
5. Decrease loss from convection (cover bed rails with blanket or bear hugger).
6. Under severe circumstances, peritoneal or hemodialysis.

What is the most common cause of hyponatremia in postoperative cardio-pulmonary bypass patients?

Fluid overload. Use diuretics; they promote free water clearance.

Why might transthoracic pacing wires not work well after 7 to 10 days?

Scar and edema can cause an insulating block to prevent conduction to the myocardium.

What is the order of removal of temporary pacing wires and chest tubes?

Wires first (if no arrhythmias), followed 1 hour later by chest tubes if less than 20 mL/hr of mediastinal chest tube drainage

What is the order of removal of IABP, endotracheal tube, chest tubes, wires, and PA catheter?

1. IABP
2. Extubate
3. PA catheter
4. Wires
5. Chest tubes

16 Renal

RENAL PHYSIOLOGY

INTRODUCTION

What 3 basic physiological features of the kidney determine renal function?

1. Blood flow
2. Glomerular filtration
3. Tubular reabsorption and secretion

What 2 factors determine the amount of blood flow to the kidney?

1. CO
2. Renal vascular resistance

What 3 factors determine the glomerular filtration rate (GFR)?

1. Hydrostatic pressure in the afferent arteriole: increased hydrostatic pressure increases the GFR.
2. Colloid oncotic pressure: decreased oncotic pressure increases the GFR.
3. Filtration coefficient.

What are the 2 principal functions of the renal tubules?

1. Reabsorption of sodium
2. Reabsorption of water

Which portion of the nephron absorbs sodium?

The distal tubule

Which portion of the nephron absorbs water?

The collecting tubule

RENAL HORMONES

What intrinsic renal mechanism sustains blood flow to the kidney when renal perfusion pressure falls?

The renin–angiotensin system

List the 5 steps of the intrinsic renal mechanism when renal perfusion pressure falls.

1. The juxtaglomerular apparatus increases the production of renin.
2. Renin stimulates increased conversion of angiotensinogen to angiotensin I.
3. Angiotensin I is converted into angiotensin II.
4. Angiotensin II increases efferent arteriole vascular resistance and peripheral vascular resistance.
5. Systemic blood pressure and renal perfusion pressure are increased.

When systolic pressure is less than 70 mm Hg, what happens to the intrinsic renal mechanism?

It fails. Afferent arterioles constrict, glomerular filtration rapidly decreases, and urine output (UO) falls.

Which hormone primarily regulates sodium reabsorption?

Aldosterone

How does aldosterone work?

Aldosterone increases the number of Na^+/K^+-ATPases in the tubular cells. This increases reabsorption of Na^+ while excreting K^+ and H^+. ATP serves as the energy source for the pump.

Which hormone primarily regulates water reabsorption?

ADH, also known as vasopressin

How does ADH work?

ADH increases the permeability of H_2O in the collecting tubule, thus increasing the reabsorption of water.

What is the function of atrial natriuretic peptide (ANP)?

ANP is released from the right atrium myocytes in response to atrial stretch (e.g., volume expansion, heart failure, pulmonary HTN). It promotes natriuresis by directly inhibiting renal reabsorption of sodium and water and indirectly inhibiting the renin–angiotensin system.

RENAL CARE AND HYGIENE IN THE ICU

What are 6 potential causes of declining renal function in an ICU patient?

1. Systemic sepsis
2. Hypotension: either immediate or in the period just before the decreased UO
3. Medications: aminoglycosides, cyclosporine, nonsteroidal anti-inflammatory drugs (NSAIDs)
4. Cholesterol embolization resulting from intra-aortic balloon pump placement or catheterization
5. Multisystem organ failure
6. Contrast nephropathy

What are 8 renal-protective measures that you should practice?

1. Maintain adequate *intravascular* volume.
2. Maintain adequate CO and MAP.
3. Monitor UO: the goal is more than 0.5 to 1 mL/kg/hr.
4. Protect the kidneys from contrast dye loads
   a. Preload with volume (0.5 normal saline is more effective than mannitol or furosemide).
   b. *N*-acetylcysteine may be protective.
5. Use diuretics sparingly and appropriately.
6. Monitor laboratory indices of urinary function: creatinine, BUN.
7. Monitor nephrotoxic drugs: amino-glycosides, vancomycin, NSAIDs.
8. Adjust drug dosages in renal insufficiency and failure states.

What is the single best parameter to determine a patient's overall fluid status?

Total body weight over time with respect to preoperative or normal body weight

True or False: Edema and excessive water-weight gain are contraindications to initial fluid administration for oliguria.

False. A patient can have excess total body fluid but still be INTRAVASCULARLY dry. Fluids (almost always) are your friends; use them wisely.

ACID-BASE BALANCE

What purpose do buffer systems serve?	Buffers minimize the change in pH associated with the addition of an acid or a base to a solution (in this case, body fluids).
Which acid serves as the buffer system for the human body?	Carbonic acid $H_2O + CO_2 \leftrightarrow H_2CO_3 \leftrightarrow H^+ + HCO_3^-$
What is respiratory acidosis?	Acidosis from increased carbon dioxide
What is metabolic acidosis?	Acidosis from an increase in acids other than carbonic acid
What are the 2 physiologic mechanisms for regulating acid-base status?	1. Respiratory: can respond in minutes with increased ventilation to eliminate excess acid (as CO_2). 2. Renal: can eliminate excess acid (as H^+) or prevent bicarbonate excretion, but this requires hours to days for response.
Acutely, a change in arterial partial pressure of carbon dioxide ($Paco_2$) change of 10 mm Hg corresponds to a pH change of what amount?	0.08 in the opposite direction. For instance, if $Paco_2$ increased to 50 mm Hg, then the pH would decrease by 0.08 (i.e., pH 7.4 to 7.32).
Chronically, a $Paco_2$ change of 10 mm Hg corresponds to a pH change of what	0.03 in the opposite direction
What is the anion gap?	The unmeasured anions in plasma. These include anionic proteins, phosphate, sulfate, and organic anions.
How is the anion gap calculated?	Anion gap = serum $Na^+ - [HCO_3^- + Cl^-]$

What is a normal anion gap?	7 to 14 mEq/L
What are some causes of metabolic acidosis with an increased anion gap?	Mnemonic **MUDPILES:** **M**ethanol intoxication **U**remia **D**iabetic ketoacidosis **P**araldehyde intoxication **I**ngestion of ethylene glycol **L**actic acidosis **E**thanol intoxication **S**alicylate intoxication
What are the 2 most common causes of metabolic acidosis with a normal anion gap (e.g. nonanion gap acidosis)?	1. Diarrhea 2. Renal tubular acidosis
What is renal tubular acidosis?	A tubular dysfunction resulting in decreased reabsorption of filtered bicarbonate, in turn resulting in excessive bicarbonate loss
What are 7 other causes of nonanion gap metabolic acidosis?	1. Carbonic anhydrase inhibitors 2. Lysine or arginine HCl 3. GI bicarbonate loss 4. Pancreatic fistula 5. Ureterosigmoidostomy 6. Addition of HCl 7. Ammonium chloride
What 2 pharmacological means can be used to manipulate acid-base status?	1. IV $NaHCO_3$ or other buffers 2. Central IV HCl or other acidic compounds
In patients with metabolic acidosis, when should sodium bicarbonate be considered?	When pH falls below 7.2 (to prevent cardiovascular collapse)
Why should bicarbonate not be routinely administered for metabolic acidosis?	An overcorrection may result, with development of metabolic alkalosis, as precursor organic anions are converted to bicarbonate.

Accumulation of lactic acid in the blood above the normal range of 0.4 to 1.3 mmol/L

What is the most common cause of lactic acidosis in the surgical ICU?

Tissue hypoxia and anaerobic metabolism because of inadequate delivery of oxygen to peripheral tissues (e.g., from heart failure, sepsis, hemorrhagic shock)

What is the significance of a lactic acid level greater than 5 mmol/L?

Mortality rate markedly increases.

What 3 factors can be increased to improve tissue oxygen delivery and, thereby, decrease anaerobic metabolism?

1. CO
2. Hematocrit
3. Arterial oxygen saturation

What 3 interventions can be used to maximize the three factors mentioned above?

1. Fluid resuscitation first, then ionotropes (if indicated).
2. Appropriate red blood cell transfusion (young and healthy, Hgb 7 g/dL; coronary artery disease, Hgb 10 g/dL); erythropoietin-α in chronic renal failure.
3. Increase F_{IO_2} and/or PEEP.

RENAL FAILURE

Define acute renal failure.

Rapid decline in the GFR over hours to weeks with retention of nitrogenous waste products, extracellular fluid, and electrolytes

Define chronic renal failure.

Renal injury of a prolonged nature leading to progressive and irreversible destruction of renal function

Define acute oliguria.

Adult: UO less than 0.5 mL/kg/hr, or 400 mL over 24 hours
Child: UO less than 1.0 mL/kg/hr

Define anuria.   UO less than 100 mL over 24 hours

What is azotemia?   Retention of nitrogenous end products
                                      of protein and amino acid metabolism
                                      (i.e., elevated BUN)

What is creatinine?   A byproduct of amino acid metabolism
                                      (molecular weight = 113 daltons). It
                                      does not bind to plasma proteins and is
                                      freely filtered by the renal glomerulus.

MEASURING AND ESTIMATING CREATININE CLEARANCE

GFR is not easily   Creatinine clearance remains the most
measured. How can it best   common clinical correlate to GFR.
be approximated?

How can creatinine   By 24-hour urine collection
clearance be measured?   Creatinine clearance =
                                      [UCr × urine vol]/[PCr × time]
                                      where creatinine clearance is in
                                      mL/min, UCr is urine creatinine
                                      (mg/dL), urine volume is in mL, PCr is
                                      plasma creatinine (mg/dL), and time is
                                      in minutes.

Name 2 ways you can   1. Urine specimen volume.
determine if you have   2. Urine creatinine content.
obtained an adequate 24-
hour urine collection?

What is considered to be   1. More than 400 mL over 24 hours in
an adequate volume for a   adults.
24-hour urine specimen in   2. Small volumes with maximal
a patient with normal renal   concentration may be adequate:
function?   high specific gravity, osmolality.

What is considered to be   Creatinine excretion correlates with
an adequate 24-hour urine   muscle mass. Compare the measured
specimen creatinine in a   creatinine excretion with the calculated
patient with normal renal   ideal excretion based on body height
function?   and ideal body weight.

How can creatinine clearance be estimated?

Collecting a 24-hour urine sample to measure creatinine clearance remains a major limitation. Therefore, numerous mathematical formulas have been developed to use serum creatinine as a reflection of the GFR. The most common is the Cockcroft and Gault formula.

What is the Cockcroft and Gault formula?

Creatinine clearance = [140 - age] × weight/[72 × creatinine] where creatinine clearance is in mL/min, age is in years, and creatinine (serum/plasma) is in mg/dL. Multiply the result by 0.85 if the patient is female.

List 3 reasons why creatinine clearance is not a perfect reflection of the GFR.

1. Small quantities of creatinine are *secreted* by the renal tubules.
2. Certain medications (e.g., cephalosporins, cimetidine) can be mistaken for creatinine and produce false overestimates of the GFR.
3. With decreasing renal function, creatinine excretion because of tubular secretion increases and falsely overestimates the GFR.

If the serum creatinine increases by 1 mg/dL above baseline levels, this correlates with what percentage decrease in GFR?

50% decrease in GFR

What are the degrees of renal impairment based on creatinine clearance using the Cockcroft and Gault formula?

Normal: Greater than 100 mL/min
Mild: 40 to 60 mL/min
Moderate: 10 to 40 mL/min
Severe: Less than 10 mL/min

ASSESSMENT AND INITIAL TREATMENT
OF ACUTE RENAL DYSFUNCTION

What 3 clinical parameters should be monitored and/or performed frequently to recognize early signs and symptoms of acute renal dysfunction?

1. UO
2. Serum creatinine
3. Physical exam

What 5 signs and symptoms should be sought during a physical exam in an acutely oliguric patient?

1. Intravascular hypovolemia: tachycardia, hypotension, flat neck veins, weak pulse
2. Poor peripheral perfusion: pale skin color, cool skin, temperature, decreased capillary refill, mental status decline
3. Poor myocardial function: distended neck veins, crackles on pulmonary auscultation, new heart murmurs
4. Urinary tract obstruction: distended bladder
5. Abdominal compartment syndrome: bladder pressure greater than 30 cm H_2O

What should be your initial algorithm for acute renal failure (oliguria and/or rising serum creatinine)?

1. Assess urinary tract patency, intravascular volume status, and perfusion status.
2. Give an IV fluid bolus.
3. Evaluate renal tubular function: prerenal, renal, mixed, postrenal dysfunction (check urine; discussed later).
4. Adjust medications and fluids appropriately.
5. Consider renal replacement therapy: hemodialysis vs. continuous renal replacement therapy (CRRT).

How do you determine the proper volume of fluid bolus?

A bolus should be approximately 10% of the estimated circulating volume. Assuming that blood makes up 7% of body weight, a true bolus is calculated as weight (kg) $\times$ 7% $\times$ 10%, or approximately 500 mL in most adults.

What 2 renal failure complications may arise that could kill your patient in the next 24 hours?

1. Hyperkalemia
2. Acid-base disorders

DIFFERENTIATING ACUTE PRERENAL, RENAL, AND POSTRENAL FAILURE

Acute renal failure can be broken down into which 3 categories?

1. Prerenal
2. Renal
3. Postrenal

Which is the most common type of acute renal failure?

Prerenal (50%–90% of cases)

What 3 tests can help to distinguish between the different causes of acute renal failure?

1. Urinary electrolytes
2. Fractional excretion of sodium (FENa)
3. Renal ultrasound

How do you determine the FENa?

FENa = ([UNa $\times$ PCr]/[PNa $\times$ UCr]) $\times$ 100
where UNa is urine Na (mEq/L) and PNa is plasma Na (mEq/L).

How can you distinguish prerenal causes from renal and postrenal causes of acute renal failure?

Prerenal: urine Na^+ less than 20 mEq/L, FENa less than 1
Renal/postrenal: urine Na^+ greater than 40 mEq/L, FENa greater than 3
Mixed or nonspecific: urine Na^+ of 20 to 40 mEq/L, FENa of 1 to 3

How can a urinalysis distinguish between prerenal and renal causes of acute renal failure?

Prerenal: high specific gravity, low pH, hyaline casts
Renal: low specific gravity, muddy brown granular casts

Urine sodium, FENa, and urinalysis are of little use if patients have received which drug class in the preceding 24 hours?	Diuretics. Check these labs BEFORE you give diuretics!

DIAGNOSIS AND MANAGEMENT OF ACUTE RENAL FAILURE

Preranal

What is the physiologic deficiency in "prerenal" acute renal failure?	Decreased renal perfusion
How do you manage a patient in prerenal acute renal failure?	1. Replace intravascular volume. 2. Monitor volume resuscitation: with or without CVP or PAWP. 3. Avoid α-adrenergic agents if inotropic support is indicated. 4. Consider adjunctive, low-dose dopamine (2–5 μg/kg/min); The effect may be trivial or profound depending on the patient and comorbidities. 5. Evaluate acute renal arterial occlusion and/or injury. 6. Evaluate for abdominal compartment syndrome. 7. Adjust medication doses appropriately. 8. Renal replacement therapy if renal dysfunction progresses.

Renal

What are 8 potential causes of renal parenchymal acute renal failure?	1. Nephrotoxic drugs 2. Ischemia 3. Radiographic contrast dye 4. Myoglobinuria 5. Syndrome of inappropriate antidiuretic hormone secretion (SIADH) 6. Hepatorenal syndrome 7. Systemic inflammatory response syndrome (SIRS)

8. Inflammatory and vasculitic causes secondary to autoimmune or postinfectious states

What are the 2 most common causes of "renal" acute renal failure?

1. Toxic injury
2. Ischemic injury

Describe the management of acute renal failure from renal causes.

1. Discontinue nephrotoxic agents when possible.
2. Avoid and/or minimize use of ionic contrast agents.
3. Maintain adequate renal perfusion.
4. Evaluate tubular function: urine creatinine, FENa.
5. Rule out SIADH, hepatorenal syndrome.
6. Adjust medication doses appropriately.
7. Renal replacement therapy if renal dysfunction progresses.

Which 2 segments of the nephron are most sensitive to ischemia?

1. Medullary thick ascending limb of the loop of Henle.
2. Pars recta of the proximal tubule.

Aminoglycoside nephrotoxicity on tubular cells is correlated best with the peak or trough levels?

Trough levels

What can be used to pro-tect against toxicity from iodinated contrast dye?

N-acetylcysteine

How can clearance of circulating myoglobin and hemoglobin be increased?

1. Crystalloid volume, volume, and more volume.
2. UO greater than 100 mL/hr until urine is clear.
3. Osmotic agents: mannitol (0.25–1 mg/kg)
4. Urine alkalinization

When would you suspect the SIADH?	Normal serum creatinine, urine Na$^+$ greater than 40 mEq/L, and normal or low serum Na$^+$
How do you treat SIADH?	Water restriction
How do you treat patients with symptomatic hyponatremia in the setting of SIADH?	Hypertonic saline (slowly)

Postrenal

What is the most common cause of "postrenal" acute renal failure?	Obstruction: ureters, bladder, urethra, Foley catheter
How can you diagnose urinary outlet obstruction?	Ultrasonography (noninvasive, can be performed at bedside), IV pyelography
Describe the management of acute renal failure from postrenal causes.	1. Decompression and drainage. a. Bladder: Foley catheter, suprapubic tube. b. Ureter: nephrostomy tube. c. Catheter: dislodge obstruction or replace catheter. 2. Measure intra-abdominal pressure to evaluate for abdominal compartment syndrome. 3. Maintain adequate renal perfusion.
How do you measure intra-abdominal pressure?	Place 50 mL of saline through the Foley catheter into the bladder, and measure the pressure through the catheter using a transducer. An intra-abdominal pressure greater than 30 mm Hg is incompatible with normal urinary function, and this pressure must be relieved.
What is the treatment of abdominal compartment syndrome?	Release the pressure within the abdominal cavity, usually by midline laparotomy or opening the surgical

incision. (Refer to the GI chapter for more details.)

PROGNOSIS FOR ACUTE RENAL FAILURE

What is the mortality rate for acute renal failure?

30% to 80%. The rate varies with comorbid factors, however, and is highest in patients with multisystem organ failure from infection or SIRS.

If a patient survives, what is the chance of complete renal recovery?

25% to 30%

What is that patient's chance of partial renal recovery?

40% to 50%

CHRONIC RENAL FAILURE

List 3 forms of chronic renal failure.

1. Nonoliguric
2. Oliguric
3. Anuric

Which form has the best prognosis?

Nonoliguric renal failure

Death related to renal failure is most often caused by what?

Infectious complications:
1. Pneumonia is the most common fatal infection.
2. Sepsis also may occur from peritonitis, urinary infection, line infection, etc.

What sequela of renal failure also contributes to death in these patients?

Bleeding diathesis because of uremia (dysfunctional platelets)

Medications and dosing intervals for renal failure should be adjusted based on which 3 principles of pharmacokinetics?

1. Desired concentration of drug
2. Volume of distribution of the drug
3. Mechanism and rate of metabolism or clearance

RENAL REPLACEMENT THERAPY

What is renal replacement therapy?	A method for providing the function of the kidneys by circulating blood through tubes made of semipermeable membranes
What is CRRT?	Continuous renal replacement therapy
How does CRRT differ from traditional "hemodialysis"?	Hemodialysis: diffusive hemodialysis CRRT: convective hemofiltration
What is diffusive hemodialysis?	Solute removal via diffusion down an electrochemical gradient. Dialysate runs countercurrent to blood flow. Solutes diffuse out of the plasma down their concentration gradients through a semipermeable membrane. This is **Brownian motion:** smaller molecules (urea) have more kinetic energy and are removed preferentially, whereas larger molecules with less kinetic energy are removed less efficiently or not at all. Diffusive hemodialysis relies on a fast dialysate flow rate, requires daily sessions, is more aggressive, and creates harsh conditions.
What is convective hemofiltration?	Solute removal via solvent drag. The dialysate (solvent) carries the plasma (solute) through a relatively high-flux or porous semipermeable membrane filter. A roller pump creates hydrostatic pressure that drives the solution through the filter. The filter removes solutes that fit through the membrane pore size. Larger molecules are more effectively removed than in diffusion dialysis. Convective hemofiltration is managed under slow flow rates, requires continuous hemodialysis, is less aggressive, and creates less harsh conditions.

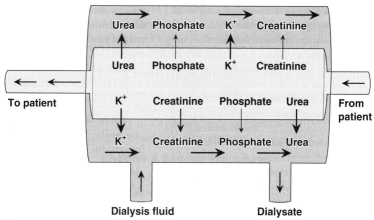

A Hemodialysis

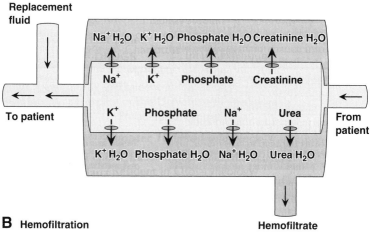

B Hemofiltration

Diffusive hemodialysis vs. convective hemofiltration.

| **When was convective hemofiltration first used clinically?** | 1977 (by Kramer and coworkers at the University of Gottingen) |

What do CVVHD, CAVHD, SCUF, CHFD, CVVHDF, and CVVH have in common?

All are modes of convective hemofiltration with or without supplemental diffusive hemodialysis
CVVHD: continuous venovenous hemodialysis
CAVHD: continuous arteriovenous hemodialysis
SCUF: slow continuous ultrafiltration
CHFD: continuous high-flux hemodialysis
CVVHDF: continuous venovenous hemodiafiltration
CVVH: continuous venovenous hemofiltration

What is the most commonly used mode of CRRT?

CVVH

What are 4 advantages of CRRT over traditional hemodialysis?

1. CRRT is slow and continuous.
2. Fluid and electrolyte shifts are more subtle.
3. Hemodynamically labile patients tend to tolerate CRRT for longer periods of time.
4. CRRT permits concomitant high-volume fluid administration.

What are the disadvantages of CRRT compared to traditional hemodialysis?

CRRT dialysate and personnel are expensive.

Often, critically ill patients do not tolerate hemodialysis because of their hemodynamic instability. What may be an alternative to hemodialysis in these patients?

Peritoneal dialysis or CRRT

True or False: Elevated levels of BUN and creatinine are absolute indications for hemodialysis.

False. Elevated BUN and creatinine values alone are not absolute indications for dialysis; however, they are indicators of declining renal function.

What are the indications for urgent hemodialysis?

Mnemonic **A E I O U:**

Acidosis: pH less than 7.1
Electrolyte disturbance: K greater than 6.5 mEq/L
Ingested insult: drug overdose with dialyzable toxin
Overload: symptomatic fluid overload
Uremic encephalopathy, pericarditis, neuropathy/myopathy

DIURETICS

List 8 adverse effects of loop diuretics.

1. Azotemia
2. Hyponatremia
3. Hypokalemia
4. Hypomagnesemia
5. Metabolic alkalosis
6. Elevation of plasma urate and cholesterol levels
7. Carbohydrate intolerance
8. Ototoxicity at high doses

Describe the adverse effects of osmotic diuretics.

Hyperkalemic metabolic acidosis, expansion of extracellular volume (ECV), and hemodilution. In extreme circumstances, volume overload, pulmonary edema, CNS depression, and severe hyponatremia can occur.

List the adverse effect of carbonic anhydrase inhibitors.

Metabolic acidosis

List 5 adverse effects of thiazide diuretics.

1. Azotemia
2. Hypokalemia
3. Hypomagnesemia
4. Elevation of plasma urate and cholesterol levels
5. Carbohydrate intolerance

List 2 adverse effects of distal potassium–sparing diuretics.

1. Hyperkalemia
2. Renal stones (Triamterene)
Avoid in patients with renal failure.

What are 3 common causes of diuretic resistance?

1. Inappropriate NaCl or fluid intake
2. Decreased renal responsiveness
3. Inadequate drug concentration reaching the tubule

List 5 causes of decreased renal responsiveness to diuretic therapy.

1. NSAIDs
2. Nephron adaptation
3. Activation of the renal angiotensin system
4. Edema: decreased effective ECV
5. Low GFR: CHF, acute renal failure, chronic renal failure, elderly, cirrhosis

FOLEY CATHETER MANAGEMENT

How can a Foley catheter that is suspected of malfunctioning be assessed?

Flush the catheter under sterile conditions using a Toomy syringe and sterile saline. If there is not free flow of saline in and out of the catheter, the Foley should be replaced.

After multiple failed attempts to place a Foley catheter in a patient who must be resuscitated, you should proceed to what technique?

A suprapubic catheter using the Seldinger technique. The bladder is just posterior and inferior to the pubic ramus.

The Foley balloon will not deflate when you attempt to remove the catheter. What substance instilled into the balloon will result in disruption of the balloon?

Mineral oil. It will destroy the integrity of the latex.

What safe, invasive procedure might be used to more quickly deflate the balloon of a defective Foley catheter?

Ultrasound-guided fine-needle puncture of the Foley balloon. Alternatively, cut the Foley catheter itself, and the balloon will likely drain.

17 Fluids and Electrolytes

NORMAL PHYSIOLOGY

BODY WATER AND FLUID VOLUMES

What percentage of body weight in an adult is water?

Total body water (TBW) is 60% of body weight, which is 42 kg in a 70-kg adult (42-L volume, because the density of water is 1 kg/L).

TBW is what percentage in infants?

TBW in newborns is higher (75%–80%) but equals adult values by 1 year of age.

Does the TBW percentage differ by gender?

Females generally have more adipose tissue; thus, the TBW percentage is lower. TBW is also lower in the obese of either gender.

What fraction of TBW is intracellular and extracellular?

Two-thirds of TBW is intracellular fluid (40% of body weight); one-third is extracellular fluid (ECF; 20% of body weight).

What constitutes extracellular fluid?

Plasma and interstitial fluid

What is the plasma volume?

Fluid in the vascular system but external to erythrocytes; approximately one-fourth of ECF (and 5% of body weight)

What is the interstitial fluid volume?

Fluid external to blood vessels and cells; approximately three-fourths of ECF (and 15% of body weight)

What is the blood volume of an adult?	Approximately 5 L, or 70 mL/kg. It consists of plasma volume and erythrocyte volume. A 70-kg person has a TBW of 42 L. The ECF is one-third of the TBW (14 L) and the plasma one-fourth of the ECF (3.5 L); assuming a hematocrit of 40% would give a red cell volume of 1.5 L, which yields 3.5 L + 1.5 L = 5 L

IONS AND OSMOLALITY

What are the major intracellular cations?	Potassium and Magnesium
What is the major extracellular cation?	Sodium
How does the body maintain the intracellular and extracellular concentration gradients of these ions?	A sodium-potassium ion pump uses adenosine triphosphate (ATP) as energy to actively pump sodium out of the cell in exchange for pumping potassium into the cell. When ATP is depleted, the ion gradient is lost, and cellular dysfunction occurs.
What is osmolality?	The concentration of a solution, as determined by the ionic concentration of the dissolved substances per unit of solvent
What is the normal osmolality of blood?	Appoximately 300 mOsm
What hormone is the main regulator of osmolality, and how does it work?	ADH. As osmolality exceeds 300 mOsm, osmoreceptor cells in the supraoptic nuclei of the hypothalamus signal the posterior hypothalamus to increase production of ADH. This increases water absorption from the distal renal tubules.

FLUID AND ELECTROLYTE REQUIREMENTS

What is the approximate daily fluid requirement for an individual?

Based on body weight, the first 10 kg require 100 mL/kg/day (or ~4 mL/kg/hr). The second 10 kg require 50 mL/kg/day (or ~2 mL/kg/hr). Weight above 20 kg requires 20 mL/kg/day (or ~1 mL/kg/hr). Each amount is added to the next as the weight increases.

How much fluid would a 10-kg infant need in a day?

1,000 mL, using the body-weight method above.

How much fluid would a 40 kg person need in a day?

1,000 mL + 500 mL + 400 mL = 1,900 mL, using the body-weight method above.

How much fluid would an average adult (70 kg) need in a day?

2,500 mL, using the body-weight method above. This results in an infusion rate of 104 mL/hr of fluid per 24 hours and accounts for the standard rate of 100 mL/hr that is frequently seen in clinical use for a maintenance fluid rate.

How much Na^+, K^+, and Cl^- are required each day?

Approximately 1 mEq/kg/day each

How much Ca^{2+} and Mg^{2+} are required each day?

Ca^{2+} = 2 g/day; Mg^{2+} = 20 mEq/day. Neither is necessary, however, in maintenance IV fluid.

What are the sources of insensible fluid loss in a healthy adult and their approximate volumes of loss?

Respiratory, 600 mL/day; skin, 400 mL/day;, and stool, 200 mL/day.

What is the effect of fever on insensible fluid loss?

Insensible loss from the skin can increase up to 250 mL per day *per degree* of fever.

What is the minimum volume of urine required to excrete the necessary solutes and waste?	Approximately 500 mL. A person who is eating must excrete 800 mOsm/day of solute, and the maximal ability of the kidney to concentrate is 1,200 mOsm/ L urine. A person who is not eating has less solute to excrete and can get by with approximately 500 mL/day.

BASIC PATIENT AND ELECTROLYTE MANAGEMENT

INTRAVENOUS FLUIDS

Which solution is used as standard maintenance fluid for a patient requiring IV fluids?	5% Dextrose (D5) with $\frac{1}{2}$ or $\frac{1}{4}$ normal saline and 20 or 30 mEq of KCl added will provide more than enough salt and just enough potassium.
What is in normal saline?	154 mEq of sodium and 154 mEq of chloride
What is in $\frac{1}{2}$ normal saline?	77 mEq of sodium and 77 mEq of chloride
What is in lactated Ringer's?	130 mEq of sodium, 110 mEq of chloride, 28 mEq of lactate, 4 mEq of potassium, and 3 mEq of calcium (i.e., similar to normal serum chemistries with lactate substituted for bicarbonate)
Which fluids are isotonic?	Normal saline and lactated Ringer's
Why does it matter which fluids are isotonic?	Isotonic fluids have electrolyte compositions similar to those of plasma and interstitial fluid and, thus, equilibrate with the extracellular compartment, not the TBW.
How much would 1 L of D5/water increase plasma volume?	D5/water equilibrates with all TBW stores. Therefore, 33 % would remain extracellular, of which 25% would remain intravascular. This translates into a volume of 80 to 100 mL.

How much would 1 L of normal saline increase plasma volume?	All would remain extracellular. Plasma volume will increase by 250 to 300 mL.
What is the meaning of "fluid resuscitation"?	To rapidly restore intravascular volume and/or total body fluid volume when there are deficits
What is a fluid bolus	A rapid infusion of IV fluid for resuscitation. "Rapid" implies that the bolus is given over minutes (15–20 min), not over an hour or more.
What is the usual volume of a fluid bolus?	Generally 500 to 1000 mL, depending on the estimated fluid deficit. Remember, a can of soda is 333 mL (usually an insufficient amount for a dehydrated individual).
Why is normal saline solution (0.9%) a better choice for fluid resuscitation than $^1/_2$ normal saline solutions?	Administration of large volumes of $^1/_2$ normal saline can lead to cellular swelling as free water from the extra-cellular space equilibrates into cells. The higher tonicity of normal saline solution minimizes this effect. Lactated Ringer's is also an acceptable choice.
Why is sterile water never given alone as an IV solution?	Because water has no tonicity, it would cause hemolysis of RBCs. Water would diffuse into the cells, causing them to swell and burst. Dextrose/water solutions are tolerated, because the dextrose provides some tonicity at the site of infusion.
How many calories are in a 1 L of D5 $^1/_2$ normal saline?	200 kcal. A 1-L amount of D5 has a mass of 1,000 g, of which 5% or 50 g is dextrose. Each gram of dextrose provides 4 kcal/g, for a total of 200 kcal.
Why is D5 included in most maintenance fluids?	The dextrose in maintenance fluids spares protein when patients are not eating. It is not intended to provide full

caloric requirements but, rather, to prevent the body from using muscle protein for glucose production.

PRINCIPLES OF FLUID AND ELECTROLYTE MANAGEMENT

What is "third spacing?"

Fluid that leaks from the vasculature and accumulates in the extracellular space. Clinically, this results in edema. Third spacing also leads to decreased intravascular fluid volume; thus, additional IV fluid is needed to maintain organ perfusion and urinary output. This commonly occurs after abdominal operations or major trauma.

What general principles guide fluid management for a patient during the first 24 hours after an elective abdominal operation?

The patient will often need resuscitation fluid running above the maintenance rate (125–150 mL/hr), with supplemental fluid as needed because of third spacing and fluid losses resulting from an open abdominal cavity during the operation.

What principles guide fluid management beginning approximately 24 hours after the operation?

Approximately 24 hours post-operatively, the IV infusion is changed to the maintenance rate (~100 mL/hr). Maintenance fluids are continued until the patient resumes oral intake, at which time they are stopped.

Why is it acceptable to give postoperative patients IV solutions that do not provide full caloric needs?

Bowel function generally resumes 4 to 6 days postoperatively, a period of time during which a lack of food intake is not harmful. However, if a patient is significantly malnourished preopera-tively or bowel function does not return after 6 or 7 days, full nutritional support is considered.

What does it mean to "mobilize" fluid?

The fluid that accumulated in the extracellular or third space postoperatively will eventually migrate (i.e., "mobilize") back into the vasculature. This usually happens around postoperative day 3.

What are the dangers of mobilizing fluid?

The fluid can reaccumulate very quickly in the intravascular space and can precipitate pulmonary edema, congestive heart failure, and MI, especially in susceptible patients.

How should the dangers of mobilizing fluid be minimized?

Reduce supplemental IV fluids on postoperative days 3 and 4, and watch for signs of volume overload in expectation of this phenomenon.

What electrolyte imbalances do you need to monitor for after starting nutritional support in a severely malnourished patient?

The "refeeding syndrome" of hypokalemia, hypomagnesemia, and hypophosphatemia is caused by an intracellular shift of these electrolytes because of increased tissue metabolism as nutritional energy becomes available.

What are 2 easy bedside measures of a patient's fluid status?

1. Hourly urinary output is an excellent acute measure.
2. Deviation from the patient's normal body weight also provides an accurate measure of the patient's overall fluid status.

What is an acceptable urine output in an adult postoperative patient?

Approximately 0.5 to 1.0 mL/kg/hr.

COMMON FLUID MANAGEMENT PROBLEMS

What 8 initial steps should be taken in the bedside assessment of a postoperative patient with low urinary output?

1. History: postoperative day, type of operation, other comorbid medical conditions.
2. General: do they appear to be "in shock" (i.e., poorly perfused; cold, clammy, anxious, dizzy, obtunded)?
3. Vital signs: is the heart rate up or BP low? Is the pulse thready (weak)?
4. Lungs: are breath sounds clear? Are oxygen saturations acceptable?

5. Cardiac: is the heart rate regular? Are there distended neck veins? Is the patient having an MI as the cause of this problem?

6. Extremities: is there peripheral edema?

7. Genitourinary: if the patient does not have a Foley, they probably need one for an accurate volume assessment. If the patient does have a Foley, it needs to be inspected for malfunction (irrigated, checked for kinks).

8. Other: is the patient bleeding from the operative site or somewhere else to cause this problem?

Your patient with a low urine output has a Foley, is postoperative day 1, has no jugular venous distension, and has clear lung sounds. What is the most likely cause of the low urine output?

Third-spacing fluids postoperatively, thus requiring a bolus of resuscitation fluid (normal saline or lactated Ringer's) of 500 to 1,000 mL.

Over what period of time should the bolus of fluid be administered?

A 500-mL bolus should take 15 minutes or less to infuse. If a patient is in shock and adequate access is obtained, the bolus can be given as fast as possible. In the trauma setting, liters of fluid can be given in minutes using special pumps.

What types of patients should be given a bolus slowly?

Patients with impaired cardiac or renal function are more sensitive to becoming overloaded, so they may require a slower infusion. However, if your assessment shows volume depletion, they should not be deprived of resuscitative fluids because of these comorbid conditions.

What if the patient's urine output does not respond to your bolus?

Reassess the patient's volume status. Likely, another bolus will be required. Although unusual, placement of a central venous catheter or PA catheter may be necessary to gain hemodynamic measurements more precise than your physical exam will allow.

What advantage does central venous pressure monitoring give you in the evaluation and treatment of a patient with low urine output?

Frequent monitoring of the central venous pressure after each bolus, allowing you to better gauge the effect of the fluid bolus. This may allow more accurate resuscitation and may prevent volume overload. The technique can be useful in patients with diseases that predispose them to volume overload (cardiac or renal disease). The catheter readings (heart pressures) also can be useful for diagnosing heart pathology (failure or infarction) as a cause for the low urine output.

Why do surgeons get upset when someone gives their patients Lasix (furosemide) the first day after an operation?

A common response to low urine output is to give diuretics to increase urine output. However, early after an operation, low urinary output is usually caused by intravascular volume depletion from third spacing or, worse, from a bleeding complication. These patients should be assessed, and most should be given extra IV fluids. Diuresis will likely worsen the problem.

How does the physical exam of a patient with chronic hypovolemia differ from a patient with acute hypovolemia?

In chronic hypovolemia, patients first manifest thirst, dry mouth, loss of skin turgor, and decreased body weight. The acute hemodynamic changes, such as increased heart rate and decreased BP, can happen as well, but not as quickly as with acute hypovolemia. In chronic hypovolemia, the body shares the loss of volume over the entire extracellular space, unlike in acute hypovolemia, in which the body loses its volume primarily from the intravascular compartment. Compare diarrhea (chronic) versus hemorrhage (acute).

What are some common GI clinical scenarios that will result in subacute hypovolemia?

Diarrhea, vomiting, bowel obstruction, and enterocutaneous fistula often present dehydration and require resuscitation. Bleeding from a duodenal ulcer or colonic arteriovenous malformation is more likely to present with acute hypovolemia.

What fluid and electrolyte abnormality occurs with frequent vomiting (or nasogastric tube suctioning)?

Hypochloremic, hypokalemic alkalosis and dehydration. The loss of a large volume of acidic (HCl) gastric juice results in alkalosis, hypochloremia, and dehydration. The kidney compensates by retaining sodium and water to preserve intravascular volume. However, this compensation produces increased excretion of potassium and hydrogen ions, which cause hypokalemia and worsened alkalosis (and paradoxical aciduria).

What fluid and electrolyte imbalances can afflict a patient with an ileostomy?

Much of the fluid and electrolyte absorption of GI secretions takes place in the colon. Patients with an ileostomy lose GI secretions and are at risk for dehydration and hypokalemia as electrolyte-rich fluid is lost.

What precautions must be taken to adequately care for patients with an ileostomy?

Accurate recording of the ileostomy output, frequent serum chemistries, and IV replacement of fluid and electrolyte losses are critical. Sampling of the electrolyte composition of the lost fluid is not necessary to provide optimal care.

ACUTE CRITICAL FLUID AND ELECTROLYTE PROBLEMS

How much acute blood loss will cause the pulse to increase?	Approximately 750 mL, or 15% of the blood volume
What common class of medications may prevent a patient from becoming tachycardic in response to a volume loss?	β-Blockers can prevent hypovolemic patients from becoming tachycardic.
How much acute blood loss will cause the BP to drop?	Approximately 1500 mL, or 30% of the blood volume
What electrolyte imbalances may occur in a patient receiving large volumes of transfused blood?	Hyperkalemia, acidosis, and hypocalcemia. Banked blood has a low pH and a high concentration of potassium. The citrate used to store the blood binds calcium, lowering its serum concentration.
What electrolyte imbalance can be precipitated by administration of succinylcholine to an immobile patient?	Succinylcholine will cause the potassium of a normal patient to rise somewhat, but immobility will magnify this effect and, thus contraindicates its use in immobile patients (e.g., ICU patients) because of the subsequent risk of hyperkalemia.

SODIUM

What is the most common cause of hyponatremia?	Excess free water administration or retention. This can be from exogenous sources (hypotonic fluids) or endogenous hormones (ADH). Stresses (e.g., surgery) can result in a transient form of the syndrome of inappropriate ADH (SIADH), which is classically seen with intracranial tumors and head injuries.

What are 7 symptoms of hyponatremia?

1. Weakness
2. Fatigue
3. Headache
4. Confusion
5. Seizure
6. Muscle cramps
7. Coma

What is hyperosmolar hyponatremia?

Excess solute, such as lipid, mannitol, glucose, protein, or radiologic contrast, in the plasma space (pseudohyponatremia) that causes an osmotic shift of water into the vascular space, causing measured Na^+ to be low.

How is the true sodium value calculated in the presence of hyperglycemia?

In general, add 1.6 mmol/L to the measured sodium concentration for every 100 mg/dL that the glucose is elevated, although newer calculations suggest this factor may even be somewhat higher.

What is the treatment of hyponatremia?

First, determine the cause. If it is mild SIADH, then restrict free water intake. If there is true Na^+ depletion from GI or renal losses and/or the patient is symptomatic, then administer isotonic or hypertonic saline to correct the Na^+ deficit. Remember also that loop diuretics cause the excretion of free water in excess of Na^+, thus raising the serum Na^+.

What is the risk of correcting a Na^+ deficit too fast?

Central pontine myelinolysis

What is an acceptable rate of correction for a Na^+ deficit?

0.5 mEq/L/hr

How does one correct a Na^+ deficit safely?

The amount of Na^+ required to increase the serum Na^+ to a desired level can be calculated: Na needed (in mEq) =

(target Na^+ - actual Na^+) $\times$ 0.6(weight, in kg). The amount of sodium needed to be infused over a certain time frame to raise the level by 0.5 mEq/hr can thus be calculated.

What are the clinical manifestations of hypernatremia?

CNS irritability: restlessness, ataxia, spasms, seizures

What are the 2 main causes of hypernatremia?

1. Excess Na^+ administration, such as using normal saline for maintenance fluids (especially in a patient with renal impairment)
2. Excess free water loss (see previous discussion); also diabetes insipidus after head injury with lack of ADH secretion

What is the risk of lowering the serum Na^+ too quickly?

Cerebral edema and brainstem herniation

What is an acceptable rate of correction for hypernatremia?

Free water should be administered at a rate such that the serum Na^+ falls at 0.5 mEq/L/hr.

POTASSIUM

What are the clinical manifestations of hyperkalemia?

1. Muscle: weakness
2. Heart: peaked T waves, widened QRS, prolonged PR interval, ventricular fibrillation, asystole

What are 3 main causes of hyperkalemia?

1. Renal failure and, therefore, the inability to excrete dietary and exogenously administered K^+
2. Cellular release: crush injuries, reperfusion of ischemic tissue, tumor lysis, succinylcholine administration
3. Excessive potassium administered in IV fluids.

What is the treatment of hyperkalemia?

1. Protect the heart: CaCl, 1 g IV, to stabilize membranes.
2. Transiently lower serum K+: 50 g of glucose (1 amp) and 10 to 20 U of insulin IV will cause uptake of K+ into cells and temporarily lower serum levels.
3. Definitively lower serum K+: Kayexalate PO or as an enema will exchange Na+ for K+ and bind it to be eliminated. Dialysis can also be used to lower K+ quickly and reliably.
4. IV NaHCO$_3$: raising pH drives potassium into cells.

What are 4 clinical manifestations of hypokalemia?

1. Muscle weakness
2. Predisposition to digitalis toxicity
3. Cardiac arrhythmias
4. Decreased intestinal motility

As blood pH increases, what happens to serum K+?

It decreases as intracellular H+ is exchanged for K+.

CALCIUM

What are the clinical manifestations of hypercalcemia?

1. Neurologic: personality disorders, confusion, coma
2. Muscular: fatigue, weakness
3. GI: nausea, vomiting, abdominal pain
4. Renal: stones
5. Dehydration (Remember: "polyuria, polydipsia and pain")

Remember: "Stones, bones, abdominal groans, and mental overtones."

Because approximately half of serum calcium is protein-bound, how can measured total serum calcium be corrected for hypoalbuminemia?

For every 1 g/dL that albumin is decreased, subtract 0.8 mg/dL from the measured serum Ca^{2+}.

What is the treatment of hypercalcemia?

Saline diuresis (normal saline at 2- to 3-fold the maintenance dose given with IV furosemide). Corticosteroids, mithramycin, and calcitonin are also effective.

What are the two major causes of hypercalcemia?

1. Hyperparathyroidism
2. Cancer with bony metastasis (especially breast cancer)

What are the clinical manifestations of hypocalcemia?

Perioral tingling, paresthesias, muscle cramps, decreased deep tendon reflexes

Chvostek's sign: tapping the facial nerve produces contraction of the facial muscles

Trousseau's sign: induction of carpal spasm by inflating a BP cuff around the upper arm for 3 minutes

What is the most common cause of severe hypocalcemia among surgical patients?

Hypoparathyroidism (usually transient) after thyroid or parathyroid surgery

GLUCOSE

What is the mechanism of diabetic ketoacidosis?

Insulin deficiency results in increased free fatty acid release from adipose tissue, increased conversion of acetyl-coenzyme A to ketoacids, and impaired metabolism of ketoacids.

When correcting this disorder, which electrolyte must be monitored closely?

Initially, the potassium may be normal, but the correction of hyperglycemia by insulin administration can induce hypokalemia as potassium is taken up by cells. Serum chemistries need to be monitored frequently and potassium replaced as needed. In addition, these patients can be very dehydrated and typically need fluid resuscitation.

18   Gastrointestinal System

What 4 GI health maintenance issues must be addressed immediately in an ICU patient?

1. Initiate enteric feeding as soon as possible.
2. Begin prophylaxis for stress ulcer.
3. Minimize the risk of large volume aspiration.
4. Make sure your patient is passing stools.

What 4 acute GI problems could kill your patient in the first 24 hours after ICU admission?

1. Hemorrhage
2. Aspiration pneumonitis
3. Intestinal necrosis
4. Intestinal perforation

What 2 measures must be taken to prevent aspiration pneumonitis?

1. If an NGT is in place, make sure that it is working properly and that gastric contents can be emptied.
2. Unless the patient is not required to lie flat (e.g., in spine trauma), keep patients in the semirecumbent position.

What is the eponymous name for aspiration pneumonitis?

Mendelson's syndrome. This is the chemical pneumonitis that occurs after aspiration of low-pH gastric contents.

ACUTE ABDOMEN AND ABDOMINAL PAIN

What is the definition of acute abdomen?

An acute illness characterized by abdominal pain as the principal symptom in which early diagnosis and treatment are important. Treatment may be surgical or nonsurgical.

What are the 3 types of abdominal pain?	1. Visceral 2. Somatic 3. Referred

What are the characteristics of each type of abdominal pain?

Visceral pain

Afferent fibers travel from irritated or stretched viscera with autonomic fibers via the splanchnic nerves to the spinal cord. Characterized by a vague, dull ache or by a cramp located deep within the abdomen, making localization to a specific area difficult.

Somatic pain

Derived from somatic innervations (spinal nerve fibers) of the abdominal wall and skin. More focused, intense, and constant than visceral pain. Results from irritation of the parietal peritoneum, thus making it easier to localize.

Referred pain

Felt at a site distant from the disease because of misinterpretation of a pain impulse traveling in an afferent fiber where multiple afferent fibers converge in the spinal cord (a shared central pathway).

What is the embryologic origin of visceral pain in the following regions?

Epigastrium

Foregut: stomach, duodenum, biliary tract, pancreas

Periumbilical region

Midgut: small intestine, right and transverse colon

Hypogastrium

Hindgut: distal transverse, descending, sigmoid colon, rectum

Where do patients with the following conditions typically feel pain?

    Cholecystitis — Epigastrium to right flank, can radiate around to the back and up to the right shoulder

    Pancreatitis or pancreatic carcinoma — Midback

    Appendicitis — Early on, the pain is periumbilical. As the inflammation worsens, the pain becomes more focal at the right lower quadrant.

    Rectal or uterine disease — Low back

    Nephrolithiasis or ureterolithiasis — Ipsilateral flank or testicle. This pain typically is migratory, affecting several dermatomes along the ureteral path.

    Ruptured aortic aneurysm — Flank, back

Where is the McBurney's point, and what is its significance? — McBurney's point is located $\frac{2}{3}$ of the distance from the umbilicus to the anterior superior iliac spine. It marks the point of maximal pain associated with appendicitis and is a surgical landmark for open appendectomy.

What is Kehr's sign? — Left shoulder pain referred from diaphragm irritation associated with splenic injury

What type of pain usually is the earliest indication of abdominal disease? — Visceral

Does visceral pain usually suggest the need for surgical intervention? — No. Visceral pain can come from many nonsurgical GI conditions, such as gastroenteritis.

What 3 stimuli can produce visceral pain?

1. Stretching of the wall of a hollow viscus or its mesentery by distension or contractions

2. Stretching of the capsule of a solid organ
3. Ischemia or inflammation within viscera

What type of pain usually suggests progressing or later intra-abdominal disease?

Somatic

Does somatic type of pain usually require surgical intervention?

If a visceral pain progresses to somatic pain, the need for surgical intervention generally is more likely.

What is the most useful method in diagnosing the acute abdomen?

History and physical exam

What 6 features of abdominal pain are important for diagnosis?

1. Location: local, referred
2. Type: visceral, somatic, referred
3. Onset: seconds, minutes, hours
4. Severity
5. Character: steady, intermittent, crampy, sharp, dull
6. Factors that initiate or relieve the pain

What is peritonitis?

Inflammation of the peritoneum

What are the 2 major types of peritonitis?

1. Chemical: gastric acid, bile, barium, stool
2. Infectious: inflammatory exudate

What 5 physical exam findings suggest peritonitis?

1. A patient lying still in bed, knees flexed, with shallow respirations
2. Localized tenderness
3. Rebound and referred tenderness
4. Pain with any maneuver causing motion of the viscera within the peritoneal cavity
5. Voluntary guarding, involuntary guarding/rigidity

How can you tell the difference in the emergency room between a patient with nephrolithiasis and one with peritonitis?

A patient with nephrolithiasis is constantly moving, changing positions to try and get comfortable. A patient with peritonitis usually lies completely still to avoid irritating other surfaces.

What are the 3 most useful imaging studies for a patient suspected of having peritonitis?

1. Plain supine and upright radiographs
2. Ultrasound
3. CT scan

Where do you find free air on a plain film?

On an upright film, look for free air under the diaphragm.

If the patient has a spinal injury, in what position can an abdominal x-ray be taken to detect free air?

Log roll the patient to the left decubitus position (left-side down), and look for free air over the right edge of the liver.

Does a patient with clear-cut peritonitis require a radiological evaluation?

NO! Further tests are not necessary and may only serve to delay the operation and needed resuscitation.

Identify 9 important, common causes of abdominal pain in the ICU patient.

1. Gastritis, gastric/duodenal ulcer, ulcer perforation
2. Cholecystitis: calculous or acalculous, cholangitis
3. Hepatitis
4. Pancreatitis
5. Bowel obstruction, mesenteric ischemia
6. Appendicitis, neutropenic enterocolitis
7. Colitis: ulcerative, bacterial, ischemic
8. Intra-abdominal hemorrhage: spontaneous (abdominal aortic aneurysm [AAA] rupture) or postoperative
9. Peritonitis from any of the above, anastomotic leak

Is the diagnosis of acute abdominal pain in the ICU patient more difficult to establish than in other patients?

YES! If you do not think about it, suspect it, and look for the subtle findings, you will miss it—and the patient may die.

Why is the diagnosis of acute abdominal pain more difficult in the ICU patient?

The history is often difficult or impossible to get in an ICU patient (the patient may be intubated, comatose, or delirious). The exam is often altered and subtle.

What 3 factors may alter the physical exam?

1. Age: the elderly often have severe disease with minimal findings.
2. Altered pain perception: a distracting injury, fresh incision, pain medications, altered sensorium, paraplegia/quadriplegia.
3. Impaired host defense: malnutrition and immunosuppression impair the inflammatory response.

GI FUNCTION AND DYSFUNCTION

Where in the brain is food intake regulated?

In two areas of the hypothalamus:
1. A lateral "feeding center"
2. A ventromedial "satiety center," which inhibits the feeding center

What is anorexia?

The lack of desire to eat

Is anorexia specific for abdominal disease?

No. Intra-abdominal inflammation, carcinoma, systemic disease, endocrinopathies, and drugs can all cause anorexia.

Is the absence of anorexia helpful in the diagnosis of acute abdominal disease?

Yes. The desire to eat generally suggests that the GI tract is ready to accept food or that a significant intra-abdominal pathologic condition is not present. The presence of hunger in a patient being worked up for appendicitis casts serious doubt on this diagnosis.

What is the treatment of anorexia?	Treat the inciting cause. No medications consistently stimulate appetite.

SWALLOWING

What is dysphagia?	Difficulty swallowing
What is odynophagia?	Painful swallowing
Swallowing is divided into what 3 stages?	1. Oral 2. Pharyngeal 3. Esophageal
Airway protection occurs during which phase?	The pharyngeal
What is the mechanism for airway protection during the pharyngeal phase?	The larynx and trachea are pulled superiorly by the suprahyoid muscles, the vocal cords close, and the epiglottis is displaced posteriorly.
From what does failure of this airway-protection mechanism in ICU patients commonly result?	Altered mental status and tubes crossing this area interfere with its proper functioning. Inappropriate bed positioning (flat) also facilitates failure.
What are 2 major categories of dysphagia?	1. Oropharyngeal 2. Esophageal
What are 3 frequent causes of oropharyngeal dysphagia in the ICU patient?	1. Odynophagia: mucositis from chemotherapy/drugs, herpetic, fungal, or other mucosal lesions; pharyngitis (from infectious causes or tube trauma) 2. Neuromuscular: head injuries, altered mental status 3. Trauma to the face/neck
What are some frequent causes of esophageal dysphagia?	Most commonly results from luminal encroachment. However, this is infrequently acute, unless it is a result of surgery. Acute esophageal dysphagia

usually is infectious (continuous, herpetic, fungal) or from direct trauma (including tubes).

What is the treatment of dysphagia?

First, treat the cause (remove tubes/ drugs, treat infections, and repair injuries). Neurologic causes may require training to relearn swallowing. Once the cause is treated, topical treatment to relieve pain is often helpful.

NAUSEA AND VOMITING

What is nausea?

A feeling of the need to vomit

Does nausea always represent an intra-abdominal process?

Often, but not always. The presence of nausea must be correlated to the clinical setting. Other causes include autonomic activation, drugs, uremia, radiation, and emotional disturbances.

What is treatment of nausea?

1. Treat the inciting cause.

2. Drugs: antihistamines, anticholinergics, phenothiazines, serotonin antagonists, dopaminergic antagonists

Are nausea and vomiting always linked?

No

What is vomiting?

The forceful expulsion of material from the GI tract through the mouth

Does vomiting always represent an intra-abdominal process?

No

Where is vomiting mediated in the brain?

The medulla

What are the 2 centers that regulate vomiting?

1. The chemoreceptor trigger zone (area postrema) is responsive to chemical stimuli in the circulation, but it is not responsive to electrical stimuli (affer-

ent impulses). It requires an intact vomiting center to induce emesis.

2. The vomiting center is responsive to visceral afferent impulses (mucosal irritation, hollow viscus distension).

How is the act of vomiting coordinated?

The medulla initiates vomiting and coordinates the respiratory, truncal, and GI musculature to cause the forceful expulsion of GI contents while protecting the airway.

Does the pattern or character of the emesis help in establishing the diagnosis?

Yes

What diagnosis is suggested by the following patterns or characteristics of vomiting?

Immediately on waking in the morning

Increased ICP, pregnancy

Not preceded by nausea

Increased ICP

Sudden and projectile

Increased ICP

Repetitive, small volumes

Toxins: food poisoning, gastroenteritis, drugs

Repetitive, large volumes of partially digested food

Gastric outlet obstruction

Feculent

Distal bowel obstruction, long-standing bowel obstruction, gastrocolic fistula

What is the typical fluid and electrolyte disturbance caused by persistent vomiting from gastric outlet obstruction?

Hypokalemic, hypochloremic metabolic alkalosis with volume depletion

If measured, what would the urinary pH be in this scenario?

Acidic. Called paradoxical aciduria, it results in worsening of the metabolic alkalosis. Potassium and hydrogen ions are excreted to allow sodium conservation to counteract the depleted circulating volume.

How should this condition be treated?

Volume repletion with IV normal saline and potassium

What are 4 measures used to treat vomiting?

1. Treatment of the underlying cause
2. NGT suctioning if appropriate
3. Antiemetic drugs
4. Aspiration precautions: elevate head of bed

DIGESTION

After a meal, the normal stomach empties within what amount of time?

3 to 4 hours

Complete passage of food into the cecum requires how many hours?

Approximately 9 hours

Name 4 reasons why intestinal transit frequently is delayed in ICU patients.

1. Intra-abdominal inflammation
2. Metabolic disturbances
3. Postoperative ileus
3. Drugs: narcotics, anticholinergics

Where is most of the water absorbed from the semiliquid chyme entering the colon?

In the cecum and ascending colon

Where is stool stored before defecation?

Sigmoid colon. Stool only passes into the rectum when defecation is about to occur.

DIARRHEA

What is the normal stool weight of an adult human per day?

Approximately 200 g

Water accounts for what percentage of normal stool weight in an adult?	Approximately 80%
What is diarrhea?	Stool weights greater than 200 g/day. Diarrhea typically is described as greater stool frequency and liquidity.
What are the 4 major pathophysiologic mechanisms of diarrhea?	1. Osmotic 2. Secretory 3. Inflammatory 4. Altered bowel motility
For all 4 major pathophysiologic mechanisms, what is the common underlying defect?	Intestinal water and electrolyte transport. This results in bowel distension, which stimulates peristalsis. The increased motility usually is secondary, not primary, in diarrhea.
What is the general cause of osmotic diarrhea?	A partially or nonabsorbed, orally ingested substance that exerts an osmotic force, drawing fluid into the intestinal lumen
What are 2 typical features of osmotic diarrhea?	1. Diarrhea ceases on cessation of oral intake. 2. Measured fecal osmolality is greater than calculated fecal osmolality (increased fecal osmotic gap).
What are 3 common, specific causes of osmotic diarrhea in the ICU?	1. Lactulose 2. Sorbitol (a common additive to many oral liquid medications) 3. Enteral feeding (tube feeds)
What are 3 general causes of inflammatory diarrhea?	1. Epithelial damage 2. Mucosal and submucosal inflammation 3. Loss of absorptive colonocytes
What are 4 typical features of inflammatory diarrhea?	1. Blood and leukocytes in the stool. 2. Inflammatory lesion on intestinal biopsy. 3. Diarrhea persists with fasting.

4. Patients frequently have fever, abdominal pain, and leukocytosis.

What are 3 common, specific causes of inflammatory diarrhea in the ICU?

1. Drugs
2. Infections (especially *Clostridium difficile*)
3. Ischemia

What is the general mechanism of secretory diarrhea?

Active ion secretion by the intestinal epithelium with the passive movement of water into the intestinal lumen

What are 3 typical features of secretory diarrhea?

1. Large volumes of usually watery diarrhea.
2. Fecal osmolality is isotonic (no fecal osmotic gap).
3. Diarrhea is unaffected by fasting.

What are 2 common, specific causes of secretory diarrhea in the ICU?

1. Drugs
2. Infections

What are the most important aspects of the patient history during the initial part of the workup for diarrhea in the ICU?

1. Drugs taken
2. Recent antibiotic use
3. Recent initiation of enteral feeds
4. Periods of hypotension: intestinal ischemia

What is the most useful initial laboratory test for the workup of diarrhea?

Microscopic examination of fresh stool for occult blood and leukocytes

What diagnosis is suggested by the presence of *both* RBCs and WBCs on a stool smear?

Inflammation with exudate (inflammatory bowel disease, invasive infection, *C. difficile* enterocolitis)

What is the next step in the workup?

Sigmoidoscopy/colonoscopy, stool for ova, parasites, and culture

What diagnosis is suggested by presence of RBCs but the absence of WBCs on a stool smear?

Epithelial damage, with no exudate (drugs, ischemia, neoplasm, *C. difficile*)

What is the next step in the workup?	Sigmoidoscopy/colonoscopy, stool for *C. difficile* culture and toxin
What diagnosis is suggested by the absence of *both* RBCs *or* WBCs on a stool smear?	Osmotic or secretory diarrhea (drugs, enteral feeds, infection)
What is the next step in the workup?	Determine fecal osmolality and fecal osmotic gap, which help to distinguish osmotic from secretory diarrhea.
Measured fecal osmolality normally approximates the osmolality of which body fluid?	Plasma (290 mOsm/L)
How is fecal osmolality calculated?	The sum of measured fecal Na$^+$ and K$^+$ multiplied by 2 (to account for anions)
How is the fecal osmotic gap calculated?	Measured fecal osmolality minus calculated fecal osmolality
A fecal osmotic gap greater than 50 mOsm/L is typical of which type of diarrhea?	Osmotic. Secretory diarrhea osmolality is close to that of plasma.
How would you treat the following types of diarrhea?	
Ischemic	Restore circulating volume and perfusion; otherwise supportive unless complications supervene.
Infectious	In the ICU patient, this is almost always *C. difficile* colitis, which is discussed below.
Osmotic	In the ICU, this is usually a drug or enteral feedings. The drug should be stopped if possible. Manipulate enteral feedings by adding fiber to the regimen.

Is most antibiotic-associated diarrhea caused by an infection?	No. Most cases appear to be caused by an alteration in intestinal flora, not by a specific infection.
How often is antibiotic-associated diarrhea complicated by infectious colitis?	Approximately 10% of the time. *Clostridium difficile* causes almost all of the cases.
How is *C. difficile* colitis treated?	Oral metronidazole, oral vancomycin, or IV metronidazole

ILEUS

What is the gut's adaptive response to severe injury?	Decreased intestinal tract perfusion, which leads to decreased intestinal secretions and decreased motility
How does this response manifest?	Food intolerance and ileus
What are the 2 types of ileus?	1. Mechanical 2. Functional: adynamic
What is a mechanical ileus?	An extrinsic or intrinsic obstruction that prevents the passage of intraluminal material
What is an adynamic ileus?	Failure of the normal peristaltic function of the intestine, thus preventing intra-luminal passage. This is very common in the ICU population.

GI BLEEDING

Define upper GI bleeding and lower GI bleeding.	Upper GI bleeding: occurs from the lips to the ligament of Treitz. Lower GI bleeding: occurs from the ligament of Treitz to the anus.
What fraction of ICU GI bleeds occur in the upper GI tract?	$^2/_3$

Define severe GI bleeding.

Documented GI bleeding accompanied by either shock or orthostatic hypotension, decrease of Hct by 8%, or transfusion of at least 2 U of packed RBCs.

In your evaluation of GI bleeding, what are 15 important elements of the history?

1. Previous GI bleeding
2. Ulcers
3. Gastroesophageal reflux disease (GERD)
4. Hepatic dysfunction
5. Cancer
6. Bleeding disorders
7. Abdominal surgery (including AAA repair)
8. Radiation to the abdomen or rectum
9. Aspirin or other nonsteroidal anti-inflammatory drug
10. Alcohol use
11. Anticoagulants
12. Weight loss
13. Abdominal pain
14. Vomiting
15. Change in bowel habits

If minimal to no changes occur in the vital signs, does this mean that the bleed was not significant?

No. Younger patients can mask severe insults because of a larger physiologic reserve than older patients.

Aside from a thorough abdominal exam, what else needs to be evaluated?

1. The rectum via digital rectal exam
2. The stomach via NGT placement and lavage

What 4 lab tests are needed?

1. CBC: repeated every 4 to 6 hours until stable
2. PT/PTT
3. Chemistry panel
4. Type and cross-match for packed RBCs

What 7 measures should be taken immediately in patients with GI bleeding?

1. Placement of two large-bore IV catheters (14- or 16-gauge).
2. NGT placement: confirms

diagnosis, helps to protect against large volume aspiration, may identify rebleeding.
3. Volume resuscitation with isotonic crystalloid.
4. Transfuse packed RBCs, platelets, or FFP as needed
5. Frequently measure vital signs.
6. Placement of Foley catheter for urine output measurement.
7. Cardiac rhythm monitoring for tachycardia and development of arrhythmias.

Who needs to be notified in the case of a GI bleed?

The gastroenterology team and/or surgical team

UPPER GI BLEEDING

What 3 signs indicate an upper GI source?

1. Hematemesis
2. "Coffee-ground" emesis
3. Positive gastric lavage

What percentage of patients with GI bleeds will have clear NG aspirates?

16%. However, a clear aspirate with bile indicates that an upper GI source is less likely or intermittent.

List the 7 major causes of severe upper GI bleeding.

1. Peptic ulcer
2. Gastric or esophageal varices
3. Erosions
4. Angioma
5. Mallory-Weiss tear
6. Tumor
7. Esophagitis

What is the mortality rate associated with severe upper GI bleeding?

10%

What percentage of patients will have a self-limited event?

80% to 85%

Of the remaining patients who continue to bleed or rebleed, what is the mortality rate?	30% to 40%
What percentage of GI bleeds are caused by peptic ulceration?	50%. Peptic ulceration is the primary cause of acute onset GI hemorrhage in the United States.
List 9 adverse prognostic factors associated with peptic ulcer bleeding.	1. Age older than 60 years 2. Comorbid medical illness 3. Shock 4. Coagulopathy 5. Onset of bleeding in the hospital 6. Multiple transfusions required 7. Fresh blood in the NGT 8. Endoscopic finding of arterial bleeding or visible vessel 9. Location of the ulcer in the posterior duodenal bulb
Can medical therapy assist in the treatment of bleeding?	Yes. Multiple trials now indicate a role for IV administration of proton-pump inhibitors (PPI) to prevent rebleeding.
What needs to be in the back of your mind concerning a patient with a GI bleed and previous AAA repair?	Aortoenteric fistula
What is a "herald bleed"?	An initial, self-limited bleeding episode that is followed by an exsanguinating hemorrhage in a person with an aortoenteric fistula

Endoscopy

What tool can be used for both diagnosis and therapy of GI bleeding?	The endoscope

Before performing endoscopy, what 3 preparatory steps should be taken?

1. Stabilize the patient with volume replacement.
2. If the airway is suspect because of encephalopathy or other aspiration risks, perform endotracheal intubation to secure the airway.
3. Correct coagulopathy and thrombocytopenia.

List 6 complications of emergency endoscopy.

1. Perforation
2. Aspiration
3. Induced hemorrhage
4. Reaction to sedative medications
5. Hypotension
6. Hypoxia

Should you perform emergency endoscopy for the patient who cannot be stabilized?

No. If the patient cannot be stabilized in the ICU, then emergent surgical exploration is required.

Name 2 commonly used techniques for endoscopic hemostasis.

1. Multipolar electrocoagulation
2. Heater-probe coagulation

STRESS ULCERS

What are stress ulcers?

Shallow, well-circumscribed, mucosal erosions that can occur in the stomach and duodenum of critically ill patients under extreme physiologic stress

What 5 factors predispose to stress ulceration?

1. Shock/hypotension
2. Sepsis
3. Prolonged mechanical ventilation
4. Burns
5. CNS trauma or tumor

What is the name for stress ulcers associated with burns?

Curling's ulcers

What is the name for stress ulcers associated with CNS trauma?	Cushing's ulcers
What strategy is employed to prevent stress ulcers?	Prophylactic treatment with H_2-receptor blockers or proton-pump inhibitors
How do stress ulcers present?	Bleeding is the most frequent mode of presentation and can be occult or massive. Pain is an infrequent complaint.
What is the most common treatment of stress ulcers?	Medical therapy if they are not bleeding, endoscopic treatment if they are bleeding
What is stress gastritis?	Multiple superficial erosions of the gastric mucosa that are associated with extremes of physiologic stress
What is a Dieulafoy's lesion?	An aberrant, large, submucosal artery that ruptures into the upper GI tract lumen and causes massive bleeding. There is no surrounding ulceration, which makes these lesions hard to identify by endoscopy.
Where do these lesions usually occur?	Within 6 cm of the gastroesophageal junction

ESOPHAGEAL VARICES

What is the etiology of esophageal variceal bleeding?	Portal hypertension
What is the acute mortality rate of esophageal variceal bleed?	Each episode is associated with a 30% mortality.
What is the long-term survival rate of patients with a history of variceal bleeding currently receiving medical management?	40%

What is the rebleed rate of esophageal varices in patients who survive their first hemorrhage?	60% at 1 year
What is the medical management of acute variceal bleeding?	Nonselective β-blockers, vasopressin, and octreotide
What is octreotide?	A long-acting analogue of somatostatin that results in selective splanchnic vasoconstriction
What 2 endoscopic methods are available to treat variceal bleeding?	1. Variceal sclerotherapy 2. Band ligation
What is a Sengstaken-Blakemore tube?	A tube with both esophageal and gastric balloons and a single aspirating port in the stomach
What is a Sengstaken-Blakemore tube used for?	Balloon tamponade of esophageal varices, which are amendable because they lie in the submucosa
What is the rebleed rate after balloon tamponade?	21% to 60% will rebleed soon after deflating the balloon.
What does TIPS stand for?	Transjugular intrahepatic portosystemic shunt
What is a TIPS procedure?	A short-term method of controlling bleeding by decreasing portal hypertension
Why is the TIPS procedure unsuitable for long-term relief?	The occlusion rate is approximately 50% at 1 year, and 20% of patients suffer worsened hepatic encephalopathy.

LOWER GI BLEEDING

What are the 3 most common causes of severe hematochezia?	1. Internal hemorrhoids 2. Colonic angiomas 3. Diverticulosis

Where are colonic angiomas most often found?	The right (ascending) colon
How are colonic angiomas treated?	Endoscopic coagulation
If, on colonoscopic evaluation, you identify normal rectal mucosa but edematous, friable tissue in the descending colon and the splenic flexure, what should you suspect?	Ischemic bowel disease

ABDOMINAL COMPARTMENT SYNDROME

What is abdominal compartment syndrome (ACS)?	Increased pressure within the abdominal compartment from an increased volume of abdominal contents
When does ACS usually occur?	ACS usually is associated with massive intestinal edema that follows laparotomy for major trauma in which there has been prolonged shock and resuscitation.
What are 3 the main contributors to ACS?	1. Crystalloid resuscitation 2. Capillary leakage (from activated inflammatory mediators) 3. Reperfusion injury
What 3 organ systems are most affected by increased abdominal pressures?	1. Renal 2. Pulmonary 3. Cardiovascular
What are 6 common manifestations of ACS?	1. Decreased urine output 2. Elevated central venous pressures 3. Increased systemic vascular resistance 4. Decreased cardiac output

5. Hypoxemia
6. Elevated peak airway pressures

How is ACS diagnosed?	Measurement of intra-abdominal pressure
How do you commonly measure intra-abdominal pressures?	Obtain bladder pressures via the Foley catheter
What pressure signifies a potential problem?	25 cm H_2O is suggestive of ACS. Greater than 30 cm H_2O is diagnostic for ACS. (Normal intra-abdominal pressure is 0 cm H_2O or subatmospheric.)
How can you prevent ACS from forming?	Anticipate the possibility, and place an alternative closure for an intensely edematous abdomen.
What is the treatment of ACS?	If ACS develops in the ICU, then the patient's abdomen must be decompressed and the wound closed with a silo closure.
What can happen if ACS is relieved too quickly?	Ischemia-reperfusion injury, causing acidosis, vasodilatation, cardiac dysfunction, and arrest, can occur. Patients should have adequate preload before compartment release.

PANCREATITIS

What is the yearly U.S. mortality rate of acute pancreatitis?	10%
What are the major etiologies of acute pancreatitis?	Biliary stone disease or alcohol abuse account for 80% of cases.

What are other causes of pancreatitis, and how can they be remembered?	Mnemonic: **BAD SHIT**: **B**: Biliary **A**: Alcohol **D**: Drugs (thiazide diuretics, steroids, valproic acid) **S**: Scorpion bites **H**: Hyperlipidemia, hypercalcemia **I**: Idiopathic and Iatrogenic (ERCP, cardiopulmonary bypass) **T**: Trauma
In blunt trauma, where is the pancreas typically injured?	At the junction of the body and the tail, which overlie the vertebrae
How does pancreatitis present?	Constant, boring pain in the epigastrium that radiates through to the back and is associated with nausea and vomiting. Commonly, patients will lean forward or pull their knees up to their chest in an attempt to partially alleviate the pain.
What is Grey-Turner's sign?	Ecchymosis in the flanks associated with hemorrhagic pancreatitis
What is Cullen's sign?	Ecchymosis in the periumbilical area associated with hemorrhagic pancreatitis
What are 6 lab findings in patients with pancreatitis?	1. Leukocytosis with a leftward shift 2. Increased Hct 3. Hyperglycemia 4. Hypoalbuminemia 5. Increased serum and urine amylase 6. Increased serum lipase
Is hyperamylasemia specific for pancreatitis?	No. It has been associated with other intra-abdominal pathologies.
What 2 plain-film findings are common?	1. On the CXR, a left-sided effusion can be seen.

2. On the abdominal x-ray, a gaseous pattern of paralytic ileus is often noted.

What is the most valuable radiologic study for pancreatitis?

CT. It is not limited by luminal air, and it can better assess the degree of pancreatic damage (necrosis).

What 3 measures are used to describe the severity of pancreatitis?

1. Ranson's criteria: each criteria met after 3 is predictive of a worsened outcome.
2. **A**cute **P**hysiology **A**nd **C**hronic **H**ealth **E**valuation II (APACHE II): worsened outcome for scores greater than 13.
3. Degree of necrosis as staged by CT: greater than 50% necrosis or air predict poor outcome.

What are the Ranson's criteria?

At presentation

1. Age older than 55 years
2. WBC count greater than 16,000 cells/mm^3
3. Glucose greater than 200 mg/dL
4. Aspartate aminotransferase (AST) greater than 250 U/L
5. LDH greater than 350 U/L

Within the first 48 hours

1. Calcium less than 8 mg/dL
2. Hct drop greater than 10%
3. Arterial partial pressure of oxygen (PaO$_2$) less than 60 mm Hg
4. Base deficit greater than 4 mEq/L
5. BUN increase greater than 5 mg/dL
6. Fluid sequestration greater than 6 L

When should a patient with pancreatitis be fed?

Early nutrition is associated with improved outcomes. As soon as possible, these patients should be given nutrition via a nasoduodenal tube or TPN through a central line.

Name 4 ways that infection can complicate severe acute pancreatitis.	1. Pancreatic abscess 2. Infected pancreatic pseudocyst 3. Acute suppurative cholangitis 4. Infected pancreatic necrosis

PANCREATIC NECROSIS

What is the incidence of infected pancreatic necrosis in patients with acute pancreatitis?	17%
What microbe is most often isolated from infected pancreatic necrosis?	*Escherichia coli*
What is the mortality rate in patients with infected pancreatic necrosis?	30%
How is infected pancreatic necrosis identified?	CT-guided fine-needle aspiration
How is infected pancreatic necrosis managed?	Administer broad-spectrum antibiotics, and undertake surgical debridement.
If bleeding is associated with pancreatic necrosis, what is the mortality rate?	50%
How should bleeding be managed in these cases?	With angiography if possible. Surgical intervention is very difficult but necessary if the angiography fails.

HEPATIC FAILURE

What is fulminant hepatic failure?	The rapid development of severe hepatic dysfunction, progressing to hepatic encephalopathy within 8 weeks of the illness in a patient without history of liver disease.

What are the 3 subdivisions of fulminant hepatic failure?	1. Hyperacute 2. Acute 3. Subacute
Those in which subdivision have the best survival?	Paradoxically, those in the hyperacute group
What are the 4 grades of hepatic encephalopathy?	I. Slowness of thought, asterixis II. Drowsiness, inappropriate behavior, confusion III. Somnolence to semistupor, some response to small stimuli IV. Coma
What are the 4 major etiologies of fulminant hepatic failure?	1. Viral infections: hepatitis 2. Toxic or idiosyncratic reactions to therapeutic drugs 3. Metabolic disorders of obscure origin 4. Toxins
What is the overall prognosis of patients with fulminant hepatic failure?	The mortality rate is 80%.
List 10 factors that indicate a poor prognosis regarding hepatic failure.	1. Age younger than 10 or older than 40 years 2. Etiology from toxins, drugs other than acetaminophen, and nonviral hepatitis 3. Stage IV encephalopathy 4. More than 1 week to development of stage III or IV encephalopathy after onset of jaundice 5. INR greater than 3.5 6. Creatinine greater than 3.4 mg/dL 7. Arterial pH less than 7.3 8. Bilirubin greater than 17 mg/dL 9. Factor V less than 20% 10. Alpha-fetoprotein less than 15 ng/mL

What type of calories should patients with fulminant hepatic failure receive?	Primarily carbohydrates, possibly branched-chain amino acids
What may be given in an attempt to treat hepatic encephalopathy?	Lactulose titrated to 2 or 3 soft stools per day
With this therapy, what can happen to the patient's water balance?	Lactulose can cause significant free-water losses and lead to hypernatremia.
What frequently happens to blood glucose in these patients?	The blood glucose drops, causing hypoglycemia.
Why do these patients become hypoglycemic?	Hepatic glycogen stores are depleted, and a concomitant loss of hepatic gluconeogenesis occurs.
Should FFP be given routinely for increases in PT?	No
When should FFP be given?	When there is evidence of spontaneous bleeding (a rare event), or when an invasive procedure is indicated
What 4 other morbid conditions are associated with fulminant hepatic failure?	1. Infection 2. Renal failure 3. Hypotension 4. Cerebral edema
In what stage of encephalopathy does cerebral edema develop?	Stage IV
What 5 clinical signs indicate its development?	1. Onset of hypertension and bradycardia 2. Increased muscle tone 3. Dilated pupils 4. Decerebrate rigidity 5. Posturing

What radiologic exam should be obtained with this clinical picture?	A non–contrast enhanced head CT
Why non–contrast enhanced?	The idea is not necessarily to confirm cerebral edema but to rule out hemorrhage, which is identified in the acute state on a non–contrast enhanced study.
Are the clinical signs of cerebral edema very reliable?	No
What can be monitored to evaluate for cerebral edema?	ICP
What ICP level should cause concern?	Greater than 25 to 30 mm Hg
What can be done to lower the ICP?	IV mannitol and, if that is ineffective, barbiturate-induced coma
Other than supportive therapy, what treatments can be considered for fulminant hepatic failure?	Hepatic transplantation should be considered early.

19

Obstetrics and Gynecology

PHYSIOLOGY OF PREGNANCY

What are the normal physiologic changes that occur during pregnancy in each of the following?

Cardiac output?	Increases by approximately 40% (1.5 L/min).
Heart rate?	Increases by approximately 15% (10 bpm).
BP?	Diastolic pressure decreases approximately 15 mm Hg during the second trimester and returns to normal by delivery.
ECG?	1. Left-axis deviation 2. Flattened or inverted T waves in III, aVF, and precordial leads 3. Increased ectopy
Blood volume?	Increases by approximately 40% to 50%.
Hematocrit?	Decreases by 5% because of hemodilution.
WBC count?	Can increase to between 10,000 and 14,000 cells/mL and be even higher during labor.
Tidal volume?	Increases by approximately 40%.
Arterial blood gases?	pH 7.40 P_{O_2} = 95 mm Hg P_{CO_2} = 32 mm Hg HCO_3 = 18.8 mEq/L

Renal blood flow and glomerular filtration rate?	Increases by 40% to 50%.
What percentage of maternal cardiac output supplies the uterus at term?	20% (500 mL/min)
List 8 hormones produced by the placenta.	1. Human chorionic gonadotropin (hCG) 2. Progesterone 3. Estrogen 4. Human placental lactogen 5. Atrial natriuretic peptide 6. Corticotropin-releasing hormone 7. Relaxin 8. Parathyroid hormone–related protein
How does progesterone affect smooth muscle, and what may be some resultant adverse effects?	Progesterone inhibits smooth muscle, which may affect the GI tract (reflux, constipation), urinary tract (infection), and biliary tract (cholestasis, cholecystitis).
When does the embryonic period end and the fetal period begin?	At 10 weeks of gestational age (8 weeks after fertilization)

HYPERTENSIVE DISORDERS OF PREGNANCY

Define preeclampsia and eclampsia.	Preeclampsia: the development of hypertension, proteinuria, and edema between the 20th week of pregnancy and approximately 7 to 10 days postpartum Eclampsia: Preeclampsia plus the occurrence of convulsions in the same time period without other etiology
What are 8 risk factors for preeclampsia/eclampsia?	1. Primigravid 2. Multiple gestation

3. Previous history of preeclampsia
4. Extremes of age
5. Obesity
6. African-American race
7. Pre-existing hypertension
8. Renal or vascular disease

What are the incidences of preeclampsia and eclampsia?

Preeclampsia: occurs in approximately 10% to 14% of primigravidas and approximately 6% of multiparas.
Eclampsia: occurs in approximately 1 in 200 preeclamptics.

How does smoking affect the risk of developing hypertension during pregnancy?

It decreases the risk! This has been demonstrated in multiple studies, but hazards of maternal smoking remain (increased risk of low birth weight, spontaneous abortion, and placental abruption).

What are the minimum criteria to establish the diagnosis of preeclampsia?

BP of 140/90 mm Hg or greater and proteinuria (>300 mg/24 hours or 1+ dipstick) after 20 weeks of gestation. Preeclampsia can also be diagnosed in patients with underlying hypertension based on increase in BP of more than 30 mm Hg systolic and 15 mm Hg diastolic or a mean pressure increase of more than 20 mm Hg.

List 11 signs and symptoms indicating severe preeclampsia.

1. Diastolic BP of 110 mm Hg or greater or systolic pressure greater than 160 mm Hg
2. Persistent 2+ proteinuria
3. Headache
4. Visual disturbances
5. Epigastric or right upper quadrant pain
6. Oliguria
7. Uremia
8. Thrombocytopenia
9. Liver enzyme elevation
10. Fetal growth restriction
11. Pulmonary edema

3. Placenta accreta
4. Retained products of conception
5. Uterine atony or rupture
6. Obstetric lacerations
7. Surgical procedures

What volume of blood loss should alert you to the possibility of significant postpartum hemorrhage?

More than 500 mL

What fraction of maternal blood volume can be lost before hypotension and inadequate tissue perfusion ensue?

$\frac{1}{4}$ of maternal blood volume (class II shock)

What 2 maternal lab values correlate with fetal distress?

1. Decreased maternal serum bicarbonate
2. Increased lactic acid levels

What 6 measures can be taken to decrease postpartum uterine bleeding (i.e., from atony)?

1. Uterine massage
2. Oxytocin IV (or intrauterine)
3. Methylergonovine IM
4. Alprostadil IM
5. Misoprostol per rectum
6. Surgical management

Name an important contraindication to methylergonovine.

Hypertension

Name an important contraindication to alprostadil.

Asthma

SEPSIS AND SEVERE INFECTION

Name 6 conditions that may lead to septic shock in obstetric and gynecologic patients.

1. Postpartum endometritis (85%) of septic shock cases in ob/gyn patients
2. Antepartum pyelonephritis
3. Chorioamnionitis
4. Septic abortion

What is HELLP syndrome?	**H**emolysis, **E**levated **L**iver enzymes, and **L**ow **P**latelets
What percentage of patients with preeclampsia develop HELLP syndrome?	Up to 20% of severe preeclamptics
Outline the treatment of preeclampsia.	1. Bed rest 2. Hospitalization 3. Magnesium sulfate 4. Antihypertensives (hydralazine, labetolol, verapamil, nifedipine, nitroprusside)
Outline the treatment of eclampsia.	1. Magnesium sulfate IM 2. Magnesium sulfate IV slowly 3. Valium 4. Intubate if needed 5. Pentathol
What is the only definitive treatment for preeclampsia/ eclampsia?	Delivery of the fetus
Does magnesium control BP?	No. It is used solely for seizure prophylaxis or treatment.
Name 6 signs of magnesium toxicity in order of increasing severity.	1. ECG changes (peaked T waves) 2. Loss of patellar reflex 3. Feeling warmth, flushing 4. Somnolence, slurred speech 5. Paresis, respiratory depression 6. Cardiac arrest

SHOCK

Define shock.	Oxygen delivery that is inadequate to meet the metabolic demands of the peripheral tissue
What is the most common cause of hypovolemic shock in obstetrics, and what are 7 conditions that cause it?	The most common cause of hypovolemic shock in obstetrics is hemorrhage, which can be caused by the following: 1. Abruptio placentae 2. Placenta previa

5. Toxic shock syndrome
6. Necrotizing fasciitis

What 8 conditions predispose the patient to postpartum infection?

1. Anemia
2. Preeclampsia
3. Prolonged rupture of the membranes
4. Prolonged labor
5. Traumatic delivery
6. Repeated examinations
7. Retention of placental fragments
8. Postpartum hemorrhage

Name the single most common bacterial pathogen isolated in obstetrical sepsis.

Escherichia coli (isolated in 50% of all cases)

What other organisms are frequently present in obstetrical sepsis?

Klebsiella, Serratia, and *Enterobacter* sp. account for 30% of cases. Others are Staphylococci, β-hemolytic streptococcus, anaerobic streptococci, *Enterococcus* sp., and *Clostridium perfringens.*

What empiric antibiotic therapy is indicated in obstetrical sepsis?

"Triple coverage": ampicillin, gentamicin, and clindamycin are the gold standard. This regimen provides coverage against aerobic *Streptococcus* sp., *Staphylococcus* sp., enteric Gram-negative organisms, and anaerobes; however, many different combinations may provide adequate coverage.

ENDOMETRITIS

What are 4 signs of endometritis?

1. Fever
2. Fundal tenderness
3. Profuse or foul-smelling lochia
4. Leukocytosis

What are the 5 most common pathogens causing endometritis?

1. Gram-positive anaerobic cocci
2. Group A and B streptococci
3. Gram-positive bacilli (*Clostridium sp., Listeria* sp.)

4. *Neisseria gonorrhea*
5. Gram-negative bacilli (*Escherichia coli, Klebsiella* sp., *Proteus* sp.)

What is the empiric antibiotic regimen for endometritis?

Clindamycin and gentamicin. Ampicillin may be added for triple therapy if no improvement occurs (5% of cases).

PYELONEPHRITIS

In addition to sepsis, what are 3 complications of pyelonephritis in pregnancy?

1. Adult respiratory distress syndrome
2. Hemolysis
3. Pulmonary edema

What is the pathophysiology of the complications of pyelonephritis in pregnancy?

Endotoxin-mediated lysis of cells

When are these complications of pyelonephritis likely to emerge?

6 to 12 hours after initiation of antibiotic treatment

What is the empiric antibiotic regimen for antepartum pyelonephritis?

Ampicillin and gentamicin

NECROTIZING FASCIITIS

What is necrotizing fasciitis?

A rapidly advancing and often lethal bacterial infection in which there is necrosis of the skin and subcutaneous tissue

Name 3 risk factors for necrotizing fasciitis.

1. Diabetes
2. Obesity
3. Hypertension

How do you manage these patients?

Stabilize rapidly (normalize electrolytes, hydrate, and cross-match multiple units of blood), perform surgical debridement immediately, and provide antibiotic treatment (usually a β-lactam and clindamycin).

TRAUMA AND PREGNANCY

What is the incidence of trauma in pregnancy?	1 in 12 pregnancies
What is the most significant contributor to both maternal and fetal death because of trauma?	Motor vehicle accidents

What is the fetal loss rate for the following?

Life-threatening maternal trauma?	40% to 50%
For minor or nonlife-threatening maternal injuries?	1% to 5%
What is the incidence of placental abruption in pregnant women who sustain severe trauma?	40% to 50%
What are 4 common findings with placental abruption?	1. Uterine/abdominal tenderness 2. Vaginal bleeding 3. Uterine contractions 4. Fetal distress Some patients exhibit no pain or bleeding, thus making uterine and fetal monitoring mandatory.
What percentage of fetal deaths occur in association with minor or nonlife-threatening maternal trauma?	50% (because of the much higher incidence of minor trauma)
What is the earliest gestational age at which viability in an extrauterine environment is possible?	24 weeks

What is the chance for intact survival of an infant born at 28 weeks of gestational age, assuming maximal care?	90%
At what gestational age is direct trauma to the uterus and developing fetus unlikely to occur because of protection by the bony pelvis?	Less than 13 weeks
Direct fetal injury complicates what percentage of pregnancies in which trauma occurs?	Less than 1%
What is the primary goal of managing trauma in pregnancy?	Maternal evaluation and stabilization
How should you position the pregnant trauma patient?	On her left side if possible. When spine injury is present or during CPR, the right hip should be elevated and the uterus manually retracted to the left.
Why this position?	The uterus compresses the vena cava, causing venous hypertension in the lower extremities and reducing cardiac output by $1/3$.
Do a normal pulse, BP, and PO_2 predict adequate resuscitation to protect the fetus?	No
Why not?	Uterine blood flow is very sensitive to catecholamines and may be reduced by 1/4 without any change in maternal BP.
What approach should be taken for the "minimally" injured pregnant patient?	Fluid resuscitation and supplemental oxygen. Consult the Ob/Gyn service for all patients and for fetal heart monitoring.

Is CT contraindicated in pregnancy?

No. Abdominal CT exposes the fetus to approximately 3.5 rads. The fetus can be exposed to 20 rads without adverse effect.

Is DPL contraindicated in pregnancy?

No. A supraumbilical, open approach is advised.

What are 5 indications for DPL after trauma in pregnancy?

1. Signs or symptoms suggesting intraperitoneal bleeding
2. Altered mental status
3. Unexplained maternal shock
4. Major thoracic injuries
5. Multiple major orthopedic injuries

What is a potential complication of fetomaternal hemorrhage in some patients, and how can it be prevented?

D (Rh) isoimmunization in D (Rh)-negative patients. D immune globulin (Rhogam) administration within 72 hours of the event provides protection.

AMNIOTIC FLUID EMBOLISM

What is the incidence of amniotic fluid embolism (AFE) in the United States?

1 in 20,000 deliveries

What are 8 signs and symptoms of an AFE?

1. Acute shortness of breath
2. Hypoxia
3. Shock
4. Mental status changes
5. Seizures
6. Hemorrhage
7. Disseminated intravascular coagulopathy (DIC)
8. Cardiopulmonary arrest

Which 3 groups of patients are at high risk for AFE?

1. Patients with an intrauterine fetal demise
2. Patients taking oxytocin
3. Patients with a short, abrupt course of labor

What are the common diagnostic and laboratory findings of AFE?

1. Arterial blood gas indicates maternal hypoxemia.
2. Coagulopathy with prolonged clotting times and elevated fibrin split products with hypofibrinogenemia.
3. CXR findings are nonspecific, with pulmonary edema frequently noted.
4. ECG findings are also nonspecific, with tachycardia, ST- and T-wave changes, and a pattern of right ventricular strain.

How is the diagnosis of AFE established?

Identification of amniotic debris in blood taken from the right side of the heart via a PAC is diagnostic. Special stains assist in identifying such material. These findings are neither sensitive nor specific, however, and the diagnosis is generally established clinically, with careful exclusion of other causes.

What is the treatment of AFE?

Therapy is supportive. Hypoxemia is corrected with supplemental oxygen and frequently requires intubation and mechanical ventilation. Pulmonary artery catheterization and inotropic support should also be considered. Coagulopathy is corrected with fresh frozen plasma and cryoprecipitate. Low-dose heparin, aspirin, and antifibrinolytic agents may also be necessary, as in the treatment of DIC from other causes.

What is the prognosis of patients with AFE?

Poor. The mortality rate remains between 60% and 90%. Overall neonatal survival rate is 70%, but almost half suffer residual neurologic impairment.

DIC IN OBSTETRICS

What is DIC?	Disseminated intravascular coagulopathy; a pathologic condition associated with inappropriate activation of coagulation and fibrinolysis because of some underlying disease state
What are the signs and symptoms of DIC?	Findings are variable but can include generalized hemorrhage, localized bleeding, purpura, petechiae, and thromboembolic phenomena. End-organ damage can result from intravascular fibrin deposits.

What 6 laboratory abnormalities occur in DIC?

1. Thrombocytopenia
2. Elevated PT and, less often, PTT
3. Elevated thrombin time
4. Elevation of D-dimer and fibrin split products
5. Decline in fibrinogen
6. Red blood cell schistocytes

What 6 obstetric complications may be associated with DIC?

1. Abruptio placentae
2. Fetal demise
3. Preeclampsia/eclampsia
4. AFE
5. Saline or septic abortion
6. Sepsis

What is the treatment of DIC?

Some aspects remain controversial.
1. Treat the inciting disease process (sometimes this is all that is required).
2. Halt intravascular coagulation: low-dose subcutaneous or IV heparin (equally effective), antiplatelet agents (aspirin), antithrombin concentrates
3. If the patient is still bleeding after the above measures, replace platelets and clotting factors (fresh frozen plasma, cryoprecipitate) based on laboratory values.

4. Finally, consider inhibition of fibrinolysis (ϵ-aminocaproic acid or tranexamic acid) only if the above measures have failed. These agents may precipitate fatal thromboses if the patient is not anticoagulated first!

THROMBOEMBOLIC DISEASE DURING PREGNANCY

What is the incidence of ante- and postpartum DVT and PE?	1 in 1000 pregnancies (50% antepartum, 50% in the puerperium)
What is the rate of PE?	1 in 6,400 pregnancies.
What is the maternal mortality rate of PE?	10% to 15% of all maternal deaths
What is the anatomic distribution of DVTs in pregnancy?	During pregnancy, thrombosis occurs in the pelvic veins more frequently than it occurs in nonpregnant women, and it occurs much more frequently in the left leg than in the right.
Why is the distribution different in pregnancy?	The gravid uterus places pressure on the inferior vena cava and iliac veins, thus creating stasis in the veins of the lower extremities. Because the inferior vena cava is normally to the right of midline, the left iliac vein has to cross over behind the left iliac artery and, therefore, is more prone to compression than compared with the right iliac vein.
What is Virchow's triad?	Virchow postulated that venous thrombosis is related to three factors: 1. Vessel endothelial injury 2. Venous stasis 3. Increased coagulability
Name 6 other predisposing factors in pregnancy.	1. Advanced maternal age 2. Traumatic delivery

3. Cesarean section
4. Thrombophlebitis
5. Endometritis
6. Smoking

How do you establish the diagnosis of DVT?

1. Classically, venography is the gold standard, but requires contrast and radiation and can itself induce venous thrombosis.
2. Real-time duplex Doppler ultrasound is now the method of choice.
3. Impedance plethysmography also can be used but generally has been replaced by ultrasound.
4. MRI can reliably detect thrombosis not only of the femoral veins but also of the pelvic veins. This option should be considered if ultrasound of the legs is negative and suspicion is high.
5. CT.

What fraction of patients with a PE will not have a detectable DVT?

$1/3$

What are the 8 most common symptoms in patients with a PE?

1. Dyspnea
2. Tachypnea
3. Chest pain
4. Cough
5. Apprehension
6. Tachycardia
7. Syncope
8. Hemoptysis

What diagnostic tests are used to confirm a PE?

The extent to which one needs to confirm the presence of a PE is controversial.
1. The gold standard is pulmonary arteriography.
2. V/Q scan.
3. CTA is now increasingly used.

What is the treatment for thromboembolic disease in pregnancy?	Heparin or LMW heparin is safe and effective and does not cross the placental barrier. Heparin should be administered to keep the PTT at 1.5- to 2.5-fold normal. Heparin should be discontinued during active labor and restarted within several hours of a normal delivery.
What about postpartum?	Postpartum patients should be converted to chronic anticoagulation on warfarin for at least 6 months.
What if a patient with a very recent PE needs to be delivered by C-section?	She should be considered for placement of a vena caval filter before surgery.
What about patients with a DVT during a previous pregnancy?	They should be maintained on low-dose heparin throughout their pregnancy.
Is warfarin contraindicated during pregnancy?	Yes! Warfarin is thought to be teratogenic in the first 8 weeks of pregnancy and may cross the placenta, thus placing the fetus at increased risk of hemorrhage. Therefore, warfarin should be avoided.

OTHER COMPLICATIONS OF PREGNANCY

What is the differential diagnosis of 3rd-trimester bleeding?	Placenta previa, abruption, and fetal hemorrhage
What is placental abruption?	Premature separation of the placenta from the uterus
What are the 3 main complications of abruption?	1. Hemorrhage 2. DIC 3. Fetal death
What are the different types of fetal heart rate decelerations and their significance?	Early, head compression Variable, cord compression Late, uteroplacental insufficiency

What is the significance of a sinusoidal fetal heart rate pattern?	Severe fetal anemia or hypoxia

ECTOPIC PREGNANCY

What is an ectopic pregnancy?	A conceptus that is implanted outside the uterus

What are 3 potential complications of an ectopic pregnancy?

1. Rupture
2. Hemorrhage
3. Maternal death

What 3 clinical parameters indicate a suspicion for ectopic pregnancy?

1. Last menstrual period more than 4 weeks ago
2. Lower abdominal pain
3. Vaginal bleeding

Sometimes, a unilateral mass is detected on pelvic exam.

How do you make the definitive diagnosis of an ectopic pregnancy?

Any one of the following:
1. Quantitative β-hCG greater than 2,000 and no intrauterine pregnancy (IUP) on transvaginal ultrasound
2. Quantitative β-hCG greater than 6,000, and no IUP on transabdominal ultrasound
3. Radiographic visualization of an extrauterine pregnancy

GENERAL GYNECOLOGY

Name 5 factors that may increase a female ICU patient's risk for developing vulvovaginal candidiasis.

1. Immunosuppression
2. Broad-spectrum antibiotics
3. Diabetes
4. Poor intertriginous hygiene
5. Immobility

Name 2 prophylactic treatments to decrease the risk of developing vulvovaginal candidiasis in susceptible patients.

1. Antifungal medication (e.g., clotrimazole per vagina)
2. Nystatin powder, liberally applied to the groin and intertriginous folds

20

Endocrine System

| What are 3 important endocrinologic maintenance issues for the critically ill patient? | 1. Be sure that stress steroids are ordered if there is any chance of adrenal suppression.
2. Monitor glucose, and have a very low threshold to use an insulin drip.
3. Have a low threshold for checking thyroid function tests. Many ill patients are hypothyroid. |

STRESS RESPONSE PHYSIOLOGY

| Which of the following are increased, decreased, or unchanged during the "normal" stress response, as would be observed in the ICU, and what is the overall physiologic effect? | This is really simple if you think about the "fight or flight" response and remember 3 basic concepts of stress response physiology:
1. Maintenance of blood pressure
2. Conservation of glucose for the brain
3. Shift of metabolism toward catabolism of protein and fat |

| Catecholamines | Increased. Secreted from sympathetic nerve terminals and adrenal medulla, catecholamines are the main component of the "fight or flight" response. They help to maintain blood pressure by producing vasoconstriction (α) and increasing cardiac output (β). The glucose available for the brain is increased by inhibition of insulin secretion (α) and stimulation of glucagon secretion (β), gluconeo-genesis, and glycogenolysis (β). Metabolism is shifted to the peripheral catabolism of fat and protein. |

| Vasopressin (ADH) | Increased. Secreted from the posterior pituitary (neurohypophysis) in response |

to high serum osmolality and hypovolemia. ADH is a potent vasoconstrictor and acts on the kidney to retain free water. Both of these functions serve to maintain blood pressure.

Renin

Increased. Stimulated by increased catecholamines, decreased renal perfusion, and decreased serum Na^+, juxtaglomerular apparatus cells in kidney release renin to preserve blood pressure. Renin converts plasma angiotensinogen to angiotensin I, followed by conversion to angiotensin II via angiotensin-converting enzyme in the lungs. Angiotensin II is a potent vasoconstrictor and stimulates aldosterone secretion, both of which serve to maintain blood pressure.

Aldosterone

Increased. Aldosterone secretion is primarily stimulated by angiotensin II and increased K^+. Adrenocorticotropic hormone (ACTH) also stimulates aldosterone release from the adrenal cortex, but to a lesser extent. Aldosterone maintains blood pressure by increasing blood volume, resulting in renal resorption of Na^+ (and, therefore, H_2O) and loss of K^+.

ACTH/glucocorticoid (cortisone) axis

Increased. Cortisone makes more glucose available for the brain by increased gluconeogenesis and increased insulin resistance, which result in decreased peripheral glucose utilization. Also, this hormone shifts peripheral catabolism/metabolism to fat and protein.

Insulin

Decreased/unchanged. This results in decreased peripheral glucose utilization, making more glucose available for the brain.

Glucagon	Increased. Increases the glucose available for the brain by increasing gluconeogenesis and glycolysis, and shifts metabolism to catabolism of fat and protein.
Growth hormone	Increased. Growth hormone decreases glucose transport into cells, causing peripheral insulin resistance. Thus, more glucose is available for the brain.
Thyroid hormones	Decreased/unchanged. It was postulated that in critical stress states, these should be elevated and that some of the pathophysiology of critical illness was caused by inappropriate euthyroidism. This hypothesis led to use of the term *sick-euthyroid syndrome.* Clinical trials have disproved this hypothesis, however, and a euthyroid or slightly hypothyroid state is normal pathophysiology for critical stress. Approximately 10% to 50% of patients will have abnormal thyroid function tests.
Testosterone	Decreased. The gonadal axis is downregulated to preserve resources needed during critical illness. Decreased testosterone results in decreased muscle mass (leading to difficulties in physical therapy and eventual mobilization), thinning of the diaphragm (difficulty clearing secretions, difficulty with independent respiration), and negative nitrogen balance (slowed wound healing, increased incidence of decubitus ulcers).

HYPERGLYCEMIA AND HYPOGLYCEMIA

How should you manage blood glucose in every ICU patient?	Maintain tight glucose control. A recent study demonstrated dramatic improvements in long-term outcomes, including survival when blood sugar

levels were maintained at 110 mg/dL or lower. Patients should be started on an insulin drip with serum glucose checks every hour, if necessary, to maintain this optimal glucose level.

What 15 symptoms and complications are associated with hypoglycemia?

1. Confusion
2. Irritability
3. Fatigue
4. Headache
5. Somnolence
6. Seizures
7. Focal neurologic deficits
8. Anxiety
9. Restlessness
10. Diaphoresis
11. Tachycardia
12. Hypotension
13. Arrhythmias
14. Angina
15. Death

How do you treat hypoglycemia?

50% Dextrose in water as an IV bolus. Resistant or more severe hypoglycemia may require a continuous 5% dextrose or a 10% dextrose drip.

What are 8 side effects associated with persistent hyperglycemia in the ICU?

1. Increased risk of nosocomial infections
2. Muscle proteolysis
3. Arrhythmogenesis
4. Electrolyte abnormalities
5. Hypovolemia
6. Poor wound healing
7. Increased incidence of wound infections
8. Prolonged ventilator wean (from increased CO_2 production)

What is diabetic ketoacidosis (DKA)?

A syndrome characterized by hyperglycemia, hyperosmolarity, dehydration, and overproduction of ketone bodies

Which patients are at risk of DKA?

Type I diabetics

What are 10 signs and symptoms of DKA?

1. Dehydration
2. Altered mental status
3. Kussmaul (deep, rapid) respirations
4. "Fruity" breath odor
5. Nausea/vomiting
6. Diffuse abdominal pain
7. Muscle weakness
8. Prerenal azotemia
9. Hypotension
10. Shock

What 4 laboratory abnormalities are seen?

1. Severe hyperglycemia
2. Anion-gap metabolic acidosis (from ketone body production, some contribution from lactic acid)
3. Hyperkalemia
4. Hyponatremia

How do you manage the patient with DKA?

1. Monitoring.
2. Fluid resuscitation with normal saline (1–2 L in the first hour, then 250–500 mL/hr) followed by $\frac{1}{2}$ normal saline.
3. IV bolus of 4 to 5 U of regular insulin, followed by 4 to 5 U/hr adjusted as necessary to lower blood glucose levels by 100 mg/dL/hr.
4. Keep a close watch on K^+ levels, and replace as necessary.
5. Give 5% dextrose once blood glucose reaches 250 mg/dL to prevent insulin-induced hypoglycemia.
6. Treat other conditions (one or more of which may have precipitated the onset of DKA)

What are 4 differences between DKA and the nonketotic hyperosmolar state (NKHS)?

1. Patients with DKA tend to be either undiagnosed or known type I (insulin-dependent) diabetics.

2. NKHS usually occurs in elderly patients with type II (noninsulin-dependent) diabetes.
3. Patients with NKHS usually do not have ketoacidosis, although they do tend to present with more severe dehydration, hyperosmolarity, and hyperglycemia (blood glucose > 800 mg/dL).
4. Neurologic symptoms are more prominent and more severe in patients with NKHS, ranging from confusion to coma and death.

How do you manage the patient with NKHS?

Similar to management of the patient with DKA, except that use of insulin is controversial.

What is an unpredictable—and often fatal—complication of DKA/NKHS?

Cerebral edema

Which patients are at risk for cerebral edema?

Patients with NKHS are at a greater risk than those with DKA. Of patients with DKA, children are more often affected than adults. Other patients at risk include those that have been subjected to a fluid resuscitation rate of greater than 4 L/m² body surface area/day.

What is the treatment of cerebral edema?

1. Mannitol, 0.25 to 1 g/kg IV.
2. Decrease the rate of other IV fluids.
3. Hyperventilation

HYPERTHYROIDISM AND HYPOTHYROIDISM

What are the 3 most common causes of hyperthyroidism in the ICU?

1. Graves' disease (thyroid stimulating hormone [TSH]-receptor autoantibodies with agonist activity)
2. Toxic nodular goiter
3. Iatrogenic hyperthyroidism (consider in patients getting iodinated contrast or on amiodarone or thyroid hormone replacement)

What is thyroid storm?

Severe hyperthyroidism manifesting as marked increases in triiodothyronine (T_3) and thyroxine (T_4), resulting in profound hypermetabolism and hyperpyrexia. Body temperatures may be so high that enzyme systems fail.

What is the treatment of thyroid storm?

1. Decrease thyroid hormone response by β-blockade with propranolol (10–40 mg PO or IV 3 or 4 times a day).
2. Decrease thyroid hormone production with propylthiouracil (100–200 mg two or three times a day) or methimazole (10–40 mg QD).
3. Decrease thyroid hormone release with iodides (Lugol's solution) or lithium.
4. Cool with cooling blankets, intubate, and paralyze to stop the heat production of shivering.

How do methimazole (Tapazole) and propylthiouracil (PTU) work?

1. Inhibit organification (conversion of unusable inorganic iodine to organic form)
2. Inhibit iodination (incorporation of iodine into thyroglobulin)

What else does PTU do?

Inhibits coupling (conversion of mono- and diiodotyrosine to T_3 and T_4) as well as peripheral conversion of T_4 to T_3. Also, PTU is the preferred drug during pregnancy, because it is less likely to cross the placental barrier.

How are β-blockers useful?

β-Blockers decrease heart rate and lessen the hypermetabolic state seen in hyperthyroid patients. There is also evidence that they decrease the rate of peripheral conversion of T_4 to T_3.

What may be seen in the ICU patient with hypothyroidism?

While unproven, a syndrome consisting of neuropsychiatric changes, hypothermia, third spacing, bradycardia, decreased respiratory drive, protracted ventilator wean, GI hypomotility, glucose intolerance, decreased free water clearance, anemia, malabsorption, and hypertriglyceridemia may be attributed to decreased T_3 and T_4 levels.

ADRENAL INSUFFICIENCY

What is the difference between primary and secondary adrenal insufficiency?

Primary adrenal insufficiency results from a dysfunction at the level of the adrenal glands (e.g., Friedrich-Waterhouse syndrome, autoimmune-mediated adrenal insufficiency) and manifests as adrenal insufficiency with hyperkalemia (from inability to produce aldosterone and cortisol). Secondary adrenal insufficiency results from a dysfunction at the level of the pituitary gland and manifests as decreased ACTH secretion (e.g., Sheehan's syndrome) and adrenal insufficiency characterized by hypokalemia.

What is an Addisonian crisis, and what are its clinical manifestations?

Adrenal insufficiency that manifests with fever, nausea/vomiting, abdominal pain, hypotension, metabolic acidosis, and altered mental status because of glucocorticoid insufficiency. Mineralocorticoid (aldosterone) insufficiency results in hyponatremia and hyperkalemia.

What is the most common etiology of an Addisonian crisis?

Inadvertent withdrawal of exogenous steroids and/or failure to provide "stress-dose" steroids after suppression of endogenous glucocorticoid production by long-term administration of steroids

What is the dose of replacement steroids for patients with adrenal insufficiency?	Hydrocortisone, 50–100 mg IV every 8 to 12 hours.
What are stress-dose steroids?	Doses of corticosteroids required to approximate the fourfold increase in production normally found during times of stress
What is a typical dosing regimen?	Hydrocortisone, 100 mg IV every 8 hours, tapered off over several days
Can oral steroids be used?	Patients capable of taking PO steroids may be switched to an equivalent dose of a prednisone taper.
Can dexamethasone be used as stress-dose steroids to prevent an Addisonian crisis?	No. It is a pure glucocorticoid and does not have mineralocorticoid effects.

SYNDROME OF INAPPROPRIATE ANTIDIURETIC HORMONE

What is SIADH?	Syndrome of inappropriate antidiuretic hormone release, which results in inappropriate retention of free water
What are 4 causes of SIADH?	1. Stress states (e.g., sepsis, infection, surgery, trauma) 2. Malignancy 3. Brain trauma 4. Surgery
What are the clinical and lab findings?	Volume overload, edema, and hyponatremia
How is SIADH treated?	By restriction of free water intake and treatment of the underlying cause

21 Hematology

OVERVIEW AND BACKGROUND

What are 9 hematologic health maintenance issues for the critically ill patient?

1. DVT prophylaxis: heparin, SCDs.
2. ASA: for patients with atherosclerotic disease.
3. Competence of the coagulation system: include vitamin K in TPN, monitor parameters.
4. Monitor platelet counts if on heparin: SQ, therapeutic, even flushes
5. Monitor PT and INR if on Coumadin.
6. Ensure platelet count greater than 50,000/mm³ for invasive procedures.
7. Ensure INR at least less than 1.5 for invasive procedures.
8. Monitor platelets if receiving antilymphocyte therapy for induction of immunosuppression.
9. When feasible, fully anticoagulate patients with atrial fibrillation, mechanical heart valves, DVT, or arterial emboli from the heart.

Name the 4 phases of hemostasis.

1. Vascular phase: vasospasm of injured vessel
2. Platelet plug phase (primary hemostasis): phospholipid surface needed for clotting cascade
3. Fibrin clot phase: secondary hemostasis
4. Clot lysis phase: fibrinolysis

What disease process causes a defect in all 4 phases of hemostasis?

Cirrhosis
1. Vascular phase: varices

2. Platelet plug phase: thrombocytopenia (splenomegaly) and platelet function
3. Fibrin clot phase: decreased hepatic synthesis of clotting factors
4. Clot lysis phase: decreased hepatic clearance of fibrin split products

How does liver disease also make one hypercoagulable?

The liver also produces endogenous anticoagulants: plasminogen, antithrombin III, protein C.

POSTSURGICAL BLEEDING AND BLOOD TRANSFUSIONS

What is the most common cause of excessive postsurgical bleeding?

Failure of local mechanical hemostasis (i.e., the surgical bleeder)

What is the treatment of excessive postsurgical bleeding?

1. Direct pressure to the site of bleeding to prevent further blood loss!
2. Re-exploration and cautery or suturing

Name 3 ways in which damaged blood vessels contribute to hemostasis.

1. Vascular spasm
2. Expression of tissue factors: potent procoagulant
3. Exposure of subendothelial collagen: potent procoagulant

What are 5 causes for abnormal mediastinal bleeding after cardiopulmonary bypass (CPB)?

1. Failure of local mechanical hemostasis: anatomic bleeder
2. Pump-induced platelet dysfunction
3. The **3 H's :**
   Hypothermia: reversible platelet and clotting factor dysfunction
   Hemodilution: thrombocytopenia, decreased clotting factors
   Heparin: inadequate reversal with protamine, "heparin rebound"
4. Fibrinolysis
5. Systemic HTN

What is the most important cause of nonsurgical bleeding after CPB?	Platelet dysfunction

RED BLOOD CELL TRANSFUSION

What are packed RBCs (PRBCs) used for?	Improving oxygen-carrying capacity without extensive volume expansion
By how much does 1 U of PRBCs raise the Hct?	3%
What are the characteristics of a unit of PRBCs?	1 U = 250 to 350 mL Hct = 50% to 80% Stored at 1 to 6°C Citrate used as anticoagulant
What is the correlation between Hgb and Hct?	An Hgb of 10 mg/dL corresponds to an Hct of approximately 30%.
What is the minimal *Hgb* level tolerated by a normovolemic, healthy adult?	Greater than 7 mg/dL. Below this level, oxygen-carrying capacity is inadequate to sustain normal cardiopulmonary function.
What is the minimal *Hgb* tolerated by elderly patients with coronary artery disease?	Greater then 10 mg/dL
What is the minimum *Hgb* tolerated by critically ill patients with coronary artery disease?	Greater than 10 mg/dL (keep Hct > 30%)
What other condition warrants keeping the Hct at a higher level?	Sepsis. Oxygen use at the tissues is impaired, so you need to increase oxygen delivery.
What 5 factors influence the decision to transfuse PRBCs?	1. Patient's age 2. Severity of anemia 3. Intravascular volume status

4. Underlying cardiopulmonary disease
5. Patient's wishes

Define massive PRBC transfusion.

Replacement of greater than 1 blood volume (5,000 mL in a 70-kg patient) during a 24-hour period

What are 8 potential complications of massive PRBC transfusion?

1. Hyperkalemia: efflux from cells (remember that stored cells have no adenosine triphosphate to run Na^+/K^+–ATPase.
2. Hypocalcemia: citrate is a calcium chelator.
3. Acid-base derangements: prolonged storage of blood promotes acidosis because of lactate production, or citrate can be metabolized to bicarbonate-producing alkalosis.
4. Dilutional thrombocytopenia.
5. Disseminated intravascular coagulation (DIC).
6. Impaired delivery of oxygen at tissue level: decreased 2,3-diphosphoglycerate levels with prolonged storage, low temperature, and alkalosis from citrate all increase the affinity of Hgb for oxygen. All are factors that shift the Hgb dissociation curve to the left.
7. Systemic hypothermia: blood stored at 1 to 6°C.
8. Iron overload: each unit of blood represents 250 mg of iron (total body store = 1 to 3 g).

What is the most common cause of bleeding following massive transfusion?

Dilutional thrombocytopenia

Should platelets routinely be given empirically during a massive transfusion?

Controversial. Older teaching advocated transfusing after every 10 U of PRBC. Ideally, platelet counts and coagulation studies should guide transfusion of platelets and FFP.

When does clinically significant hypocalcemia occur?

In normal patients, when the transfusion rate exceeds 1 U of PRBC every 5 minutes.

In what patients is this not true?

In patients with hypothermia or hepatic dysfunction, citrate may not be metabolized as quickly. A calcium infusion may be necessary.

What is the most common acid-base derangement following massive transfusion?

Metabolic alkalosis, which occurs once normal perfusion is restored. Lactate and citrate are converted to bicarbonate.

What are 3 other adverse effects of blood transfusion?

1. Transfusion reactions
2. Viral transmissions
3. Immunomodulation

TRANSFUSION REACTIONS

What is the frequency of transfusion reactions?

10% to 15% of all patients receiving blood

What is the most common type of transfusion reaction?

Febrile reactions: fever, chills, flushing, urticaria

What causes a febrile reaction?

1. Minor leukocyte antigens in the donor blood.
2. Recent evidence also indicates that cytokines released in storage play a role.

What is the treatment for a febrile transfusion reaction?

1. Always confirm that more serious reactions are not present (assess the patient).
2. Tylenol and diphenhydramine if mild; epinephrine or steroids if severe.

What is the option for patients with recurrent febrile reactions?

Leukocyte-reduced or filtered blood products are available.

Which is the most severe type of transfusion reaction?

Acute hemolytic transfusion reaction ($\sim$1 in 6,000)

What causes acute hemolytic transfusion reaction?

ABO incompatibility (most commonly a clerical error)

What are 9 clinical features of an acute hemolytic transfusion reaction?

1. Fever: earliest sign (why you need to investigate febrile reactions closely)
2. Flushing
3. Anxiety
4. Chest pain
5. Flank or back pain
6. Reddish discoloration of urine: hemoglobinuria
7. DIC: release of thromboplastin
8. Renal failure: pigment nephropathy
9. Vascular collapse

What is the treatment of acute hemolytic transfusion reaction?

1. Stop transfusion immediately!
2. Vigorous IV fluid administration.
3. Insert urinary catheter.
4. Include $NaHCO_3$ in IV fluids to alkalinize urine and mitigate effects of free Hgb on kidneys: pigment nephropathy.
5. Mannitol: osmotic diuresis.
6. Vasopressors: if necessary to support circulation.

What 5 laboratory values correspond to intravascular hemolysis?

1. Falling Hct
2. Low serum haptoglobin (protein that binds free Hgb)
3. Elevated serum and urine free Hgb levels
4. Elevated LDH
5. Schistocytes and other RBC fragments on peripheral smear

What is a delayed hemolytic transfusion reaction?	Hemolysis that occurs several days (3–10 days) after a transfusion. Consider this diagnosis with an unexplained drop in Hct.
What causes delayed hemolytic reaction?	Minor RBC antigen incompatibility

INFECTIOUS COMPLICATIONS

What is the current risk of viral transmission from 1 u of blood?	Hepatitis B: 1 in 60,000 Hepatitis C: 1 in 200,000 Human immunodeficiency virus: 1 in 500,000 Human T-cell lymphotropic virus type I (HTLV-1): 1 in 650,000
What hematologic malignancy is associated with HTLV-1?	Adult B-cell lymphoma
What is the most common transfusion-associated hepatitis infection in the United States?	Hepatitis C
Overall, what virus is most commonly transmitted through blood transfusions?	Cytomegalovirus (CMV; 50% of all donor units contain CMV)
In what patient populations is CMV clinically significant?	Immunosuppressed patients and transplant recipients who are seronegative for CMV

PLATELETS AND DISORDERS OF PRIMARY HEMOSTASIS

What is primary hemostasis?	Formation of a primary platelet plug
What role, if any, do RBCs play in primary hemostasis?	RBCs facilitate transport of platelets to the site for platelet plug. (Anemia causes platelet dysfunction.)

Disorders of primary hemostasis are divided into what 2 general classes?

1. Platelet dysfunction
2. Thrombocytopenia

PLATELET DYSFUNCTION AND INHIBITION

What is platelet dysfunction?

A qualitative defect in platelet adhesion, activation, secretion, or aggregation, regardless of the platelet count

What are the signs of primary hemostatic disorders?

Usually mild, superficial mucocutaneous bleeding that is easily controlled and begins immediately after minor trauma or an invasive procedure. Examples include:
1. Bleeding into skin: easy bruisability, petechiae, ecchymoses, purpura
2. Bleeding after minor mucous membrane trauma/surgery: epistaxis
3. Oozing from skin incisions or sites of percutaneous catheters

What are the 3 most common causes of platelet dysfunction in the ICU patient?

1. Drugs are the primary cause! Some (ASA and other nonsteroidal anti-inflammatory drugs) inhibit the action of platelets; others inhibit platelet production or trigger an immune response in which platelets are the innocent bystander (β-lactam antibiotics, furosemide, nitroglycerin, H_2-blockers).
2. Uremia: interference with von Willebrand factor (vWF)–mediated platelet adhesion.
3. Hypothermia: cold blood does not clot.

What percentage of the normal pool of platelets is found within the spleen?

$1/3$

How does ASA affect platelets?

Irreversibly acetylates and inhibits cyclo-oxygenase, thereby inhibiting

	thromboxane A_2 production and its platelet aggregatory effects
What is the onset of action of ASA?	2 hours
What is the duration of action of ASA?	The entire life of the platelet (7–9 days)
What is the lab test to establish the diagnosis of platelet dysfunction?	Bleeding time (prolonged)
What is normal bleeding time?	Less than 5 minutes
What are glycoprotein IIb/IIIa inhibitors?	Antibodies or peptides that bind to and block the platelet receptor IIb/IIIa
What does the platelet IIb/IIIa receptor do?	It binds fibrinogen and enables platelets to cross-link, forming the initial hemostatic plug.
When are platelet IIb/IIIa inhibitors indicated?	These inhibitors are widely used in acute coronary syndromes and following coronary stenting procedures (level I evidence in these patient populations).

How should one treat platelet dysfunction for each of the following causes?

Drugs	Discontinue the offending agents. Transfuse platelets for severe or persistent bleeding.
Uremia	Dialysis, desmopressin (DDAVP), cryoprecipitate
Hypothermia	Warming blankets/lights, warm fluids and respiratory gases

Von Willebrand Syndromes

What is the most common, inherited cause of platelet dysfunction?

Von Willebrand syndromes, which are also the most common group of serious inherited hemostatic disorders in general

What is vWF?

Von Willebrand factor; a glycoprotein that binds platelets to subendothelial collagen and serves as a carrier/stabilizer of factor VIII.

What are the von Willebrand syndromes?

Genetic disorders with multiple subtypes characterized by a qualitative or quantitative defect in vWF (autosomal recessive as well as dominant forms exist)

What type of von Willebrand syndrome is most common?

Type I (phenotype is half the normal amount of vWF)

What are the lab tests to establish the diagnosis of von Willebrand syndromes?

1. Prolonged bleeding time: low vWF
2. Elevated PTT: low factor VIII activity

What is treatment for von Willebrand syndromes?

1. DDAVP: for type I only
2. Cryoprecipitate, factor VIII concentrate: depends on the subtype

What causes acquired von Willebrand disease (vWD)?

Antibodies that inhibit vWF function: multiple transfusions, autoimmune conditions

Tumors that absorb vWF: Wilm's tumor classically, lymphomas

What is DDAVP?

1-Deamino-8-D-arginine vasopressin or desmopressin; an ADH analogue with hemostatic properties (stimulates release of preformed vWF and factor VIII from endothelial cells)

When is DDAVP used in ICU patients?

1. To control clinically significant bleeding from acquired platelet dysfunction (especially uremia), type

I vWD, and mild hemophilia A and after CPB.
2. To treat central diabetes insipidus: look for this in head traumas and neurosurgical patients

What are 6 side effects of DDAVP?

1. Tachyphylaxis
2. Hyponatremia
3. Seizures
4. Facial flushing
5. Headache
6. HTN

THROMBOCYTOPENIA

How is thrombocytopenia defined?

Usually, a platelet count of less than $100,000/mm^3$ is used to define thrombocytopenia, because the bleeding time is prolonged below this level.

What are the signs of thrombocytopenia?

The same as those of other primary hemostatic disorders, except that spontaneous internal hemorrhage can occur when platelet counts fall below $20,000/mm^3$ (including lethal intracranial hemorrhage)

What are 3 common causes of thrombocytopenia in the critical care patient?

1. Decreased platelet production (marrow suppression), typically from drugs (H_2-blockers are very common offenders in the ICU) or sepsis
2. Platelet sequestration from splenomegaly, as in a patient with portal HTN
3. Increased destruction as a result of:
   a. Immunologic destruction: drugs (heparin, quinidine, sulfa) and autoimmune disorders
   b. Increased utilization: DIC, sepsis, severe hemorrhage with massive blood transfusion

c. Mechanical destruction: prosthetic cardiac valves, vascular prostheses, intra-aortic balloon pump

What is the most common cause of a deficit in platelet function or number?

DRUGS!

What are lab criteria to establish the diagnosis of thrombocytopenia?

Platelet counts of 50,000 to 100,000/mm³ (minor), 20,000 to 50,000/mm³ (moderate), and less than 20,000/mm³ (severe)

What platelet count is considered to be adequate to safely undergo surgery or an invasive procedure?

50,000/mm³ or greater

PLATELET TRANSFUSION

What are 3 indications for platelet concentrate transfusions?

1. All patients with platelet counts less than 20,000
2. Before, during, or after surgery or invasive procedure with platelet count of less than 50,000
3. Significant bleeding in the setting of platelet dysfunction, regardless of the platelet count (e.g., mediastinal bleeding after CPB)

Why is a platelet count of 20,000 the threshold for transfusion in a patient who is not bleeding?

Below that value, there is an increased risk of spontaneous hemorrhage.

What is the volume contained in 1 U of random-donor platelet concentrate?

50 mL

What is the number of random-donor units in 1 U of single-donor platelet concentrate?

6 to 8. This is why a unit of platelets is sometimes referred to as a "6-pack."

By how much does 1 random-donor unit raise the platelet count?

5,000 to 10,000/mm³

What are 3 adverse effects of platelet transfusions?

1. Transfusion reactions: up to 30% have a nonhemolytic febrile reaction (the highest of any blood product).
2. Bacterial transmission: samples must be stored at room temperature (remember that cold platelets are dysfunctional).
3. Platelet-specific antibodies: platelets are the most immunogenic of all blood products

What can be done to minimize the formation of platelet-specific antibodies?

Administer human leukocyte antigen–specific platelet concentrates or single-donor platelets to decrease overall exposure to antigens

HEPARIN-INDUCED THROMBOCYTOPENIA

What is HIT?

Heparin-induced thrombocytopenia; an autoimmune destruction of platelets by cross-reacting immunoglobulin G antibodies to heparin

What is the incidence of HIT?

2% to 5% of all patients exposed to heparin

What are 3 clinical features of HIT?

1. Thrombocytopenia (often <50,000/mm³) develops approximately 1 week after exposure to heparin of any dose via any route and may develop sooner if previously exposed to heparin.
2. 1% of patients with HIT develop arterial and/or venous thrombi as part of the syndrome (life-threatening in 30%).
3. Excessive bleeding is a rare complication.

How is HIT diagnosed?

Usually as a clinical diagnosis, because detection of heparin-platelet-antibody complexes in a patient's serum has low sensitivity and specificity

What is the treatment of HIT?

1. Discontinue all heparin (including catheter flushes and heparin locks).
2. Use alternative anticoagulation if necessary.

What form of heparin is more likely to induce HIT?

Unfractionated heparin is more immunogenic than LMW products.

What is the prognosis for a patient who is diagnosed with HIT?

Excellent if diagnosed before the onset of severe thrombocytopenia or thromboses. Therefore, the platelet count should be monitored daily in all patients after the institution of heparin therapy.

What other serious complication can occur following prolonged heparin exposure?

Heparin-induced osteopenia. It is thought that heparin activates osteoclasts.

COAGULATION, ANTICOAGULATION, AND DISORDERS OF SECONDARY HEMOSTASIS

What is secondary hemostasis?

Formation of a cross-linked fibrin clot

What are the pathways of the coagulation cascade?

Classical pathway: extrinsic (factor VII), intrinsic (factors XII, XI, IX, VIII)

Common pathway: factors V, X, XIII, thrombin, fibrinogen

Recent evidence shows that factor VIIa–tissue factor complex can also activate factor XI directly, thus creating an overlap of the classical extrinsic and intrinsic pathways.

PROTHROMBIN TIME, PARTIAL THROMBOPLASTIN TIME, AND CLOTTING FACTORS

What does PT measure?
Activity of the extrinsic pathway

What is INR?
International normalized ratio; another means of expressing the activity of the extrinsic pathway. It simply normalizes the patient's PT to the normal PT range from the same laboratory. This eliminates the wide variability in PT measurements between different laboratories that results from different lab techniques and reagents.

Name 5 things that prolong the PT.
1. Warfarin
2. Vitamin K deficiency
3. Liver disease: decreased factor VII synthesis
4. DIC
5. Supratherapeutic heparin doses: common pathway

What does PTT measure?
Activity of the intrinsic pathway

Name 8 things that prolong the PTT.
1. Heparin
2. Inherited factor deficiencies: hemophilia A and B
3. Liver disease
4. DIC
5. Severe vitamin K deficiency: common pathway
6. Supratherapeutic warfarin doses: common pathway
7. vWD
8. Lupus anticoagulant

Which clotting factors are unstable at temperatures above 4°C?
Factors V and VIII. Therefore, these factors are found at low levels in whole blood (stored at ~4°C); in FFP (stored at <0°C), they are present at adequate levels for therapeutic replacement of these factors.

Which is the only clotting factor not produced by the liver?

Factor VIII, which is made by endothelial cells

The factor VIII level helps to differentiate which two clinical conditions?

1. DIC
2. Decompensated liver disease
Bleeding from DIC will have low factor VIII levels. These levels will be normal in cirrhotic patients.

What is the most common inherited hypercoagulable state?

Factor V Leiden (activated protein C resistance)

What is the prevalence of factor V Leiden?

2% to 4% of the population

Heparin

What is heparin?

A naturally occurring, mucopolysaccharide polymer that is obtained from bovine and porcine sources for clinical use

How does heparin work?

By potentiating the effects of antithrombin III, which degrades several clotting factors (including thrombin and factor X)

Name 4 ways to administer heparin.

1. IV infusion: systemic anticoagulation
2. SQ: DVT prophylaxis
3. Intra-arterially: vascular surgery
4. Catheter flushes: to maintain patency

How are the effects of heparin monitored?

PTT or activated clotting time. Heparin elevates both at therapeutic doses.

What is heparin's duration of action?

The half-life is approximately 90 minutes. If the patient is on heparin drip, stop at least 4 hours before surgery or invasive procedure.

Can the effects of heparin be reversed or neutralized?	Yes. Use IV protamine sulfate.

Warfarin and Vitamin K

How does warfarin work?	By inhibiting vitamin K reductase
What 6 clotting factors depend on vitamin K for production?	1. Factor II 2. Factor VII 3. Factor IX 4. Factor X 5. Protein C 6. Protein S
Which of these 6 factors have the shortest half-life?	Protein C and protein S. Therefore, patients treated with warfarin are transiently hypercoagulable before reaching therapeutic anticoagulation levels.
Why is the PT affected more than the PTT by warfarin?	Of the procoagulant vitamin K–dependent proteins, factor VII (extrinsic pathway) has the shortest half-life and, therefore, is more dependent on continued production to maintain serum levels. Inhibition of its synthesis will thus affect PT more than PTT.
How long does it take to see the full effect of warfarin activity?	48 to 72 hours
How long does it take for the INR to normalize on cessation of warfarin therapy?	5 to 7 days (assuming no other coagulopathy exists)
What are the clinical uses of warfarin?	Long-term prophylactic anticoagulation (e.g., mechanical valves, atrial fibrillation) or therapeutic (e.g., DVT)
How is warfarin administered?	Orally

How are the effects of warfarin reversed?	1. Immediately with FFP. Rule of thumb: 1 U of FFP decreases the PT by 2 seconds. 2. Slowly (within 4 hours) with vitamin K: SQ, IM, or IV.
What class of antibiotics have a warfarin-like effect?	Cephalosporins inhibit reduction and recycling of vitamin K.
What is the typical dose of vitamin K?	10 mg (can be repeated every 8–12 hours if necessary)
What are 4 common causes of vitamin K deficiency?	1. Malnutrition 2. Malabsorption: interruption of the enterohepatic circulation of bile acids (i.e., acalculous cholecystitis in the ICU patient, terminal ileal disease) 3. Broad-spectrum antibiotics: eradication of endogenous vitamin K–producing gut flora 4. Normal neonate: no gut flora

HEMOPHILIA

What clotting factor is deficient in hemophilia A?	Factor VIII
What clotting factor is deficient in hemophilia B?	Factor IX (Christmas factor)
Which type of hemophilia is more common?	Hemophilia A (~85% of all hemophiliacs)
What are the recommendations for factor replacement for an acute bleeding episode in hemophiliacs?	25% to 50% factor level should be maintained for at least 72 hours.
What are the recommendations for factor replacement perioperatively in hemophiliac patients?	Hemophilia A: Goal is 100% factor level preoperatively and maintenance of at least 40% postoperatively. Hemophilia B: Goal is 60% factor level preoperatively and maintenance of

20% to 30% for 10 to 14 days post-operatively (less severe bleeding diathesis)

How can factor VIII be replaced?

Administer FFP, cryoprecipitate, or factor VIII concentrate.

How much factor VIII is in each?

FFP: 1 U/mL
Cryoprecipitate: 5 to 10 U/mL
Factor VIII concentrate: 40 U/mL
Each unit of factor VIII raises levels by 2% per kilogram and must be dosed every 8 to 12 hours.

DEEP-VEIN THROMBOSIS

What is Virchow's triad?

1. Intimal injury
2. Stasis
3. Hypercoagulability
These three factors conspire to cause DVT.

What are 13 common risk factors for DVT?

1. Age older than 40 years
2. History of DVT
3. Major surgery: particularly lower extremity orthopedic or vascular procedures
4. Malignancy
5. Obesity
6. Trauma
7. Varicose veins/superficial thrombophlebitis
8. Cardiac disease
9. Hormones
10. Prolonged immobilization/paralysis
11. Pregnancy
12. Central venous catheterization: be particularly wary of femoral lines
13. Hypercoagulable states

Overall, what is the most common condition associated with DVT?

Pregnancy

Which anticoagulation therapy is safe in pregnancy?	Heparin (warfarin crosses the placenta, is teratogenic, and may cause fetal demise)
What is the most significant complication of DVT?	PE
What are 3 long-term sequelae of DVT?	1. Postphlebitic syndrome: venous insufficiency, venous stasis ulcers 2. Recurrent DVT 3. Recurrent PE
Where do most DVTs begin?	In the deep veins of the calf
What is the source of most PEs?	The iliac and femoral veins (50% will have a PE, although most are asymptomatic)
What is the intent of DVT prophylaxis?	To prevent the potentially life-threatening sequelae of PE
How do sequential compression stockings prevent DVTs?	1. Rheologic mechanisms: prevents stasis of blood 2. Release of tissue plasminogen activator: systemic fibrinolytic effect 3. Prevention of anesthesia induced intimal injury: anesthesia damages intima through venodilation
What is adequate prophylaxis for the following patients?	
A patient at low risk for thromboembolism (minor surgery, age < 40 years, no risk factors)	None suggested in the International Consensus Study. Other studies recommend early ambulation.
A patient at moderate risk for thromboembolism (major surgery, age > 40 years, no risk factors)?	One of the following: low-dose heparin, LMW heparin, ASA, elastic stockings, or intermittent pneumatic compression (International Consensus Study)

A patient at high risk for thromboembolism (major surgery, age greater than 60 years, or additional risk factors)

Low-dose heparin or LMW heparin plus elastic stockings or pneumatic compression devices (International Consensus Study)

Special-risk patients (major orthopedic procedures, polytrauma or spinal injury)

Low-dose or LMW heparin or therapeutic warfarin

What is Homan's sign?

Pain on forced dorsiflexion of the foot. Suggests a DVT, but is present only in $1/3$ of patients.

What is phlegmasia cerulea dolens?

A cyanotic hue to an extremity affected by DVT (deoxygenated static blood)

What is phlegmasia alba dolens?

Pallor of an extremity affected by DVT. This indicates that the interstitial pressure in the extremity now exceeds the arterial perfusion pressure (risk of venous gangrene).

How are DVTs diagnosed?

Duplex ultrasonography is the initial procedure of choice and is considered by many to be the "gold standard" for diagnosing peripheral DVT.

What is meant by "duplex study"?

Two components are analyzed. Real-time B-mode ultrasound is used mainly to determine the compressibility of the vein (less compressible with clot present). The other component is pulsed Doppler capability (analyzes flow characteristics).

What is the evidence that duplex scanning may be the new "gold standard" of DVT diagnosis?

Compared to venography, B-mode ultrasound using lack of compressibility as the sole determinant of a positive ultrasound shows sensitivities of at least 91% and specificities of 97% or better.

Compared to venography, Doppler flow criteria also has a sensitivity of 91% and a specificity of 99% in patients with venography-confirmed DVT.

What is still considered to be the absolute "gold standard" for DVT diagnosis (both peripheral and central DVTs)?

Contrast venography. Note, however, that not all patients are candidates for venography based on previous history of contrast reactions or renal insufficiency. The test is also very expensive. Most clinicians would use this in high-risk patients with equivocal findings on ultrasound.

What is the standard therapy for DVT?

Anticoagulation with heparin while warfarin takes effect (generally 5 days), followed by at least 3 to 6 months of warfarin therapy (goal INR 2–3). For recurrent DVT, lifetime warfarin is used.

What is the evidence in favor of using LMW heparin in treating DVTs?

Several randomized trials show that LMW heparins are at least as effective and as safe as the traditional, unfractionated heparin.

What are the 2 main advantages of LMW heparin therapy?

1. No need to follow PTT: very reliable bioavailability
2. Can be given SQ BID.

What are 2 indications for placement of a vena cava (Greenfield) filter?

1. Patient at high risk for thromboembolism in whom anticoagulation is contraindicated
2. PE while receiving adequate anticoagulation therapy

What is the recommended treatment of a patient with DVT and PE who has significant bleeding complications with anticoagulation therapy?

1. Stop the heparin immediately. Consider protamine reversal if the bleeding is severe.
2. Place a vena cava filter.

DISSEMINATED INTRAVASCULAR COAGULATION

What is DIC?

Disseminated intravascular coagulation; a systemic syndrome characterized by both hemorrhage and intravascular thrombosis. It is triggered by a variety of clinical situations and disease processes, and it often results in end-organ dysfunction.

What is the most significant cause of morbidity and mortality from DIC?

End-organ dysfunction from diffuse vascular thromboses (not hemorrhage, although this is the most obvious manifestation)

What is most common cause of DIC?

Infection (sepsis)

Name 10 conditions associated with DIC.

1. Obstetric catastrophes: amniotic fluid embolus, retained fetus, abruptio placentae
2. Massive transfusion
3. Hemolytic transfusion reaction
4. Bacterial sepsis: Gram-negative or Gram-positive
5. Viremia: human immunodeficiency virus, CMV, varicella zoster virus (VZV), hepatitis
6. Malignancy: metastatic solid tumors and leukemias
7. Trauma: especially crush injuries associated with extensive soft-tissue devitalization
8. Liver disease
9. Cardiovascular disorders: giant hemangiomas, aortic aneurysms
10. Intravascular prostheses/devices: intra-aortic balloon pumps, vascular grafts

What is the common pathway for the initiation of blood coagulation activation?

All of the above conditions upregulate endothelial cell expression of tissue factor.

What key inflammatory cytokine has been shown to induce DIC?

Interleukin-6 (given to human cancer patients and shown to induce thrombin generation)

What is the test to establish the diagnosis of DIC?

No single test has been proven as a gold standard. DIC is a clinical diagnosis.

What 7 tests support the diagnosis of DIC?

1. Elevated PT and PTT: rapid consumption of clotting factors
2. Thrombocytopenia: platelet-trapping in diffuse microvascular fibrin clots
3. Hypofibrinogenemia: plasmin mediated
4. Increased fibrin degradation product (FDP) titers
5. Increased D-dimer fragments: the most reliable test
6. Increased bleeding time
7. Decreased antithrombin levels

Which 2 enzymes must both be active in the systemic circulation for DIC to develop?

1. Thrombin
2. Plasmin

What are the end results of circulating thrombin?

Diffuse intravascular thromboses

What are the 2 effects of increased circulating plasmin?

1. Impaired hemostasis
2. Diffuse hemorrhages

What are FDPs?

Breakdown products of plasmin's enzymatic action on fibrinogen and fibrin monomers

How are D-dimer fragments formed?

Plasmin-mediated cleavage of cross-linked fibrin

What is the treatment of low-grade DIC?

1. Treat underlying cause: often the only therapy needed

2. Antiplatelet agents: ASA
3. SQ heparin: if no response to the above measures

What are 4 steps in the treatment of fulminant DIC?

1. Treat the inciting process.
2. Halt intravascular coagulation. Administer low-dose SQ or IV heparin (equally effective), antiplatelet agents, and antithrombin concentrates.
3. If bleeding persists after the above measures, replace platelets and clotting factors (FFP, cryoprecipitate) based on lab values.
4. Finally, consider inhibition of fibrinolysis (ϵ-aminocaproic acid or tranexamic acid) only if the above measures have failed. These must be given with heparin, or they may precipitate fatal thromboses.

No supportive measure (i.e., replacement of platelets or factors) has been shown to decrease overall mortality in DIC patients.

What indicates the efficacy of heparin therapy?

Increasing levels of fibrinogen and decreasing FDPs (NOT the PTT value, which is completely unreliable in the setting of DIC). FDPs should decline in 1 to 2 days. Improvement of platelets lags 1 week behind control of coagulopathy.

FIBRINOLYTIC PHARMACOTHERAPY

What is the mechanism of action of fibrinolytic agents?

Activates plasminogen to plasmin, which dissolves the fibrin clot. Unlike heparin/warfarin, these agents act to dissolve an already formed clot.

What 4 fibrinolytics are available for therapy?

1. Recombinant tissue plasminogen activator

2. Pro-urokinase: from melanoma cell cultures
3. Urokinase: renal cell cultures
4. Streptokinase: β-hemolytic streptococci

What are the main differences pharmacologically among these fibrinolytics?

Pro-urokinase and recombinant tissue plasminogen activator are more specific. They only activate plasminogen associated with clots and, thus, localize the lytic process to sites that contain clots; other products break down other plasma proteins, including coagulation factors.

What is the difference in efficacy among these fibrinolytics?

The efficacy and toxicity are equal between "specific" and "nonspecific" fibrinolytic agents. Fibrin specificity does not have clinical benefit.

What are 7 indications for fibrinolytic therapy?

1. Acute MI
2. Thrombotic stroke
3. Life-threatening DVT/PE
4. Acute arterial occlusion
5. Axillary-vein thrombosis
6. Occluded AV shunts or dialysis catheters
7. Veno-occlusive disease of the liver

What are 2 complications associated with fibrinolytic therapy?

1. Bleeding: intracranial hemorrhage is the most devastating; incidence of 0.5% in patients with MI treated with fibrinolytics.
2. Allergic reactions: most patients have antibodies to streptokinase, which is a natural protein of group B streptococci. Of those patients with allergic reactions, fever, rash, and bronchospasm occurs in 5% of people on streptokinase and anaphylaxis in less than 0.5%.

What are the contraindications to fibrinolytic therapies?

Absolute contraindications:

1. History of hemorrhagic stroke at any time
2. History of nonhemorrhagic stroke or other cerebrovascular event within the past year
3. Marked HTN (systolic BP >180 mm Hg; diastolic BP >110 mm Hg)
4. Suspicion of aortic dissection
5. Active internal bleeding (excluding menses)

Relative contraindications:

1. Current use of an anticoagulant (INR >2–3)
2. Recent (within 2 weeks) invasive or surgical procedure or prolonged (>10 min) CPR
3. Known bleeding diathesis
4. Pregnancy
5. Active peptic ulcer disease
6. History of severe HTN

22

Skin

FUNCTIONS OF SKIN

Name 4 functions of the skin.

1. Protective barrier
2. Sensory receptor
3. Immune system regulator
4. Body temperature controller

What is the normal core temperature in humans?

36 to 37.5°C

Describe the normal diurnal variation in core temperature.

There is a temperature nadir in the early morning hours and a temperature peak around 4:00 to 6:00 PM.

Name 4 physiologic adaptations you might observe that limit heat loss or gain.

1. Sweating
2. Shivering
3. Peripheral vasodilatation
4. Vasoconstriction

What 5 interventions can be used in the ICU to increase body temperature?

1. Heat lamps (be sure they are not placed too close to the skin)
2. Warm air blankets (i.e., Bair Huggers)
3. Warm IV fluids
4. Blankets
5. Heated ventilator gases

What interventions can be used in the ICU to decrease body temperature?

Sponge baths, ice packs, and fans. More aggressive measures include gastric or colonic lavage with iced saline or cooling blankets.

COMMON SKIN REACTIONS OR FINDINGS

How do you avoid or treat dry skin in the ICU?

"Soak and grease." It is appropriate to bathe the skin, but emollients should be applied immediately after the skin is patted dry.

What is intertrigo?

An inflammatory eruption occurring in the skin folds (e.g., groin, axilla, beneath a pannus). Clinically, it appears as a red, macerated plaque with secondary fissuring.

Is intertrigo infectious?

No. Intertrigo is caused by moisture and friction; however, these areas may become secondarily infected by yeast or bacteria.

How is intertrigo treated?

Keep the skin in the affected area cool and dry. This may involve repositioning the patient to open up skin folds or placing towels or blankets in skin folds to prevent the skin from directly apposing itself. If secondary infection with yeast occurs, an antifungal agent should be added.

What is contact dermatitis?

An inflammatory skin reaction caused by either an allergen or an irritant. Irritant reactions are the most common.

What does contact dermatitis look like?

Vesicles on an erythematous base. These are often seen in "streaks" or linear arrangements (think "poison ivy"). The eruption is localized to the area of the contact.

What are 6 common causes of contact dermatitis in the ICU?

1. Tape
2. Latex
3. Laundry detergents
4. Plastic tubing
5. Creams (e.g., steroid, antibiotic)
6. Betadine

How is a contact dermatitis treated?

Discontinue the causative agent. If the lesion is oozing, apply wet dressings followed by a topical steroid ointment.

Oral steroids are indicated when an acute contact dermatitis is widespread. Antihistamines may help to relieve itching.

What is miliaria?

A condition caused by obstruction of the eccrine sweat ducts. Commonly referred to as "heat rash," it appears as tiny vesicles with varying amounts of erythema. It is NOT isolated to hair follicles; it is often seen on the backs of bed-bound patients. Treatment is to keep the patient cool.

When should topical steroid be applied to a "rash"?

Topical steroids should be applied to inflammatory lesions only after infectious etiologies have been ruled out!

WOUND CARE

Should wounds be kept dry?

No. Wounds heal best in a moist environment (e.g., antibiotic ointment and a semiocclusive dressing). This enhances epithelialization.

How often should wounds be inspected?

At least daily

Do surface cultures of wounds have any value?

No. Positive cultures do not warrant antibiotic treatment unless there are signs of wound infection.

Why do positive wound cultures not warrant antibiotic treatment?

Colonization of skin and the external surface of wounds is normal. Treatment for wound colonization with antibiotics is unnecessary, alters the patient's normal bacterial flora, and applies selective pressure favoring multidrug-resistant organisms.

How should an infected wound or ulcer be managed?

1. The wound should be **opened and drained**.

2. Additionally, **systemic antibiotics** are important in treating true wound infections.

DECUBITUS ULCERS

What are decubitus ulcers?

Pressure-induced ulcers that develop when soft tissue is compressed between a bony prominence and an external surface. This pressure results in tissue ischemia with subsequent tissue necrosis.

What percentage of all hospitalized patients get decubitus ulcers?

3% to 5%

What percentage of ICU patients get decubitus ulcers?

30% to 50%

Name the 6 most common areas for decubitus ulcers.

1. Sacrum
2. Greater trochanter
3. Ischial tuberosity
4. Calcaneus
5. Lateral malleolus
6. Occiput

Name 4 risk factors for the development of decubitus ulcers in the ICU.

1. Immobility: sedated and ventilated patients, debilitation, and paralysis (spinal cord injuries or cerebrovascular accident [CVA])
2. Vascular disease: sacrum after aortobifemoral bypass or calcaneus of patients with poor peripheral perfusion
3. Low cardiac output: CHF or patients on vasopressors
4. Equipment: tubes, cervical collars, restraints, backboards

How long does it take a decubitus ulcer to develop?

It can develop rapidly! In animal models, it takes only 2 hours of continuous pressure for an ulcer to develop.

How may decubitus ulcers be prevented?

Decubitus ulcers should virtually never happen. They can be prevented as follows:
1. Frequent turning schedules: every 1–2 hours in an immobile patient.
2. Primary pressure relief: pillow between legs to avoid pressure ulcers at the knees and ankles; padding areas around pressure points.
3. Air mattresses.
4. Good skin hygiene: keep skin clean and dry.
5. Aggressive nutritional support.
6. The patient's backside and all pressure points should be examined daily.

Define the 4 stages of pressure ulcers.

Stage I

Persistent erythema over a bony surface; intact epidermis.

Stage II

Partial-thickness skin loss involving epidermis, dermis, or both; characterized by blister or shallow ulcer formation.

Stage III

Ulceration through the epidermis and dermis into subcutaneous fat; does not extend to muscle, fascia, or bone.

Stage IV

Ulcerations extend to musculoskeletal structures, including muscle, tendons, ligaments, bone, and fascia.

When should pressure ulcers be debrided?

Debridement is necessary for stage III and IV ulcers with nonviable tissue covering tissue that can potentially granulate.

What function does debridement serve in the care of ulcers?

Necrotic tissue is a medium for bacterial overgrowth that prolongs the inflammatory process and delays granulation. It needs to be removed for proper wound healing.

What 5 signs/symptoms should alert the physician to a possibly infected ulcer?	1. Fever 2. Tachycardia 3. Elevated WBC count 4. Zone of erythema around the ulcer 5. Purulent drainage from the ulcer
Are decubitus ulcers downstaged as they heal?	No. The healing granulation tissue of an ulcer is physiologically different from normal tissue and cannot be compared. Therefore, a wound maintains its original "stage" designation even as it heals.

SKIN MANIFESTATIONS OF SYSTEMIC DISEASE

What are 6 skin manifestations associated with cirrhosis of the liver?	1. Jaundice 2. Spider angiomata 3. Palmar erythema 4. Caput medusa 5. Alopecia 6. Spoon nails
What 3 cutaneous signs may be associated with thrombocytopenia?	1. Petechiae 2. Purpura 3. Ecchymoses
Name the cutaneous signs associated with hemorrhagic pancreatitis.	Grey-Turner's sign (flank ecchymosis) and Cullen's sign (periumbilical ecchymosis). These occur in 1% of cases and suggest severe hemorrhagic pancreatitis.

CUTANEOUS DRUG REACTIONS

What percentage of all medical inpatients are affected by skin eruptions?	Approximately 2% to 6%
Name the 4 most common morphologic patterns of cutaneous drug reactions.	1. Morbilliform 2. Urticarial 3. Fixed drug eruptions 4. Erythema multiforme (EM)/Stevens-Johnson syndrome (SJS)/toxic epidermal necrolysis (TEN)

Which medications are most commonly associated with the development of skin eruptions?

The greatest incidence occurs with sulfonamides, antibiotics, anti-convulsants, and nonsteroidal anti-inflammatory drugs (NSAIDs).

Name a patient population particularly at risk of drug eruptions.

Human immunodeficiency virus–positive patients (mechanism unknown)

MORBILLIFORM ERUPTIONS

Describe the typical morbilliform eruption.

Fine, pink-red macules and papules. It initially occurs on the trunk or in dependent areas. The rash is symmetric and tends to become confluent.

When associated with medications, how long before the rash appears?

The typical eruption begins within 1 to 2 weeks of starting a new medication and usually fades within 1 to 2 weeks after its discontinuation.

How are morbilliform eruptions treated?

If feasible, the offending agent should be discontinued. Pruritus may be treated with topical antipruritics, such as hydrocortisone cream or Sarna lotion. Oral antihistamines may also be helpful to relieve the itching. If the reaction is severe, oral steroids may hasten resolution of the rash; however, the patient's other comorbidities must be considered before prescribing steroids.

Is anaphylaxis likely if an agent that causes a skin eruption is continued?

Probably not. A drug may be continued in the face of a morbilliform eruption with little fear of an anaphylactic episode.

URTICARIAL ERUPTIONS

Describe an urticarial eruption.

Erythematous, edematous wheals with accompanying pruritus. The dermis is infiltrated with fluid, giving the skin a "peau d'orange" appearance. Lesions typically resolve within 24 hours, leaving no residual scar.

What is the usual time course of urticarial drug reactions?

The time course depends on the mechanism of the drug reaction. Such eruptions may occur within minutes of administration (e.g., an anaphylactic reaction), within 12 to 36 hours (e.g., an immunoglobulin E–dependent accelerated reaction), or up to 7 to 10 days (e.g., as a serum sickness syndrome).

How is an urticarial eruption managed?

Identify and discontinue the offending medication. Oral antihistamines of the H_1 type are the mainstay of therapy. H_2-Blockers may also be helpful. Severe cases associated with wheezing, laryngeal edema, and circulatory collapse may require subcutaneous epinephrine, tracheal intubation, and systemic steroids.

FIXED DRUG ERUPTIONS

Describe a fixed drug eruption.

A fixed drug eruption is a reaction pattern consisting of well-circumscribed, erythematous or dusky-colored macules. The area may blister. Lesions are often preceded by a burning sensation, and they often heal with hyperpigmentation.

What are the 2 most common areas where fixed drug eruptions occur?

1. Mouth
2. Genitals

What are the 4 drugs that most commonly to cause fixed eruptions?

1. Sulfa
2. Phenopthalein
3. Tetracycline
4. NSAIDs

ERYTHEMA MULTIFORME, STEVENS-JOHNSON SYNDROME, AND TOXIC EPIDERMAL NECROLYSIS

Are EM, SJS, and TEN distinct disease processes?

Most people consider EM, SJS, and TEN to be along a continuum.

What is EM?

A syndrome characterized by symmetrically distributed, round lesions with concentric color changes (e.g. "targetoid"). These lesions are self-limited.

Name 2 precipitants of EM other than a drug reaction.

1. Herpes infections
2. Mycoplasmal infection

What is SJS?

A severe form of EM with marked oral mucosal and ocular involvement. These patients often develop extensive epidermal necrosis with large denuded areas (>10% body surface area). They often are systemically ill and may have a fever that precedes the rash.

What is TEN?

The most severe form of this reaction pattern spectrum. Most people define TEN as when more than 30% of the total body surface area is sloughed. TEN is almost always secondary to a drug reaction.

How is the diagnosis of SJS/TEN established?

The syndromes are diagnosed clinically. The histologic picture may not be diagnostic, but a biopsy should be performed to rule out other blistering processes.

Are systemic corticosteroids useful in SJS and TEN?

The use of systemic corticosteroids in the treatment of SJS and TEN is controversial. They may be useful in SJS early on in the disease, but they have also been associated with a higher complication rate and prolongation of disease if used too late. In frank TEN, steroids are contraindicated. New evidence suggests that IV immunuglobulin (IVIG) might be a better treatment for SJS/TEN.

What 3 conditions most commonly account for the mortality in SJS?

1. Bacterial septicemia
2. Fluid–electrolyte abnormalities
3. Organ failure

This condition is considered to be the equivalent of a large burn.

23

Musculoskeletal System

What are the 3 primary musculoskeletal concerns of the critically ill patient?	1. Early stabilization of broken bones 2. Management of soft-tissue injuries 3. Prevention of deleterious effects of immobilization

IMMOBILIZATION

What are 3 major problems associated with immobilization?	Patients are at increased risk of DVT, pressure ulcers, and contractures.
What can be done to prevent DVT?	SQ heparin (either unfractionated or LMW, if high risk); SCDs
How can the chance of developing contractures be lessened?	1. Keep muscles moving, even if passively 2. Apply splints to keep joints in neutral positions
What patient population is most susceptible to the untoward effects of immobilization?	The elderly

BONE FRACTURES

Which 3 types of bone fractures are most likely to be lethal or to significantly prolong hospitalization?	1. Pelvic fractures 2. Lower extremity long bone fractures 3. Spinal fractures
How much blood can a patient lose from a pelvic fracture?	The entire blood volume can be lost!

How can a pelvic fracture be diagnosed by clinical exam?

Screening pelvic radiographs should be obtained for all blunt trauma patients with a significant mechanism of injury. The practice of assessing pelvic stability by bimanual manipulation of the iliac crests is condemned by many, because it fails to identify 75% of all pelvic fractures and is painful (at best) for the alert patient.

What strategies can be used to minimize bleeding from pelvic fractures?

Pelvic stabilization with military antishock trousers (MAST), although this practice has fallen out of favor recently.

How should bleeding from a pelvic fracture be addressed if simple sta-bilization does not work?

Early angiography with embolization and operative fixation

What bones should be examined during the secondary or even tertiary radiographic surveys in trauma patients?

Any bone with an overlying skin abnormality (e.g., erythema, edema) or any area demonstrating tenderness on exam

What physical exam findings are associated with femur fractures?

The affected limb appears to be shortened, with the foot everted.

COMPLICATONS OF FRACTURES

What are 2 potentially lethal complications associated with lower extremity long bone fractures?

1. Fat emboli (immediately)
2. DVT or PE (later)

How can the risk of pulmonary complications from long bone fractures be reduced?

Early fixation (within 24–48 hours)

What is the incidence of DVT following trauma, and how can this risk be reduced?

The incidence of DVT in trauma patients is 8.8%. This risk is reduced to 2.9% when the patient is treated prophylactically with SQ heparin and SCDs.

What about DVT in patients with spinal cord injuries?

Patients with spinal cord injuries have a 27% incidence of DVT. This risk is reduced to 10% with use of *prophylactic* SQ heparin and SCDs.

What is fat embolism syndrome?

A constellation of signs and symptoms that occurs after major bone injury in which the lungs are showered with fat released from the bone marrow. In severe cases, it can result in ARDS or disseminated intravascular coagulation (DIC).

What is the classic triad for diagnosis of fat embolism syndrome?

1. Hypoxia
2. Confusion
3. Petechiae over the upper body

SOFT-TISSUE INJURIES AND PATHOLOGY

COMPARTMENT SYNDROME

What is compartment syndrome?

Increased pressure within a fascial compartment leading to inhibition of venous outflow and decrease of arterial inflow. Tissue ischemia and necrosis result if the syndrome is not recognized and treated immediately.

What are 5 specific etiologies of extremity compartment syndrome?

1. Trauma (most common)
2. Revascularization procedures with prolonged ischemia
3. DVT
4. External compression (MAST or dressings)
5. Bleeding secondary to anticoagulation

Where in the body are compartment syndromes most common?

Calf, forearm, and thigh

What are the 5 "P's" of compartment syndrome?	1. **P**ain out of proportion to physical exam 2. **P**aresthesias 3. **P**aralysis 4. **P**oikelothermia 5. **P**ulselessness
What is the first manifestation of compartment syndrome?	Pain out of proportion to physical exam
Why are decreased pulses and decreased capillary refill unreliable findings in compartment syndrome?	They occur late in the evolution of the condition, because flow through major vessels is usually maintained. Distal pulses may remain palpable even after irreversible muscle necrosis has occurred.
What are the 3 clinical "hallmarks" of compartmental hypertension?	1. Increased tissue tension 2. Neurologic and muscular dysfunction 3. Occlusion of venous outflow within the compartment
How is the diagnosis of compartment syndrome established?	By directly measuring the pressure within the compartments in question. This is done by attaching a simple hypodermic needle to a standard pressure monitor (typically used in the ICU to measure CVP or arterial pressure). The needle is advanced through the skin into the compartment, and the pressure can then be measured.
What compartment pressure is consistent with compartment syndrome?	30 mm Hg
When should compartment syndromes be treated?	Immediately!
How are compartment syndromes treated?	Open fasciotomy of all compartments in question (see Chapter 8)

RHABDOMYOLYSIS

What is rhabdomyolysis? Acute destruction of skeletal muscle

What are 8 major causes of rhabdomyolysis?
1. Crush injuries
2. Electrical burns
3. Acute muscular ischemia
4. Seizures
5. Infections
6. Hypokalemia
7. Toxins
8. Hypophosphatemia

How is rhabdomyolysis dangerous to the patient's cardiac status? Electrolyte and acid-base disturbances secondary to washout of injured muscle (e.g., lactic acid, K^+, etc.) can cause cardiac dysrhythmias.

What is the effect of rhabdomyolysis on the kidney? Resultant myoglobinuria can lead to acute tubular necrosis (ATN) and renal failure.

How is the diagnosis of rhabdomyolysis established?
1. Urinalysis positive for blood
2. No urinary erythrocytes
3. Urinary myoglobin assay

What is the treatment of rhabdomyolysis?
1. Prevent further muscle destruction.
2. Reduce the risk of ATN by producing a brisk diuresis with IV fluids. Additionally, the urine is alkalinized with IV sodium bicarbonate, which helps to prevent precipitation of myoglobin in the renal tubules.
3. Treat acidosis and hyperkalemia aggressively.
4. In extreme cases, early amputation may be considered to protect the patient's life.

Section 3   Pathologic Processes

24 Malnutrition

BASIC PRINCIPLES

Which patients are at highest risk for malnutrition?

Those with:
1. Pre-existing health problems
2. Poor socioeconomic conditions
3. Severe injury or illness

What are the human body's basal caloric needs?

25 to 35 kcal/kg/day (unless stressed)

How many kcal do carbohydrates, proteins, and fats provide?

Carbohydrates: 3.4 kcal/kg
Protein: 4 kcal/kg
Fat: 9 kcal/kg

What is the Harris-Benedict equation, and how is it used?

The equation used to determine basal metabolic rate (BMR) based on height, weight, age, and gender. Conversion factors are used for metabolic stressors (e.g., sepsis = 1.3 × BMR).

How does one calculate a BMR using the Harrison-Benedict equation?

Males: $66 + (13.7 \times wt) + (5 \times ht) - (6.8 \times age)$
Females: $655 + (9.6 \times wt) + (1.7 \times ht) - (4.7 \times age)$
Weight in kilograms, height in centimeters, age in years

In what 3 settings might actual body weight be unreliable when making nutritional calculations?

1. Obesity
2. Stressed or malnourished patients
3. Edema
In these settings, use a patient's ideal body weight (IBW).

How does one calculate IBW?

Males: 50 kg for the first 5 feet of height, 2.3 kg for each additional inch

Females: 45.5 kg for the first 5 feet of height, 2.3 kg for each additional inch

What constitutes obesity? Weight greater than 125% of IBW

What constitutes morbid obesity? Weight greater than 200% of IBW

What is corrected IBW (CIBW)? An equation used to calculate weight for nutritional purposes when the patient's actual weight is greater than 125% of IBW

How is CIBW calculated? $CIBW = IBW + (actual\ wt - IBW) \times 0.25$

What is the Fick method for determining caloric needs? Indirect calorimetry via PAC that calculates O_2 consumption and converts to kilocalories per day

What is the metabolic profile, and what information does it provide? Indirect calorimetry via alveolar gas analysis to determine caloric needs and a respiratory quotient (RQ).

What is RQ, and how is it used? RQ is the ratio of CO_2 production to O_2 consumption. It provides insight regarding substrate utilization: RQ = 1.0 with carbohydrate use and 0.7 with lipid use.

What is the preferred fuel of the colon? Short-chain fatty acids

What is the preferred fuel of the small bowel? Glutamine

What 4 supplements may improve immune function when included in nutritional formulations?
1. Arginine
2. Glutamine
3. Nucleotides
4. Omega-3 fatty acids

CARBOHYDRATES

Which tissues preferentially use glucose as an energy substrate?

Brain, RBCs, and renal medulla use glucose exclusively when it is available.

How does the body store carbohydrates?

300 g of glycogen are stored in liver and skeletal muscle and are converted to glucose by glucagon. This amount provides approximately 1,200 kcal in the unfed state, which lasts for approximately 24 hours.

At what rate should carbohydrates be administered?

1 kcal/kg/hr will maintain nitrogen balance. Lesser rates lead to glycogenolysis and gluconeogenesis, whereas greater rates lead to lipogenesis (all of which expend energy).

What is insulin resistance, and when does it occur?

Hyperglycemia despite elevated insulin levels. It is often seen in sepsis and severe trauma.

PROTEIN

What are the protein requirements of patients?

Normal patients: 1.0 g/kg/day
Stressed or critically ill patients:1.5 to
    2.0 g/kg/day
This is necessary to counteract protein
    catabolism.

What is the nitrogen balance?

Metabolic status with respect to protein turnover. The difference between nitrogen intake and output, it is used to approximate protein balance. Nitrogen balance is calculated as (protein intake)/6.25 − [(UUN × 0.8) + 1], where UUN is urinary urea nitrogen excretion (gm/24 hrs). Positive balance indicates anabolism; negative balance indicates catabolism.

How do you convert protein intake to nitrogen intake?

Protein is 16% nitrogen. Therefore, 1 g of nitrogen is in 6.25 g of protein.

What are 4 characteristics of protein malnutrition?	1. Poor wound healing 2. Anergy 3. Decreased transferrin, albumin, prealbumin, and lymphocytes 4. Easily pluckable hair Warning: The patient may look well nourished and still have protein malnutrition.
How do branched-chain amino acids benefit patients with hepatic failure/dysfunction?	Branched-chain amino acids (valine, leucine, isoleucine) are metabolized by skeletal muscle and, thereby, avoid hepatic processing for energy production. They also lessen encephalopathy by decreasing aromatic amino acid transport across the blood-brain barrier.

LIPIDS

Lipids should provide what portion of a patient's nonprotein calories?	Approximately 30% to provide a 70:30 ratio of carbohydrate calories to lipid calories unless the patient is in respiratory failure, in which case the lipid percentage should be higher
Why should the lipid percentage be higher for patients in respiratory failure?	Lipids have a lower RQ and produce less CO_2 per O_2 consumed compared to glucose.
Excessive infusion of omega-6 lipid solutions (linoleic acid/soybean oil) can lead to what clinical problem?	Omega-6 fatty acid causes an increase in prostaglandin E_2 levels, which suppresses monocyte function. Use of omega-3 fatty acid solutions does not increase prostaglandin E_2 levels and produces fewer immune-related complications.

INTENSIVE CARE UNIT NUTRITION

Where does nutritional support lie among patient care priorities in the ICU?	Airway, breathing, circulation, tissue oxygenation, acid-base balance, electrolyte balance, nutritional support

What are 4 relative indications for nutritional support in ICU patients?

1. Pre-existing malnutrition
2. When nutrition is not received for 5 to 7 days
3. An illness with an expected course of 7 to 10 days or longer
4. Hypermetabolic conditions: sepsis, burns, pancreatitis

What 4 proteins may be measured to assess nutritional status/protein catabolism?

1. Serum albumin
2. Transferrin
3. Prealbumin
4. Retinal-binding protein

What are the approximate half-lives of these proteins?

Albumin: 20 days
Transferrin: 9 days
Prealbumin: 2 days
Retinal-binding protein: 10 to 12 hours

In what 3 clinical settings might visceral protein measurements prove to be unreliable?

1. Decreased synthesis from causes other than malnutrition: liver failure
2. Increased losses from burns/wounds/ascites
3. Increased losses from some cancers that alter albumin/transferrin production

What are 4 indications of malnutrition?

1. Progressive loss of 10% of a patient's IBW during a 4- to 6-month period.
2. IBW less than 90%.
3. Rapid weight loss of more than 6% of body weight: this may mean a direct loss of muscle protein, which may be insufficient to maintain caloric needs.
4. Objectively: a serum albumin of less than 3.0 g/dL; albumin is an indicator of long-term nutritional status; serum prealbumin has a shorter half-life and is an indicator of short-term nutrition and, thus, replenishment.

When should an ICU patient undergo a nutritional status assessment?	On ICU day 2 and every 4 to 5 days thereafter

MODALITIES OF NUTRITIONAL SUPPORT

What are the 3 modalities of nutritional support that can be used?	1. Enteral nutrition 2. TPN 3. Peripheral parenteral nutrition (PPN)
What is the golden rule of surgical nutritional support?	If the gut works, use it.

ENTERAL NUTRITION

What is the preferred route of nutritional support?	Enteral feedings. They are cheaper, equally effective, and pose fewer complications than TPN and PPN. Also, they reduce villous atrophy and bacterial translocation.
When is supplemental enteral nutrition considered to be routine care?	1. Protein–calorie malnutrition, with inadequate oral intake of nutrients over the previous 5 days 2. Normal nutritional status but less than half the required oral intake of nutrients for the previous 7 to 10 days 3. Severe dysphagia 4. Major full-thickness burns 5. Massive small-bowel resection in combination with administration of TPN 6. Low-output enterocutaneous fistulas
Name 4 settings in which supplemental enteral nutrition usually is helpful.	1. Major trauma 2. Radiation therapy

3. Mild chemotherapy
4. Liver failure and severe renal dysfunction

Name 4 settings in which enteral nutrition is of limited or undetermined value.

1. Intensive chemotherapy
2. Immediate postoperative period or poststress period
3. Acute enteritis
4. More than 90% resection of small bowel

Name 8 contraindications to enteral nutrition.

1. Complete, mechanical intestinal obstruction
2. Ileus or intestinal hypomotility
3. Severe diarrhea
4. High-output external fistulas
5. Severe, acute pancreatitis
6. Shock
7. Aggressive nutritional support not desired by the patient or legal guardian
8. Prognosis not warranting aggressive nutritional support

What are 3 complications associated with enteral nutrition?

1. Aspiration: this complication can kill your patients. Be careful!
2. Diarrhea.
3. Metabolic abnormalities: hyperkalemia, hypokalemia, hyponatremia, hyperglycemia, hypophosphatemia.

What is the most frequent complication seen in patients receiving enteral nutrition?

Diarrhea. This can be treated by changing rate or osmolality. Opiates are useful after infectious etiologies are excluded.

What is the major risk when initiating enteral feedings in an ICU patient?

Aspiration and subsequent aspiration pneumonitis

What 4 conditions place the ICU patient at high risk for aspiration?	1. Endotracheal intubation 2. Sedation or obtundation 3. Nasogastric intubation 4. Supine positioning Remember, a tube in the airway does not prevent aspiration. Patients aspirate around cuffs.
What can be done to reduce the incidence of aspiration in patients receiving enteral nutrition?	Transpyloric or jejunal feedings. When using the gastric route, elevate the head to 45°. Stop if gastric residuals are more than 150 mL or if gastric dilation seems to be present on examination or CXR.
What is the top priority in enteral nutrition?	To be as certain as you possibly can to keep the food in the gut, preferably beyond the pylorus. The lungs are a very poor place to absorb nutrients!

TOTAL PARENTERAL NUTRITION

Name 5 settings in which TPN is considered to be routine care.	1. Malabsorption from:
	  a. Massive small-bowel resection
	  b. Impaired intestinal motility and absorption associated with small-bowel diseases
	  c. Radiation enteritis
	  d. Protracted diarrhea
	2. Bone marrow transplant patients receiving high-dose chemotherapy or radiation
	3. Moderate to severe pancreatitis
	4. Patients who have lost more than 10% of usual body weight
	5. Catabolic patients with or without evidence of malnutrition when the GI tract cannot be used for 5 to 7 days

Name 8 settings in which TPN usually is helpful.	1. After major surgery when an adequate enteral diet will not be resumed within 7 to 10 days

2. After stresses, such as moderate trauma or burns of 30% to 50% of body surface area, when an enteral diet cannot be resumed for more than 7 to 10 days
3. Enterocutaneous fistula
4. Inflammatory bowel disease
5. Hyperemesis gravidarum
6. In patients for whom adequate enteral nutrition cannot be initiated within 7 to 10 days of hospitalization
7. Small-bowel obstruction secondary to inflammatory lesions
8. Preoperatively: over 7 to 10 days

Name 3 settings in which TPN is of limited value.

1. Functional GI tract within a 10-day period in a well-nourished patient who endures minimal stress or trauma
2. Untreatable disease
3. Immediate postoperative period

What are 3 contra-indications to TPN?

1. A functional and usable GI tract
2. During a period of nutritional support estimated to be fewer than 5 days
3. When the risks of TPN are believed to exceed the potential benefits

What components can be ordered in TPN solution?

Dextrose, amino acids, lipids, electrolytes, vitamins, minerals, trace elements, and/or insulin, heparin, and H_2-blockers.

What lab studies are used to monitor ICU patients receiving TPN?

Daily electrolytes, BUN, and creatinine; blood glucose; Chem20 and magnesium daily for 3 days and twice weekly thereafter.

What change in TPN can be made for a ventilator-dependent patient with an RQ greater than 1.0?

Reduce the carbohydrate-to-lipid ratio to lower CO_2 production and ease the respiratory burden of CO_2 clearance. In other words, use more lipids.

Complications of Total Parenteral Nutrition

Complications	Possible Causes
Hematologic	Deficiencies of iron, vitamin B12, copper, or folic acid
GI	
Gallstone sludge	Prolonged (4–6 weeks) continuous parenteral nutrition
Increased LFTs	Overfeeding (fatty liver)
Pancreatitis	Hypertriglyceridemia; hypercalcemia
Mechanical	
Air embolism	Air enters open needle or catheter during insertion
Catheter embolism	Venous catheter sheared as it is pulled through the introducer needle
Catheter misplacement	Subclavian catheter into ipsilateral jugular vein, etc.
Pneumothorax	Insertion needle penetrates apical pleura
Thoracic duct laceration	Attempt to catheterize left subclavian vein
Venous thrombosis	Location of catheter (femoral vein); prolonged use of vein
Metabolic	
Azotemia	Renal insufficiency; too much protein
Hyperchloremic metabolic acidosis	Excess chloride content of crystalline amino acids
Hypocalcemia	Inadequate administration; hypoalbuminemia; after phosphorus repletion without calcium
Altered coagulation	Hypertriglyceridemia
Cyanosis	Altered pulmonary diffusion capacity
Essential fatty acid deficiency	Lack of essential fatty acids (linoleic acid, linolenic acid) in TPN
Pyrogenic reaction	Secondary to Intralipid (fat emulsion)
Hypertriglyceridemia	Rapid fat infusion; decreased clearance
Hyperglycemia (glycosuria, osmotic diuresis, ketoacidosis, hyperosmolar non-ketonic coma)	Inadequate endogenous or exogenous insulin; excess dose or rate of infusion of dextrose
Hypoglycemia	Persistence of exogenous insulin production secondary to prolonged stimulation of islet cells of high carbohydrate loads when TPN is stopped

Complications	Possible Causes
Metabolic (continued)	
Hypomagnesemia	Inadequate administration; cisplatin
Hypermagnesemia	Excess administration; renal failure; antacids or laxatives
Osteomalacia	Excess aluminum in casein hydrolysates
Hypophosphatemia	Inadequate administration, especially when patient becomes anabolic after starvation (refeeding syndrome); diabetic ketoacidosis; intracellular shift secondary to excess dextrose
Hypokalemia	Diuresis; inadequate intake; increased protein anabolism (refeeding)
Hyperkalemia	Excess administration; renal failure; metabolic acidosis
Night blindness	Deficiency of vitamin A (long-term TPN, Crohn's disease)
Refeeding syndrome	Aggressive TPN in malnourished patient; excess carbohydrate and sodium; hypophosphatemia
Sepsis	
Candidemia	Phagocyte dysfunction in patient with hypophosphatemia; overgrowth of Candida sp. in gut
Culture of catheter tip yields 1,000 organisms	Most common organisms are *Staphylococcus epidermidis, S. aureus, Klebsiella pneumonia,* and *Candida albicans.*

PERIPHERAL PARENTERAL NUTRITION

What are 2 limitations of PPN?

1. Difficult to meet 100% of nutritional needs
2. Increased risk of phlebitis and thrombosis if infused with high-osmolality solutions

What is the maximum total osmolality that can be used with PPN?

900 mOsm/L

What is the maximum allowable dextrose concentration for PPN?

10% dextrose. Greater concentrations will sclerose peripheral veins and, therefore, require central venous access.

What 2 actions can be taken to improve tolerance of PPN and avoid thrombosis and sclerosis of the utilized peripheral veins?	1. Administer subtherapeutic doses of heparin through the line to prevent thrombosis. 2. Low-dose hydrocortisone may reduce local inflammation.

NUTRITION IN SPECIAL POPULATIONS

Name 5 special accommodations that must be made in the nutritional planning for patients with renal insufficiency.	1. Fluid restriction 2. Low potassium/magnesium/phosphate 3. Lower protein 4. Calcium supplementation 5. Adequate provision of carbohydrate calories to maintain nitrogen balance in the face of low protein input.
Name 3 special accommodations that must be made in the nutritional support for prenatal patients.	1. Increased protein 2. Increased folate 3. Increased vitamin requirements
Name 4 special accommodations that must be made in the nutritional support for patients with hepatic failure.	1. Low protein: to avoid encephalopathy/hyperammonemia 2. Low salt/fluid: in the setting of ascites 3. Use of branch-chain amino acids 4. Metabolic changes with liver failure: may affect carbohydrate/lipid metabolism
Name 3 special accommodations that must be made in the nutritional support for patients with diabetes mellitus.	1. Close monitoring of blood sugar 2. Use of short-acting insulin regimens initially 3. Monitoring for "pseudohyponatremia," which can accompany elevated serum glucose

NUTRITIONAL END POINTS

What 3 considerations should guide nutritional supplementation?	1. Transition from PPN/TPN to gut feeding as soon as possible. 2. Start thinking about transitioning the patient to the most physiologically normal route of feeding they will tolerate from day 1. 3. Swallow/gastric-emptying studies/speech consults may be necessary to aid in this progression.

KEY EVIDENCE-BASED DATA YOU SHOULD KNOW

Veteran Affairs Total Parenteral Nutrition Cooperative Study. N Engl J Med 1991;325:525–532.	Showed similar rates of postoperative complications in patients receiving parenteral nutrition (PN) versus those who did not. The complications were, however, different in the two groups, with infectious complications more frequent in the PN group and noninfectious complications more common in the non-PN group. Concluded that preoperative PN improves postoperative course in patients with severe malnutrition, but also concluded that in mild to moderately malnourished patients, use of PN may outweigh benefits.
Muller J, et al. Preoperative parenteral feeding in patients with gastrointestinal carcinoma. Lancet 1982;i:68–71.	Demonstrated significantly decreased mortality in 125 patients with GI cancer when used PREOPERATIVELY.
Battistella FD, et al. A prospective, randomized trial of intravenous fat emulsion administration in trauma victims requiring TPN. J Trauma 1997;43:52–60.	IV infusions of fat emulsion during the early postinjury period increased susceptibility to infection, prolonged pulmonary failure, and delayed recovery in critically injured patients.

Davies AR, et al. Randomized comparison of nasojejunal and nasogastric feeding in critically ill patients. Crit Care Med 2002;30(3):586–590.

Demonstrated (n = 73) that postpyloric feedings significantly reduced gastric residual volume and improved tolerance of enteral feeding with very low requirement for parenteral nutrition.

Beale RJ, et al. Immunonutrition in the critically ill: a systematic review of clinical outcome. Crit Care Med 1999;27(12):2799–2805.

Meta-analysis of 15 randomized, controlled trials demonstrating that although present in all populations, the benefits of immunonutrition are most pronounced in surgical patients. Significant reductions in infection rates, ventilator days, and hospital length of stay were noted with the use of immunonutrition.

25 Infection

What 6 health maintenance issues related to infectious disease should be addressed frequently in your patients?

1. Vital signs: temperature, heart rate, blood pressure, finger stick blood glucose.
2. Cultures, WBC count, and differential when clinically indicated.
3. Antibiotics: review daily (trying to reduce number and duration).
4. Antifungal overgrowth control: consider nystatin powder and solutions.
5. Antifungal treatment: consider for unexplained sepsis, re-explorations, and immunosuppressed patients.
6. Wounds: check all, including line sites, daily.

DIAGNOSIS

What is the standard workup for fever?

1. History and physical exam
2. Examination of wounds, suture lines, line sites
3. Blood cultures from 2 sites (at least one peripheral)
4. Sputum culture
5. Urine culture
6. CXR
7. Change or rewiring of indwelling central lines if not done in the previous 3 to 5 days

What are the 5 W's of postoperative fever?

Wind: atelectasis, aspiration, pneumonia.
Water: urinary tract infection.
Wound: look at wound every day, starting with postoperative day 2 (or earlier if dehiscence is suspected).

Walking: DVT, pulmonary embolism.
Wonder drug: drug reactions.

A differential diagnosis of fever can be made by organ systems. What is the most common cause of fever in each of the following?

CNS	Meningitis
Respiratory system	Pneumonia, pulmonary embolism
Cardiovascular system	Endocarditis
GI system	Cholecystitis, colitis
Genitourinary system	Urinary tract infection
Hematologic system	Transfusion reaction
Wounds	Wound infection
Skin	Decubitus ulcers
Monitoring equipment	Intravascular catheter-related infection

What are 8 risk factors for infection in the ICU?

1. Immunocompromised patient
2. Multisystem organ failure (MSOF)/severity of illness
3. TPN
4. Broad-spectrum antibiotic usage
5. Hyperglycemia
6. Malnutrition
7. Ventilator dependence
8. Age

What 3 relatively unusual sites of infection are more prevalent in the ICU?

1. Central lines
2. Sinuses
3. CNS

Why are sinuses at risk?

Because of tubes, such as NGTs. The worst offenders are nasotracheal tubes.

What 3 etiologies most often account for persistent fever in the ICU?

1. An undiagnosed site of infection: lines, sinuses, CNS, abdomen
2. Noninfectious etiology: drugs

3. Organisms not treated by current antibiotics: resistant bacteria, viruses, and fungi (if a patient remains persistently febrile in the ICU, especially a diabetic who has a central line and is receiving TPN, assume fungus until proven otherwise)

WOUND INFECTIONS

What are 9 common causes of impaired host defenses in surgical patients?

1. Diabetes mellitus
2. Malnutrition
3. Uremia
4. Trauma
5. Burns
6. Steroids
7. Malignancy
8. Chemotherapy
9. Radiation therapy

What are 4 categories of surgical wounds?

1. Clean: no trauma; no entry into GI, genitourinary, or respiratory tract
2. Clean-contaminated: GI tract, respiratory tract, or oropharynx entered; sterile biliary/GI tract entered; minor break in technique
3. Contaminated: acute inflammation, infected bile or urine, gross GI tract spillage
4. Dirty: established infection

What antibiotic prophylaxis should be used to prevent surgical wounds?

Cefazolin will cover skin organisms, enteric Gram-negative organisms, and some oral anaerobes. Use combination therapy, cefoxitin (biliary and colonic) or cefuroxime (head and neck), in procedures requiring better anaerobic coverage.

When should antibiotic prophylaxis be given?

30 minutes before incision

Do clean wounds or procedures require antibiotic prophylaxis?	No
What is the threshold bacterial load at which contamination and subsequent wound infection are thought to occur?	100,000 colony-forming units per gram of tissue
How should heavily contaminated wounds be closed?	By delayed primary closure after 3 to 5 days
What organisms can cause infections presenting in the first 24 hours after surgery?	β-Streptococci and clostridial infections
What constitutes appropriate sterile technique for a bedside patient procedure?	1. Wear a mask and eye shield (to comply with universal precautions). 2. Prep thoroughly with antiseptic solution. 3. Prep an area many times larger than seems to be necessary. 4. Use towels to block off the site. 5. Don a sterile gown and gloves. 6. Cover everything with 3 to 4 feet of sterile drapes if possible. 7. Do not let the back end of J-wires hit nonsterile objects.

INTRA-ABDOMINAL INFECTIONS

What is bacterial translocation?	The movement of enteric bacteria into normally sterile body spaces (e.g., lymph nodes, portal vein) despite an intact GI tract
What 4 conditions are felt to predispose to translocation?	1. Severe trauma 2. Burns 3. Sepsis 4. Absence of food in gut

Which bacteria most commonly translocate?

Gram-negative rods

What is the clinical relevance of translocation?

Unknown. Translocation may predispose patients to the hematogenous spread of infection.

Name 3 ways that enteral nutrition might improve immune defenses.

1. Decreases bacterial translocation by employing bacteria in lumen in digestion; alters diffusion gradient.
2. Improves blood flow to the gut.
3. Provides immune-enhancing elements for enterocyte metabolism (glutamine).

What should be considered in a patient with fever and diarrhea, and/or leukocytosis?

Clostridium difficile diarrhea

How is *C. difficile* diarrhea diagnosed?

C. difficile toxin is found in stool.

What is the relationship between antibiotic administration and development of *C. difficile* diarrhea?

Antibiotic use decolonizes the gut of its normal flora, allowing *C. difficile* organism and toxin overgrowth. Clindamycin has the highest incidence of associated *C. difficile* diarrhea, but almost any antibiotic can be to blame.

What is the treatment of *C. difficile* diarrhea?

1. IV or oral metronidazole or oral vancomycin
2. Stopping other antibiotics, if possible
3. Recolonization of bowel
4. Enteral feeds

What serious complications are associated with *C. difficile* diarrhea?

Pseudomembranous colitis progressing to toxic megacolon and colonic perforation

Name 5 situations in which peritonitis should be suspected.	1. Prolonged ileus 2. Continued sepsis despite antibiotics 3. Drainage from abdominal wound 4. Unexplained fever, tachycardia, or leukocytosis 5. Increasing abdominal pain and distension
How can peritonitis be diagnosed in an intubated, unresponsive patient?	Obtain an abdominal CT scan to locate fluid collections and evidence of organ inflammation.
What is tertiary peritonitis?	Recurrent or persistent peritonitis following previous intervention for intra-abdominal infection. It carries a high rate of mortality.
What 5 organisms are commonly associated with tertiary peritonitis?	1. Yeast 2. *Staphylococcus epidermidis* 3. *Pseudomonas* sp. 4. *Enterobacter* sp. 5. *Enterococcus* sp.
How is tertiary peritonitis treated?	1. Administer broad-spectrum antibiotics, including antifungal treatment. 2. Repair or divert source of infection in GI tract. 3. May require frequent re-operations to decontaminate diffusely diseased peritoneal cavity.
Name 4 common sites of intra-abdominal abscess.	1. Subdiaphragmatic 2. Sub-hepatic 3. Interloop 4. Pelvic
What are 5 principles of managing intra-abdominal abscess?	1. Place a percutaneous drain if possible, and culture drainage. 2. Start empiric antibiotics that cover Gram-positive organisms, Gram-negative enteric organisms, and anaerobes.

3. Change antibiotics as dictated by culture sensitivities.
4. Remove drain when sepsis resolves or drainage is less than 25 mL/day
5. Rescan if improvement occurs within 72 hours.

NECROTIZING SOFT-TISSUE INFECTIONS

How can necrotizing fasciitis be recognized?

Severe pain out of proportion to local findings (red, hot, shiny, and swollen without sharp demarcation), along with systemic toxicity. A plain radiograph may illustrate gas in the "soft tissue, suggesting clostridial infection.

What are 5 risk factors for developing necrotizing fasciitis?

1. Peripheral vascular disease
2. IV drug use
3. Immunosuppression from diabetes, malignancy, or alcoholism
4. Obesity
5. Malnutrition

What organism is most commonly isolated in necrotizing fasciitis?

It is usually polymicrobial: Gram-positive staphylococci, streptococci, and clostridia; Gram-negative enteric bacteria and anaerobes. Monomicrobial infections are most often streptococci, staphylococci, or clostridia.

What is the definitive treatment of necrotizing fasciitis?

Aggressive surgical debridement to healthy, bleeding tissue combined with broad-spectrum antibiotic therapy

What are the antibiotics of choice for necrotizing fasciitis?

Coverage should be broad spectrum:
Penicillin G to cover clostridia
Vancomycin or semisynthetic penicillin to cover Gram-positive organisms
Aminoglycoside or monobactam to cover Gram-negative organisms

Clindamycin or metronidazole to cover anaerobes

What is the mortality rate of necrotizing fasciitis?

At least 20%. This infection advances rapidly, with delay in treatment being associated with progressive MSOF and poor outcomes.

What is the term for necrotizing infection of the perineum?

Fournier's gangrene. This condition is seen most often in diabetic patients.

FUNGAL INFECTIONS

Which fungus is most commonly isolated in the ICU?

Candida albicans

What 7 conditions are believed to predispose to fungal infection?

1. Long-term antibiotic use
2. Diabetes
3. Fistulae
4. Central venous catheters
5. Severe illness
6. Burns
7. Immunosuppression

What are the 3 most common indications for the treatment of fungus in the ICU?

1. Multiple (>2) sites of fungal colonization
2. Persistent fever
3. Leukocytosis despite adequate antibacterial coverage

What are 5 common sites of fungal colonization?

1. Urine
2. Sputum
3. Wound
4. Nasopharynx
5. Intertriginous folds

What is the rationale for treating multiple sites of fungal colonization?

Retrospective studies have shown an association between more than 2 sites of colonization and eventual fungemia.

From simplest to most aggressive, what are the 4 options for treating candiduria?	1. Removal Foley, and reculture in 48 hours 2. Intracystic instillation of amphotericin B for 3 to 5 days 3. IV fluconazole 4. IV amphotericin B
What is the usual dose of amphotericin B used to treat fungal infections in the ICU?	5 to 8 mg/kg total, given as 0.3 to 1.0 mg/kg/day
How is amphotericin usually administered?	In a daily dose
What are 5 side effects associated with amphotericin?	1. Nausea 2. Vomiting 3. Fever 4. Rigors 5. Vasodilatation
Name 2 ways in which these side effects of amphotericin can be avoided.	1. Administration of amphotericin as a continuous infusion 2. Pretreatment with antihistamine
Name 2 other serious side effects associated with amphotericin.	1. Anemia 2. Nephrotoxicity with associated renal tubular acidosis, increased creatinine and decreased potassium
What should be done in the setting of renal dysfunction?	Use liposomal or lipid complex amphotericin B or another antifungal agent (e.g., fluconazole) if possible.
Name 4 ways in which the sites of fungal overgrowth can be managed to attempt to decrease fungal infections.	1. Nystatin mouth rinse 2. Nystatin in gut 3. Mycostatin powder for intertriginous folds 4. Nystatin suppositories in vagina and rectum

Name 3 settings in which amphotericin should be given empirically.

1. Persistent fever or sepsis in ICU patients thought to be covered with antibiotics
2. Re-explorations of immunocompromised patients
3. Recurrent bowel perforation

HOSPITAL-ACQUIRED INFECTIONS AND RESISTANT ORGANISMS

What 8 factors place patients at risk for hospital-acquired infections?

1. Advanced age
2. System or organ failure
3. Loss of barrier function: injury/surgery to skin or mucosa
4. Presence of foreign body: indwelling devices (urinary catheter, central line, endotracheal tube)
5. Immunodeficiency
6. Anesthesia/sedation
7. Antibiotics
8. Colonization with opportunistic or resistant bacteria/fungi

What are the most common organisms exhibiting antibiotic resistance?

Staphylococcus aureus: methicillin
Enterococcus sp.: vancomycin
Pseudomonas sp.: β-lactams, cephalosporins, aminoglycosides
Klebsiella sp., *Escherichia coli*: penicillins and cephalosporins (because of extended-spectrum β-lactamases)
Enterobacter sp., *Acinetobacter* sp.: 3rd-generation cephalosporins
Candida sp: fluconazole

How should the physician control the spread of resistant organisms?

1. Barrier methods: contact isolation, use of gloves
2. Hand hygiene: washing, alcohol hand gels
3. Formulary restriction: limited access to broad-spectrum antibiotics
4. Selection of empiric antibiotics on a rotating schedule: antibiotic cycling

5. Narrowing antibiotic coverage when possible
6. Following cultures carefully to identify patterns of resistance

Which 2 organisms may require "double-coverage" (i.e., 2-drug antibiotic therapy)?

1. *Pseudomonas* sp.
2. *Enterococcus* sp. (particularly for endocarditis)

Enterobacter sp. and *Acinetobacter* sp. may also qualify.

What is the importance of *Pseudomonas aeruginosa*?

It is the second most common cause of nosocomial pneumonia (after *Staphylococcus aureus*) and the most common Gram-negative rod.

Which 6 antibiotics have significant antipseudomonal activity?

1. Antipseudomonal penicillins: piperacillin
2. Imipenem/meropenem
3. Ciprofloxacin
4. Ceftazidime
5. Cefepime
6. Aztreonam

Are aminoglycosides effective?

They still have reasonable activity against *Pseudomonas* sp., but not against *Enterococcus* sp., and the risk of nephro- and ototoxicity mandates careful blood-level monitoring.

What is the treatment for significant *Enterococcus faecalis* infections?

High-dose ampicillin plus gentamicin, or vancomycin

What about vancomycin-resistant *Enterococcus* sp.?

Most isolates reflect colonization, which is not generally treated. Infection can be treated with linezolid.

What is the treatment of significant *Enterobacter cloacae* or *E. aerogenes* infections?

An aminoglycoside, imipenem/meropenem or (possibly) piperacillin-tazobactam. Never use a 3rd-generation cephalosporin because of the rapid development of resistance.

What are the 4 classic criteria for the diagnosis of hospital-acquired pneumonia?

1. A single or a predominant organism on adequate sputum culture obtained more than 48 hours after admission
2. Leukocytosis
3. Pyrexia or hypothermia
4. New infiltrate on CXR

Some hospitals require quantitative cultures.

What is the approximate mortality rate of hospital-acquired pneumonia in nonimmunocompromised, mechanically ventilated patients?

20% to 40%

What 2 central venous line locations have the greatest incidence of infection?

1. Femoral
2. IJ

The femoral location has a higher incidence of infection than the IJ location.

What central venous line locations have the lowest incidence of infection?

Subclavian

If a line is suspected of being infected, what do you do?

Rewire, and send the tip of catheter for culture. With a high suspicion of infection, consider inserting a new catheter at a new site instead of rewiring.

What culture result requires insertion of a new line at a new site?

More than 15 colonies of bacteria

What 4 factors contribute to line infections?

1. Lipid-based IV solutions
2. High-concentration dextrose solution
3. Manipulations
4. Difficult sites for dressings

Name 4 measures that may decrease line infections.

1. Employ strict sterile technique when inserting, manipulating, or using a line for infusions or draws.
2. Use chlorhexidine, not betadine, for skin prep.
3. Remove the line as soon as it is not required for care.
4. Maintain clean, well-dressed sites.

SEPSIS

What is the difference between SIRS, sepsis, and septic shock?

SIRS is the systemic inflammatory response syndrome, a generalized immune response to severe illness. SIRS can be called "sepsis" if the etiology is infectious. Septic shock is sepsis with hypotension, organ failure, and perfusion abnormalities despite fluid resuscitation.

What are the criteria for diagnosing SIRS?

2 or more of the following must be present and represent a change in the patient's condition:
1. Temperature greater than 38°C or less than 36°C
2. Heart rate greater than 90 bpm
3. Respiratory rate less than 20 breaths per minute or an arterial partial pressure of carbon dioxide ($PaCO_2$) less than 32 mm Hg
4. WBC greater than 12 $10^3/mm^3$ or less than 4 $10^3/mm^3$ or left shift (>10% bands)

What changes in coagulation can you expect to see in SIRS?

Procoagulant state: consumptive coagulopathy associated with decreases in antithrombin III and protein C

How can coagulopathy be treated?

1. Correct hypothermia.
2. Transfuse fresh frozen plasma to correct INR/PTT
3. Give platelets if platelet count is less than 100,000/mm^3

4. Administer vitamin K in the setting of Coumadin use or liver disease.
5. Rule out other causes: renal failure, drugs such as aspirin that inactivate platelets
6. IF patient has severe sepsis, use activated protein C.

Which 2 cytokines most closely reproduce the septic response in animal models?

1. Interleukin-1
2. Tumor necrosis factor

Which cytokine is most consistently elevated in clinical sepsis and is correlated with a bad outcome?

Interleukin-6

What is MSOF?

Multisystem organ failure; a condition associated in some cases with the end stage of sepsis and other systemic inflammatory syndromes. Multisystem organ dysfunction syndrome indicates a lesser degree of organ impairment and may precede MSOF.

What 5 organ systems are most commonly affected by multisystem organ dysfunction syndrome, and how does organ failure present?

1. Respiratory: respiratory insufficiency with difficulty in oxygenation and ventilation
2. Cardiovascular: hypotension, shock
3. Renal: oliguria, anuria
4. Hepatic: hepatic liver enzyme dysfunction, hepatic synthetic function
5. Immune: untreatable sepsis

What are the approximate mortality rates associated with increasing numbers of systems involved?

1 system: 10%
2 systems: 30%
3 systems: 70%
4 or 5 systems: 80%

26 Immunosuppression

GENERAL

What are the anatomic components of the immune system?

Primary lymphoid organs (bone marrow and thymus) and secondary lymphoid organs (lymph nodes, spleen, Peyer's patches, bronchial-associated lymphoid tissue, and mucosa-associated lymphoid tissue)

What 2 types of patients are very immunosuppressed?

1. Transplant patients
2. Patients with acquired immune deficiency syndrome (AIDS)

What 3 types of patients are relatively immunosuppressed?

1. Patients with autoimmune diseases treated using immunosuppressive agents (arthritics treated with methotrexate)
2. Patients taking steroids (lung disease)
3. Severely injured patients (trauma, burns)

What 3 types of patients are somewhat immunosuppressed?

1. Patients with diabetes
2. Patients who have just been on cardiopulmonary bypass
3. Patients at the extremes of age

What are 4 categories of defective immunity and their causes?

1. Anatomic barrier breakdown: burns, mucus membrane ulceration
2. Defective phagocytosis: leukemia, cytotoxic agents, neutropenia
3. Altered humoral immunity: lymphoma, hypogammaglobulinemia, splenectomy, multiple myeloma
4. Impaired cell-mediated immunity: human immunodeficiency virus

(HIV), antirejection medications (cyclosporine, azathioprine)

What category of pathogens takes advantage of defective humoral immunity?

Encapsulated bacteria (*Streptococcus pneumoniae, Haemophilus influenzae, Neisseria meningitidis*)

What 5 categories of pathogens take advantage of defective cell-mediated immunity?

1. Viruses (varicella, herpes, cytomegalovirus)
2. Protozoa (*Pneumocystis carinii, Toxoplasma gondii*)
3. Fungi (*Candida* sp., *Cryptococcus neoformans, Histoplasma capsulatum*)
4. Mycobacteria (*Mycobacterium avium-complex, Mycobacterium tuberculosis*)
5. Intracellular (*Listeria* sp., *Salmonella* sp., *Legionella* sp.)

What are 3 reasons why it is important to have an idea of a patient's immune competency?

1. They may have infections or tumors that are difficult to find.
2. They may have unusual infections with organisms of low intrinsic pathogenicity, and they may have rapidly growing tumors.
3. They may have difficult-to-treat (resistant) infections or tumors.

What are 6 health maintenance guidelines for patients who are known to be immunosuppressed?

1. Follow blood counts to watch for marrow suppression.
2. Follow cyclosporine levels.
3. Monitor blood pressure and creatinine in a patient receiving cyclosporine.
4. Review prophylactic medications, such as Bactrim and acyclovir, to be sure they are being administered properly.
5. Pay extra attention to potential sites of occult infection (e.g., perineum, CNS).

6. Monitor for possible exposure to pathogens, such as from contaminated water or exposure to people with communicable diseases.

What type of tumors do immunosuppressed patients have?

1. Transplant patients: can have explosive or resistant growth of any type of tumor, but the most common tumor associated with immunosuppression is lymphoma. Other tumors are usually epithelial (skin, cervix, etc.).
2. AIDS patients: can have many tumors, but Kaposi's sarcoma is the classic AIDS-related tumor.

What type of infections can immunocompromised patients (including those on therapeutic steroids) have?

1. Any type, and even usually benign agents can be virulent in these patients.
2. Viral infections are common, especially with the DNA viruses (cytomegalovirus, herpes simplex virus).
3. Also prone to contract *Pneumocystis carinii,* resistant tuberculosis, and toxoplasmosis.
4. Fungal infections are prevalent.

What sort of workup should you do for immunocompromised patients (including those on therapeutic steroids) who may have an infection?

1. Get a good history (exposures, animals in house, symptoms, prophylactic drugs being taken, history of the current illness, etc.).
2. Examine the patient. (The abdominal examination will be less reliable than in the usual patient.)
3. Round up the usual suspects (blood, urine, sputum, CXR).
4. Consider moving quickly to less common tests (LP, chest and abdominal CT, sinus films, stool culture) guided by the clinical situation.

5. Remember that a patient taking steroids may have a normal abdominal examination, even in the situation of a perforated viscus; thus, obtain plain films of the abdomen, including an upright film to look for free air.

HUMAN IMMUNODEFICIENCY VIRUS

How do you measure the severity of immunodeficiency in patients with HIV?

Measure CD4 lymphocytes.

What is the normal range of CD4 lymphocytes?

800 to 1,200 cells/mL

What level of CD4 lymphocytes signifies severe immunocompromise and possible inability to heal wounds?

50 cells/mL

What are the 3 primary reasons why patients with HIV are admitted to the ICU?

1. Pneumonia
2. Cryptococcal meningitis
3. Toxoplasmic encephalitis

What is the classic cause of pneumonia in a patient with HIV, and how is it treated?

Pneumocystis carinii. Treat with Bactrim or dapsone.

Will a patient with HIV and cryptococcal meningitis present with signs of meningeal irritation?

Only approximately 25% present with meningismus. Many will only have fever. Therefore, have a high index of suspicion, and consider LP sooner than you would in an immunocompetent patient.

27

Neoplasia

OVERVIEW AND EPIDEMIOLOGY

Where does cancer rank as a cause of mortality in the United States?

Second. It accounts for 22% of all deaths.

List the 3 most common cancers in men.

1. Lung
2. Prostate
3. Colorectal

List the 3 most common cancers in women.

1. Breast
2. Colorectal
3. Uterine

What are the approximate overall 5-year survival rates for cancer patients?

Men: 30%
Women: 50%

Name 4 epidemiological factors associated with cancer.

1. Geographic and ethnic patterns
2. Dietary, chemical, viral, and physical agents
3. Hormonal factors
4. Familial influences

BIOLOGY OF NEOPLASIA

Do most tumors arise from groups of transformed cells or from single cells?

Most tumors arise from a single transformed (or mutated) cell.

Name the 3 stages of carcinogenesis.

1. Initiation
2. Promotion
3. Progression

What is the term for the cumulative acquisition of mutations leading to invasive cancer?

Multistep carcinogenesis

Name 2 fundamental properties of mutated cells.

1. Escape from normal growth regulation
2. Passage of the transformed genome to daughter cells

Approximately how many doublings does it take for a solid tumor originating from a single cell to become clinically detectable (1 g or 1 cm³)?

Approximately 30

What is the growth fraction of a tumor?

The percentage of tumor cells in the tumor mass undergoing replication (i.e., S phase)

Why is the growth fraction important?

Along with the cell loss fraction, it is a primary determinant of the clinical growth of a tumor.

What are the 4 principle ways in which tumors may metastasize?

1. Direct extension
2. Spread through a cavity
3. Lymphatic dissemination
4. Hematogenously

Describe the components of the TNM staging system.

T: size and extent of primary tumor
N: degree of nodal involvement
M: presence and extent of distant metastases

What is the function of the p53 gene?

The p53 gene induces growth arrest after DNA damage and helps to direct cell towards apoptosis.

What are the rate and significance of p53 mutations?

p53 is mutated in approximately 55% of tumors, which may contribute to resistance to apoptosis-inducing therapies.

Tumor Markers, Antigens, and Hormones

Tumor Markers, Antigens and Hormones	Associated Cancer
Carcinoembryonic antigen	Colorectal, pancreatic, gastric, and breast cancer
Alpha-fetoprotein	Hepatoma and nonseminomatous testicular cancer
Prostate-specific antigen	Prostate cancer
CA 15-3	Breast, ovarian, and lung cancer
CA 19-9	Pancreatic, colon, and gastric cancer
CA 125	Nonmucinous ovarian cancer
B-HCG	Gestational trophoblastic and nonseminomatous testicular tumors
Her2-neu	Breast cancer
BRCA1	Breast and ovarian cancer
BRCA2	Breast cancer (male and female)
APC	Colorectal cancer
DCC	Colorectal cancer
RET proto-oncogene	Medullary thyroid cancer

TREATMENT PRINCIPLES

SURGICAL DIAGNOSIS AND TREATMENT

Name the 4 different types of biopsies.
1. Fine-needle aspiration
2. Core biopsy
3. Incisional biopsy
4. Excisional biopsy

What type of biopsy should be used for extremity sarcomas?
Excisional for those less than 4 cm; otherwise, longitudinal incisional biopsy (less lymphatic disruption and easier excision of the scar)

Name 4 situations in which a biopsy not needed.
1. When it would not alter the extent of the operation
2. When it carries unacceptable risk
3. When it complicates subsequent extirpative therapy
4. When it is not easily obtained

List the 4 factors that determine margins of resection for primary tumors.

1. Location
2. Capacity for local spread
3. Potential for multifocal disease
4. Blood supply to the organ to be resected

Is surgery ever indicated for metastatic disease?

Yes

Name 3 indications for surgery for metastatic disease.

1. When there is a low likelihood of additional occult metastases
2. When there is a low morbidity to the operation
3. When medical therapies are not available or effective

What 2 metastatic tumors have had the best outcomes with regard to resection?

1. Liver metastases from colorectal cancer
2. Pulmonary metastases from sarcoma

RADIATION THERAPY

How does radiation therapy work?

By direct effects (chromosomal DNA breaks) and by indirect effects (generation of free radicals)

How does hypoxia affect radiation therapy?

Hypoxic tumors are relatively radioresistant.

What is a gray?

The energy absorbed per unit of mass (1 gray = 100 rads)

How does cell cycle affect radiation therapy?

Cells in mitosis (i.e., M phase) are most sensitive to radiation therapy.

List the potential acute and late complications of radiation therapy.

Acute: injury to rapidly proliferating tissues (e.g., the GI tract, skin, and lymphoid tissues)
Late: necrosis, fibrosis, fistula formation, and organ-specific damage

GI reactions occur when cumulative radiation doses exceed what levels?

>4,000 to 5,500 cGy

What 3 types of GI reactions are common in patients receiving radiation treatment?	1. Esophagitis 2. Gastritis 3. Enteritis
Name 6 symptoms of GI reactions in patients receiving radiation treatment.	1. Pain 2. Nausea 3. Vomiting 4. Diarrhea 5. Bleeding 6. Loss of appetite
What side effect may occur after radiation is delivered to a significant lung volume?	Radiation pneumonitis. This usually occurs 2 to 3 months after treatment and is characterized by cough, dyspnea, and chest pain.
What is the treatment of radiation pneumonitis?	Corticosteroids

CHEMOTHERAPY

Chemotherapy is most effective for what type of tumor burden?	Micrometastatic disease (in which all the clinically evident cancer has been removed and metastases are too small to be apparent)
What are 4 different methods of timing chemotherapy?	1. Induction: chemotherapy as the primary treatment; curative or palliative 2. Salvage: for patients who have failed previous chemotherapy regimens 3. Adjuvant: therapy after the primary tumor has been treated by excision and/or radiation therapy for patients with high risk of developing recurrent disease 4. Neoadjuvant: therapy before surgery and/or radiation to improve resectability and organ preservation
How is response to chemotherapy characterized?	1. Complete: regression of all evident disease for at least 4 weeks or 1 treatment cycle

2. Partial: reduction of the tumor by 50% to 99% for at least 4 weeks or 1 treatment cycle
3. Minor: less than 50% reduction in size or less than 4-week duration of response

What is the major advantage to combination chemotherapy?

The increased chance to overcome drug resistance by using agents with different modes of action

PATIENT MANAGEMENT

What is the most common cause of death in patients with metastatic cancer?

Organ failure from tumor invasion

Is bleeding a common cause of death in patients with cancer?

Yes. Bleeding is the third most common cause of cancer death in patients with metastatic cancer, following organ failure from tumor invasion and infection. It is the second most common cause of death in patients with hematologic neoplasms.

List 3 conditions that are likely to end a cancer patient's life suddenly or prematurely.

1. PE
2. Blood loss: hemoptysis from lung cancer
3. Pericardial tamponade from malignant pleural effusion

GASTROINTESTINAL ISSUES

What are the 3 most common GI problems requiring operation in patients with cancer?

1. Obstruction
2. Hemorrhage
3. Perforation

Obstruction and Ileus

What is the most common cause of bowel obstruction in cancer patients?

Primary or metastatic malignancy, followed by benign causes such as adhesions and radiation enteritis (as opposed to the predominantly benign causes of obstruction seen in the overall population with bowel obstruction)

What is the most common type of obstructing tumor?

Adenocarcinoma of the colon or rectum

How is bowel obstruction typically treated?

Initially, resuscitation involves making the patient NPO (nothing through the mouth), administration of IV fluids, and insertion of an NGT. In the case of an obstructing tumor, this may be followed by resection of the tumor.

What are 5 factors resulting in the syndromes of ileus and pseudo-obstruction in oncology patients?

1. Narcotics
2. Anticholinergic medications: many antiemetics
3. Chemotherapeutic agents: particularly vincristine
4. Electrolyte imbalance
5. Tumor-related disruption of autonomic supply

GI Hemorrhage

What are the most common sources of GI bleeding in patients with cancer?

Peptic ulcer disease and gastritis, often exacerbated by thrombocytopenia, coagulopathy, and corticosteroid use. Hemorrhage from tumors is less common.

What are 4 other causes of bleeding in the cancer patient?

1. Thrombocytopenia
2. Abnormalities in plasma levels of coagulation factors
3. Circulating inhibitory factors
4. Drugs

What types of drugs may cause bleeding, and how?

Aspirin, other nonsteroidal analgesics, corticosteroids, chemotherapy, and antimicrobials can cause GI mucosal ulceration or have direct effects on the level of platelets, their function, or the circulating coagulation factors.

What is the most common cause of thrombocytopenia in the cancer patient?

Chemotherapy

Is acute life-threatening GI hemorrhage common in the cancer patient?

No. Most episodes of bleeding are minor and not of hemodynamic significance.

Acute life-threatening GI hemorrhage in the cancer patient results from what?

Hemorrhage can result from hemostatic abnormalities or structural pathology, such as mucosal chemotoxicity, radiation enteritis, or erosions and ulcerations because of neoplasm or infection.

Which 3 types of neoplasms are most commonly associated with upper GI bleeding in which bleeding is directly caused by the neoplasm?

1. Gastric lymphoma
2. Gastric leiomyosarcoma
3. Gastric carcinoma

Is gastric carcinoma a common cause of upper GI bleeding?

No. It only accounts for approximately 5% of all upper GI bleeding.

What are 4 other, less common causes of acute upper GI bleeding in the cancer patient?

1. Mallory-Weiss syndrome
2. Esophageal varices secondary to:
   a. Cirrhosis and portal hypertension
   b. Massive hepatic replacement by tumor
   c. Acute portal vein thrombosis
3. Acute erosive fungal or viral esophagitis
4. Biliary tract hemorrhage

How is Mallory-Weiss syndrome related to the cancer patient?

Several authors have reported Mallory-Weiss syndrome in cancer patients with chemotherapy-induced vomiting.

In patients presenting with massive lower GI bleeding, what percentage of cases are the result of a cancer or polyp?

Approximately 10%

Enterocolitis

Describe the clinical syndrome of neutropenic enterocolitis.

Neutropenic enterocolitis, also known as typhlitis, affects patients who are neutropenic from chemotherapy and usually is seen in the setting of hematologic malignancies. It consists of febrile neutropenia, abdominal pain (principally right lower quadrant), distention, and diarrhea. The diagnosis is one of exclusion, and CT findings of bowel wall thickening affecting the ileum and right colon, often with pneumatosis, are helpful but inconstant and nonspecific.

What is the treatment of neutropenic enterocolitis?

Complete bowel rest with total parenteral nutrition and broad-spectrum antibiotics. Indications for surgery include progressive symptoms, sepsis, hemorrhage, or perforation. Surgery generally requires right hemicolectomy and ileostomy.

PULMONARY ISSUES

Embolism

Name 3 causes of PE in the cancer patient.

1. Hypercoagulable state induced by the neoplasm or chemotherapy
2. Compression of vessels or obstruction of venous blood flow by tumor
3. Surgery: immobility, hypercoagulable state, etc.

PEs that result in sudden death usually occlude more than what percentage of the pulmonary vascular bed?

50%

Why are prompt recognition and treatment so important in the patient with suspected PE?

75% to 90% of those who die do so within the first few hours of the embolic event.

What is the overall mortality rate of PE?	If unrecognized and untreated, 30% to 35%
Where do most PEs originate?	In the deep venous system of the proximal lower extremities and, less commonly, in the pelvis
What are the "classic" ECG findings in a patient with a PE?	The classic S_1Q_3 pattern with right-axis deviation and right bundle branch block. The ECG may actually be normal but often shows sinus tachycardia, inverted T waves, or nonspecific ST-T wave abnormalities.
What should be the initial diagnostic test in a patient with suspected PE?	High-resolution CT (CTPA)
What other diagnostic tests could be performed in a patient with suspected PE?	V/Q scan and pulmonary angiogram
Does a normal V/Q scan rule out PE?	A normal scan suggests a less than 1% chance of a major embolus.
What is the chance of an embolus with a high-probability scan?	A high-probability scan suggests a more than 85% chance of an embolus.
What is considered to be the "gold standard" in establishing the diagnosis of a PE?	Pulmonary angiography
In what 2 situations should a pulmonary angiogram be obtained?	1. To make a definitive diagnosis when the patient is at risk for complications from anticoagulation 2. If the clinical picture is uncertain
What are the initial supportive measures?	1. Supplemental oxygen 2. Mechanical ventilation (if required) 3. IV access and fluid administration

4. Possibly vasopressors (if the patient remains hypotensive)

How is PE initially treated?

A 10,000 to 20,000 U bolus injection of IV heparin should be administered, followed by a continuous infusion of 1,000 to 1,500 U/hr. Minimal delay should occur in giving heparin after PE is suspected.

What laboratory tests should be obtained in monitoring heparin therapy?

A baseline PTT should be obtained before initiation of heparin therapy, followed by additional measurements on a regular basis to follow the adequacy of anticoagulation. The heparin should be maintained at a rate that achieves a PTT of 1.5- to 2.0-fold that of control values.

What is the major acute complication of heparin therapy?

Hemorrhage. This is very rare, however, with continuously infused heparin.

Is the cancer patient at special risk for such complications?

The cancer patient may be at increased risk of bleeding caused by thrombocytopenia from chemotherapy or antibiotics, known or unknown vascular invasion by neoplasm, brain or epidural metastases, or GI ulcerations.

Are there any absolute contraindications to anticoagulation?

Yes. Patients with known bleeding diatheses as well as patients with known neoplastic disease of the CNS should not be anticoagulated.

What can be done for patients with contraindications to anticoagulation in the event of a PE?

In the case of massive or life-threatening PE, a sternotomy and pulmonary embolectomy may be required. Such patients require a vena caval filter or umbrella to prevent subsequent emboli.

What can be done for the patient who has failed anticoagulation therapy or is at high risk from anticoagulant therapy?

Such patients are candidates for caval interruption procedures or vena caval filters.

Is pulmonary thrombo-embolectomy commonly performed?

No. Patients with emboli massive enough to require this procedure often do not survive to reach the operating room.

What is the operative mortality rate of pulmonary thromboembolectomy?

Approximately 50%

Hemoptysis

Define massive hemoptysis.

Expectoration of at least 600 mL of blood in a 24-hour period, or intrabronchial bleeding at a rate that presents a threat to life

Do patients with massive hemoptysis usually die of exsanguination?

No. The actual cause of death usually is flooding of the bronchial tree with blood, causing asphyxiation by interference with gas exchange.

What is the most common cause of massive hemoptysis in patients older than 40 years?

Bronchogenic carcinoma

Patients with which histo-logic type of bronchogenic carcinoma are most likely to present with massive hemoptysis?

Squamous cell carcinoma

What procedure should all patients with massive hemoptysis undergo to determine the site and cause of bleeding?

Bronchoscopy

Which type of bronchoscopy is considered to be the technique of choice?

Rigid bronchoscopy has been the traditional technique of choice for the evaluation of massive hemoptysis because of its larger diameter and better ability to suction, administer oxygen, and control the airway. **Rigid bronchoscopy requires general anesthesia** and does not allow visualization of the upper lobe bronchi. **Flexible bronchoscopy has become more popular recently** because of its lack of requirement for general anesthesia and its ability to inspect a much larger area of the bronchial tree. Drawbacks include difficulty in suctioning large amounts of blood and in maintaining oxygenation.

What is the initial treatment for massive hemoptysis?

Once the bleeding site is identified, the patient is placed bleeding-side down to avoid aspiration into the nonbleeding lung. Oxygen, IV fluids, and blood products are given as appropriate. Selective bronchial intubation may be performed to protect the patient's airway, and a balloon catheter (Fogarty) may be passed through the rigid bronchoscope to tamponade the bleeding site.

What is the definitive treatment of massive hemoptysis?

Surgical resection of the bleeding pulmonary segment

What is the mortality rate of conservative, nonsurgical management?

50% to 100%. Therefore, a thoracic surgical consult should be obtained in all cases of massive hemoptysis.

What options exist for patients who are not surgical candidates?

Prolonged balloon tamponade with a Fogarty catheter and arteriography with therapeutic embolization of bronchial (not pulmonary) arteries. Radiation therapy may be helpful in controlling bleeding tumors, but its effect may be delayed by several days.

Effusions

What is a malignant pleural effusion?

A collection of fluid in the pleural cavity caused by any form of cancer

Which 2 malignancies commonly produce malignant pleural effusions?

1. Carcinomas of the lung, breast, ovaries, and GI tract
2. Lymphomas

What is the pathophysiology of a malignant pleural effusion?

Decreased lymphatic outflow secondary to malignant obstruction and increased capillary permeability resulting in an exudative effusion

What is the most common cause of massive pleural effusion (>2 L)?

Cancer typically can cause larger effusions than congestive heart failure, cirrhosis, or pneumonia.

How is the diagnosis of pleural effusion established?

Initially by physical exam with decreased breath sounds and dullness to percussion over the affected area. The diagnosis is then confirmed by CXR.

What 5 chemotherapeutic agents have been implicated as causing pleural effusions?

1. Methotrexate
2. Procarbazine
3. Cyclophosphamide
4. Mitomycin
5. Bleomycin

What 4 "remote" effects of a neoplasm may result in pleural effusion?

1. Hypoproteinemia
2. Mediastinal lymphatic obstruction
3. Superior vena caval obstruction
4. Pericardial tamponade

What else should be considered in the differential diagnosis of pleural effusions?

1. Congestive heart failure
2. Fluid overload
3. Pneumonitis
4. Tuberculosis
5. PE
6. Autoimmune disease
7. Drug toxicity

Name 4 common symptoms of malignant pleural effusions.	1. Dyspnea 2. Orthopnea 3. Cough 4. Chest pain
To what aspect of the effusions are symptoms most closely related?	Symptoms appear to be more closely related to the rate of fluid accumulation than to the total volume.
How often are malignant pleural effusions bilateral?	Approximately 1/3 of patients have bilateral effusions.
Blunting of the costophrenic angle represents how much pleural fluid?	300 to 500 mL of pleural fluid
What specific radiograph is useful in cases when the diagnosis is in question or in cases of subpulmonic effusion?	The lateral decubitus CXR may detect as little as 100 mL of pleural fluid.
How is the diagnosis of malignant pleural effusion typically established?	By thoracentesis and cytology
Which patients should undergo therapeutic thoracentesis?	Patients with any of the following should undergo thoracentesis promptly: 1. Significant dyspnea 2. Hypoxemia 3. Mediastinal shift 4. Hemodynamic instability 5. Evidence of empyema
Why should total drainage during the first 12 hours not exceed approximately 1500 mL?	To avoid the risk of unilateral expansion pulmonary edema because of rapid changes in pressure gradients
What are 3 treatment options for patients with malignant pleural effusions?	1. Tube thoracostomy with chemical pleurodesis 2. Thoracoscopy with talc pleurodesis

3. Pleurectomy or pleuroperitoneal shunt: rare

Does the development of a pleural effusion necessarily signify incurable disease?

In most circumstances, an effusion signifies advanced, incurable disease. However, with certain malignancies, such as lymphoma, the patient may still be effectively treated and even cured of disease even if a true malignant effusion is present.

What is the survival of patients with malignant pleural effusions at 6 months?

The overall prognosis is poor. The survival rate at 6 months is less than 25%. Survival is slightly better in patients with lymphoma and breast cancer.

FLUIDS, ELECTROLYTES, AND NUTRITION

What is the syndrome of cancer cachexia?

The catabolic state present in many cancer patients that is believed to be secondary to tumor–host interactions and resulting in the release of cytokines, particularly tumor necrosis factor and interleukin-6. It consists of weight loss, anorexia, muscle wasting, weakness, hyperlipidemia, glucose intolerance, and hepatic gluconeogenesis despite adequate intake of protein and calories.

SYNDROME OF INAPPROPRIATE ANTIDIURETIC HORMONE SECRETION

What is SIADH?

The syndrome of inappropriate ADH secretion, resulting in hypervolemic hyponatremia. Findings include hyponatremia with an inappropriately high urine sodium and an osmolality of urine greater than that of the plasma.

What is the most common malignancy associated with SIADH?

Small-cell lung cancer

What is the treatment of SIADH?	Severe hyponatremia should be treated with normal saline and furosemide with a slow (<1 mEq/L/hr) correction in sodium. The overall treatment is directed at the primary cancer. Otherwise, the first-line therapy is free-water restriction. Demeclocycline, an ADH antagonist, can be used in resistant cases.

Hypercalcemia

Hypercalcemia develops in what percentage of patients with malignancy?	10% to 20%
What is the mechanism of malignancy-associated hypercalcemia?	The most common cause is tumor production of a parathyroid hormone–like (not parathyroid hormone itself) peptide, resulting in bone resorption. Less common causes are generation of osteoclast-activating factor or the production of other bone-mobilizing peptides, such as interleukin-1 and tumor necrosis factor, by tumors.
Solid tumors account for what percentage of cases of malignancy-associated hypercalcemia?	Solid tumors, particularly lung and breast carcinoma, account for approximately 80% of the total cases.
Describe 6 symptoms of full-blown hypercalcemic crisis.	1. Somnolence or lethargy 2. General weakness 3. Abdominal pain 4. Dehydration 5. Renal failure 6. Nausea and vomiting
How does hypercalcemia affect renal function?	Elevated serum calcium impairs the kidney's ability to concentrate urine, resulting in polyuria and polydipsia. An ensuing contraction alkalosis with

dehydration leads to further renal impairment and frank renal failure.

How is hypercalcemia treated acutely?

Levels greater than 13 mg/dL require prompt treatment, including hydration with normal saline to restore intravascular volume, followed by diuresis (furosemide) that enhances calciuresis by facilitating a provoked natriuresis.

What 4 parenteral medications are effective in treating acute hypercalcemia?

1. Plicamycin
2. Calcitonin
3. Gallium nitrate
4. Hydroxyethane biphosphonate

OTHER ISSUES

What are 2 mechanisms of tumor-related hypo-glycemia?

1. Insulin production by insulinomas
2. Production of insulin-like peptides, such as insulin-like growth factor (IGF)-1 and IGF-2, and somatomedins by tumors, such as hepatocellular carcinomas, some sarcomas, and mesotheliomas

What is the most common complaint in patients with malignant spinal cord compression?

Pain, which may be exacerbated by movement, coughing, or valsalva. The majority of patients also have weakness, sensory deficits, and autonomic dysfunction.

Section 4

Special ICU Populations

28

Pediatric Patients

AIRWAY MANAGEMENT

What are 3 important anatomic considerations in maintaining an airway in infants?

1. An infant has a large head, predisposing to neck flexion. Keep extension maintained until the ETT is placed.
2. The larynx is more anterior in neonates and infants compared to older children.
3. The tongue is relatively larger in infants and is prone to obstructing the airway. The chin lift–jaw thrust or the sniffing position may be used to open an obstructed airway.

ENDOTRACHEAL TUBES AND TRACHEOSTOMIES

What are the 2 methods of estimating the appropriate-size ETT for an infant or child?

1. Infant: tube diameter equals nostril or the smallest finger
2. Child: size in mm = 4 + age in years/4

What are appropriate-size ETTs for infants and children?

1. Premature infant: 2.5 to 3.0 mm
2. Infant: 3.0 to 3.5 mm
3. Toddler: 4.0 to 4.5 mm
4. Young school-aged child: 5.0 to 5.5 mm
5. Older children: 6.0 to 7.0 mm

When are cuffed ETTs used?

Usually only in children beyond the toddler and preschool years

Why are cuffs avoided in infants and toddlers?

To avoid trauma to the airway and subsequent subglottic stenosis. This is especially true in premature and term infants.

How long may premature and term infants be intubated with an ETT?	Almost indefinitely with adherence to the following principles: 1. Appropriate-size uncuffed tube. 2. Tube should allow leakage around it at 20 cm H_2O positive pressure. 3. Secure the ETT so it does not move (to avoid airway trauma).
When are tracheostomies used?	Essentially never in premature infants. Infants may require a tracheostomy when long-term airway access is needed secondary to neurologic damage or congenital defects (e.g., severe micrognathia or cleft palate). Older children usually will need tracheostomies for long-term care in cases of severe neurologic damage from primary disease or trauma.
What is the first step in resuscitating a child with a tracheostomy who has respiratory distress?	The tracheostomy should be examined for patency and appropriate position. Because of the small size of a child's airway, they are especially vulnerable to mucous plugging and malposition of tracheostomies.
What procedure do you perform to provide an airway for a child with significant facial trauma?	A needle cricothyroidotomy. A 14- or 16-gauge needle may be used and connected to a jet ventilator. This will oxygenate well, but it will not ventilate well.

RESPIRATORY MANAGEMENT

What are 6 signs of respiratory distress in infants and children?	1. Tachypnea 2. Stridor 3. Grunting 4. Nasal flaring 5. Retraction of the chest wall 6. Cyanosis

What adjunct may be used to improve respiratory insufficiency in premature infants or very low-birth-weight babies?	Surfactant administration into the ETT
What complication following general anesthesia is especially worrisome in babies younger than 50 weeks of gestational age?	Apneic episodes. For this reason, elective surgeries are postponed until the age of 50 weeks, or the child is admitted to the hospital for ECG and pulse oximetry monitoring postoperatively.

MECHANICAL VENTILATION

What mode of mechanical ventilation is typically used in children?	Pressure control. This is less likely to produce barotrauma than ventilating with preset tidal volumes.
What alternative ventilation strategy may be used in children instead of conventional pressure-control ventilation?	High-frequency oscillatory ventilation (HFOV) delivers smaller volume at rates ranging from 180 to 900 breaths per minute.
List 3 advantages that may be seen with HFOV.	1. Oxygenation and ventilation are possible when conventional strategies fail. 2. HFOV minimizes barotrauma secondary to high airway pressures. 3. HFOV can be useful in patients with air leaks, such as patients with bronchopleural fistulas.
What is the most likely cause of right upper lobe (RUL) lung collapse in a child maintained on mechanical ventilation?	Right mainstem bronchus intubation or edema at the RUL branch secondary to an ETT being too low in the trachea. The trachea in children is very short, and the appropriate placement for the tip of the ETT has a range of approximately 1 cm in children younger than 4 years.

What are 2 side effects of prolonged high oxygen content administered during mechanical ventilation in infants (especially premature infants)?	1. Bronchopulmonary dysplasia (a type of lung fibrosis) 2. Retrolental fibroplasia (retinal damage)

STRIDOR

What is stridor?	Harsh noise heard on breathing caused by obstruction of the trachea or larynx. Stridor is often accounted for in newborns by congenital malformations causing airway obstruction.
List 3 symptoms and signs of stridor.	1. Dyspnea 2. Cyanosis 3. Difficulty with feedings
What is the differential diagnosis of stridor?	1. Laryngomalacia: the primary cause of stridor in the infant. Results from inadequate development of supporting structures of the larynx. It is usually self-limited, and treatment is expectant (unless respiratory compromise is present). Laryngomalacia causes inspiratory stridor. 2. Tracheobronchomalacia: similar to laryngomalacia, but involves the entire trachea. Tracheobronchomalacia causes expiratory stridor. 3. Vascular rings and slings: abnormal development or position of thoracic large vessels resulting in obstruction of the trachea/bronchus.
What are 3 symptoms of vascular rings?	1. Stridor 2. Dyspnea on exertion 3. Dysphagia
How are vascular rings diagnosed?	1. Barium swallow, revealing typical configuration of esophageal compression 2. Echocardiogram 3. Arteriogram

How are vascular rings treated?	Surgical division of the ring (if the patient is symptomatic)

CIRCULATION

ACCESS

What 2 routes of vascular access are available in pediatric patients that are not available in adult patients?	1. Intraosseous venous access in children younger than 8 years. 2. Access to umbilical vessels in neonates
How is an intraosseous line placed?	Intraosseous lines are most frequently placed in the proximal, medial tibia with a specialized intraosseous needle or a rigid bone marrow–aspiration needle. A sturdy 16- or 18-gauge needle may be used. This allows access to the bone marrow that drains into the venous system.
When is an intraosseous line appropriate?	In patients younger than 8 years who are severely volume depleted and in whom placement of any other peripheral IV line is not possible
How long may an intraosseous line be kept in place?	No longer than 24 hours, because the infection rate increases the longer the line is in place. Convert to a standard IV line or central venous catheter when able.
Central lines are placed using what type of technique in premature or small-for-gestational-age infants?	Venous cutdown techniques are used to place central access in small babies.

FLUIDS

What are maintenance fluid requirements for infants and small children?	1. 100 mL/kg/day for the first 10 kg, 50 mL/kg/day for the next 10 kg,

and 25 mL/kg/day for each 10 kg thereafter

2. This may be calculated by the "4, 2, 1" rule: 4 mL/kg/hr for the first 10 kg, 2 mL/kg/hr for the next 10 kg, and 1 mL/kg/hr for each 10 kg thereafter.

What types of IV fluids are recommended for repletion and maintenance of intravascular volume in children?

Lactated Ringer's is the closest crystalloid solution to the composition of blood and is used for fluid boluses. Because renal function is less mature in infants, $\frac{1}{2}$ normal saline (NS) is sometimes used in smaller quantities for resuscitation to avoid acute sodium and fluid overload. Dextrose (5%), $\frac{1}{4}$ NS, and 20 mEq KCl is recommended for maintenance fluids.

Why do premature infants have even greater water requirements than term infants?

Their skin is extremely thin, which allows potentially twice the insensible loss of water that would normally be expected for their surface area.

SHOCK

What is the definition of shock?

Inadequate end-organ perfusion

What are 5 causes of shock?

1. Hypovolemia (especially trauma, severe enteritis)
2. Spinal cord injury
3. Cardiac failure
4. Sepsis
5. Anaphylaxis

What is important to remember about the infant's and child's cardiovascular response to hypovolemia?

Adequate blood pressure will be maintained until approximately 25% of volume is lost! Tachycardia and decreased urine output are earlier signs of hypovolemia.

| What is appropriate urine output for infants and children? | 1. Infant: 2 mL/kg/hr
2. Toddler: 1 to 2 mL/kg/hr
3. School-aged child: 1 mL/kg/hr
4. Adolescent: 0.5 mL/kg/hr |

What is appropriate urine output for infants and children?

1. Infant: 2 mL/kg/hr
2. Toddler: 1 to 2 mL/kg/hr
3. School-aged child: 1 mL/kg/hr
4. Adolescent: 0.5 mL/kg/hr

How do a child's fluid resuscitation needs differ from an adult's, and why?

Children have a relatively greater total body water content than adults. Most of this is contained in extracellular fluid. Renal function in childhood is also less efficient, and children are less able to concentrate their urine, thus wasting electrolytes and water during periods of dehydration. These factors make children less able to tolerate fluid and electrolyte losses.

At what rate should fluids be replaced?

In boluses of 20 mL/kg until adequate urine output is obtained

What amount of blood is normally given to pediatric patients when they need a transfusion?

After 10 mL/kg have been given, the patient is reassessed to determine need for additional blood.

PEDIATRIC ADVANCED LIFE SUPPORT

What drugs may be administered via an ETT?

Mnemonic: **LEAN**
Lidocaine
Epinephrine
Atropine
Naloxone

How should chest compressions be performed in infants and toddlers?

For infants and toddlers younger than 1 year, one or two fingers are used to compress the sternum. The rate of compressions is from 100 to 120 per minute. The depth of compressions is adequate when a palpable pulse over the brachial artery is obtained. Five compressions are done for each breath administered.

How should chest compressions be performed in school-aged children?	For children younger than 10 years, one hand is used for compressions, and a rate of 100 compressions per minute is the goal.
Is it appropriate to wait to perform cardiac countershock in a child who has arrested?	Yes. Unlike advanced life support in adults, resuscitation of an arrested child involves a trial of ventilation with 100% oxygen before cardiac countershock is performed.

EXTRACORPOREAL MEMBRANE OXYGENATION

What is ECMO?	A form of cardiopulmonary bypass
What does ECMO do?	Provide an external membrane for oxygenating blood independent of native lung function
What are the indications for ECMO therapy?	In general, ECMO is used in patients with reversible pulmonary disease who are unable to oxygenate or ventilate adequately with maximal conventional or HFOV. Specific indications include: 1. Meconium aspiration 2. Sepsis 3. Diaphragmatic hernias 4. Severe pneumonia 5. Cardiac failure The criteria used to determine the need for ECMO vary from hospital to hospital, but such criteria should predict an 80% to 90% mortality rate without ECMO.
In what patient population is ECMO most frequently used?	Neonates
How does ECMO work?	A central artery and vein are cannulated. The right common carotid artery and the right internal jugular vein are the vessels most commonly

used in children. The baby's blood volume is then pumped past an oxygenating membrane and warmer. This provides respiratory support for days to 2 to 4 weeks, allowing the original problem to resolve.

Is anticoagulation necessary during ECMO?

Yes. Systemic heparinization must be maintained to prevent clotting.

GASTROINTESTINAL MANAGEMENT

What does bilious vomiting in an infant signify?

Suspect malrotation with volvulus until proven otherwise! Approximately 90% of patients with malrotation present with bilious vomiting before their first year of life. An immediate diagnostic study should be done.

What is the best diagnostic study for malrotation and volvulus?

Upper GI study (UGI)

What is the key radiographic feature in patients with malrotation?

Abnormally placed ligament of Treitz on the UGI. The normal position of the duodenojejunal junction is to the left of midline, rising to approximately the level of the pylorus and displaced posteriorly.

NECROTIZING ENTEROCOLITIS

What is necrotizing enterocolitis (NEC)?

Necrosis of the intestinal mucosa, often with bleeding. This may progress to transmural intestinal necrosis, shock/sepsis, and death.

What are predisposing conditions for NEC?

Stress: shock, hypoxia, respiratory distress syndrome, apneic episodes, sepsis, exchange transfusions, patent ductus arteriosus and cyanotic heart disease, hyperosmolar feedings, polycythemia, and indomethacin treatment. It is generally associated with prematurity (>90%).

What is the pathophysiologic mechanism for NEC?

Probable splanchnic vasoconstriction with decreased perfusion, mucosal injury, and (probably) bacterial invasion

What is NEC's claim to fame?

The most common cause of emergent laparotomy in the neonate

What are 6 signs and symptoms of NEC?

1. Abdominal distention
2. Vomiting
3. Heme positive stool or gross rectal bleeding
4. Fever or hypothermia
5. Jaundice
6. Abdominal wall erythema (consistent with perforation and abscess formation)

What are 4 radiographic findings in NEC?

1. Fixed, dilated intestinal loops
2. Pneumatosis intestinalis (air in the bowel wall)
3. Free air
4. Portal vein air (sign of advanced disease)

What are 3 laboratory findings in NEC?

1. Low hematocrit
2. Low glucose
3. Low platelets

What is the treatment of NEC?

75% of cases are managed medically:
1. Cessation of enteral feedings
2. Orogastric tube
3. IV fluids/TPN
4. IV antibiotics (triple antibiotics)
5. Ventilator support as needed
6. Serial abdominal exams and abdominal films

What are surgical indications in NEC?

Intra-abdominal free air caused by perforation and a positive peritoneal tap revealing transmural bowel necrosis. Relative indications include abdominal wall erythema, significant abdominal tenderness, or a fixed, dilated loop on serial plain films.

What are the indications for a peritoneal tap?

Severe thrombocytopenia, distended abdomen, abdominal wall erythema, and unexplained clinical downturn in the face of maximal medical therapy

What complications may occur with NEC?

Complications are common and include further bowel necrosis, Gram-negative sepsis, disseminated intravascular coagulopathy, wound infection, cholestasis, short bowel syndrome, strictures, and late small bowel obstruction.

What is the prognosis of patients with NEC?

Greater than 80% overall survival

NUTRITION

Do healthy children have nutritional needs that differ from those of adults, and if so, why?

Yes, children have tremendous metabolic needs. This is caused by rapid cell division and growth. They also have fewer nutritional reserves in the form of glycogen and fat.

What are the baseline nutritional requirements of children?

Infants need 110 kcal/kg/day. This need gradually decreases to 40 kcal/kg/day in adulthood.

What routes are available to feed children who cannot eat?

Peripheral parenteral nutrition, TPN, and enteral tube feedings. These routes are very similar to those available for adults, including modes of access and types of complications that may result.

TEMPERATURE REGULATION

Why are infants and children so prone to hypothermia?

They have a greater ratio of body surface area to volume, so more heat escapes through their skin. They also have a lower percentage of body fat to help insulate against heat loss.

What measures are taken to prevent this loss of heat?

The infant's or child's ambient temperature is kept appropriate with incubators, warming lights, OR temperature, and blankets. Care is taken to reduce exposure of abdominal or thoracic cavity contents for protracted periods, and IV fluids and ventilator gases are warmed before administration.

At what weight can an infant begin to self-regulate his or her body temperature?

Approximately 1,800 to 2,000 g

MISCELLANEOUS

What does TORCHES stand for?

Nonbacterial fetal and neonatal infection:
TOxoplasmosis
Rubella
Cytomegalovirus
HErpes
Syphilis

What are 6 potential signs of child abuse?

1. Cigarette burns
2. Rope burns
3. Scald to posterior thighs and buttocks
4. Multiple fractures/old fractures
5. Genital trauma
6. Delay in accessing the health care system

Is child abuse a major problem?

Abuse is the leading cause of death in children between the age of 6 and 12 months.

29

Pediatric Cardiology

GENERAL KNOWLEDGE

DIAGNOSIS AND PATHOPHYSIOLOGY

What are 3 signs of heart disease in the newborn?

1. Cyanosis
2. CHF
3. Shock

Does every newborn with heart disease have signs or symptoms?

No, many are asymptomatic.

Why do children present with heart disease after discharge from the nursery?

Critical heart disease occurs after ductal closure, which occurs days to weeks after birth.

What are the cardiac causes of cyanosis in the newborn?

The 5 T's:
1. Tetralogy of Fallot
2. Transposition of the great arteries
3. Tricuspid atresia
4. Total anomalous pulmonary venous connection
5. Truncus arteriosus (pulmonary atresia with or without a ventricular septal defect [VSD])

What are 6 signs and symptoms of heart failure in neonates and infants?

1. Tachypnea.
2. Tachycardia.
3. Sweating.
4. Poor feeding.
5. Gallop rhythm: may be present along with hepatomegaly and dependent edema.
6. Rales: rarely auscultated in neonates.

What are 3 causes of heart failure in neonates?	1. Coarctation of the aorta 2. Aortic stenosis 3. Hypoplastic left heart syndrome
What is the cause of heart failure in infants?	Left-to-right shunting lesions, such as VSD or AV canal defects
What are the initial studies for a newborn suspected of having congenital heart disease?	ECG and CXR. An oxygen challenge test should be performed in patients with suspected cyanotic heart disease. The definitive test is the cardiac echocardiogram.
What is the oxygen challenge?	A test to distinguish cyanotic heart disease from pulmonary disease in newborns. Infants are placed on 100% oxygen. A PO_2 of greater than 150 mm Hg on ABG should rule out cyanotic heart disease. It may be inaccurate in certain cyanotic heart lesions, such as tetralogy of Fallot.
What are 8 cardiovascular complications of Kawasaki syndrome?	1. Coronary artery aneurysm 2. Associated coronary artery stenosis or rupture of aneurysm with hemopericardium 3. Myocardial infarct 4. Myocarditis 5. Pericarditis 6. Pericardial effusion 7. Valvulitis (usually mitral) 8. Systemic arterial aneurysm

PROSTAGLANDIN THERAPY

What is prostaglandin E_1 used for?	To maintain ductal patency. For patients with ductal-dependent pulmonary or systemic blood flow, it may be life-saving.
What are 6 side effects of prostaglandin E_1?	1. Apnea 2. Hypotension

3. Fever
4. Irritability
5. Edema
6. Cutaneous flushing

VASCULAR RESISTANCE AND CARDIAC OUTPUT

What is the definition of vascular resistance?

The mean pressure difference across a vascular bed of interest divided by the amount of flow

What is the natural history of changes in PVR during the perinatal period?

Before birth, PVR is suprasystemic. With the first breath of life, the PVR falls to subsystemic levels. The PVR continues to fall for the first few weeks of life, but the vast majority of that fall occurs during the first 24 hours after birth.

Why is PVR important in VSDs?

Infants with large VSDs may have a later fall in PVR. By 2 to 4 weeks of life, this drop in PVR will lead to a significant increase in left-to-right blood flow (or Qp/Qs, the ratio of pulmonary to systemic blood flow). If the VSD is large enough, CHF will develop at this time.

What are short- and long-term results of uncontrolled pulmonary shunting?

Large left-to-right shunts cause CHF (short term) and pulmonary hypertension (long term).

What is Eisenmenger's syndrome?

Chronic pulmonary overcirculation leading to irreversible pulmonary hypertension. When the pulmonary resistance becomes suprasystemic, intracardiac shunts become right to left, causing progressive cyanosis.

What is the Fick principle?

CO is directly proportional to oxygen consumption and inversely proportional to the difference between the arterial and mixed venous blood oxygen content.

What are the 3 most common methods for determining CO?

1. The Fick principle (comparing arterial and mixed venous oxygen saturations)
2. Thermodilution
3. Indicator dye dilution

Which method is favored for low-CO states?

The Fick principle. It provides less sampling error in situations with a higher arterial to mixed venous oxygen difference.

What is meant by "balancing" pulmonary and systemic blood flow?

In patients with single-ventricle physiology, optimal hemodynamic outcome is thought to occur when the amount of pulmonary blood flow is equal to the amount of systemic blood flow. A systemic oxygen saturation of 75% to 85% occurs when the pulmonary and systemic flows are balanced.

OPERATIVE CARE

What are 2 guiding principles of operative care of congenital heart disease?

1. Completely correctable lesions (e.g., tetralogy of Fallot, transposition of the great arteries, coarctation) should be done early, before vital organs are damaged.
2. Palliate-only lesions (e.g., hypoplastic left heart syndrome, single ventricles and variants) should be done with minimal trauma to the child to minimize vital organ damage.

Describe the difference between open heart surgery and closed heart surgery.

Open heart surgery is surgery performed on cardiopulmonary bypass. Closed heart surgery may include ligation of patent ductus arteriosus (PDA), repair of coarctation of the aorta, systemic to PA shunt, and PA band.

What are 3 common causes of stridor in the perioperative pediatric cardiac patient?

1. Subglottic edema or stenosis, vocal cord paralysis (recurrent laryngeal nerve palsy) or dysfunction (edema)
2. Infantile laryngomalacia
3. Tracheomalacia

How is an atrial septal defect (ASD) diagnosed?

Systolic ejection murmur and wide fixed split second heart sound. Many cases are asymptomatic.

How do you treat an ASD?

Close surgically or in the cath lab. The type of repair is dependent on the anatomy.

How do you diagnose a PDA?

By a continuous murmur in the left infraclavicular area. In premature infants, a large PDA may cause heart failure and respiratory compromise.

How do you treat PDA?

Surgically ligate or close during a cardiac catheterization.

How do you diagnose a vascular ring?

Neonates and infants present with stridor.
Barium swallow is the test of choice.
Echocardiogram, MRI, CT, or cardiac catheterization may be helpful.

How do you treat a vascular ring?

Surgical division of the ring

What are 3 stages in palliating single-ventricle physiology?

1. Augment pulmonary blood flow, usually with a systemic to PA shunt.
2. Reduce volume overload of the ventricle with a SVC to PA anastomosis (bidirectional Glenn shunt or hemi-Fontan procedure).
3. Fontan operation, in which the single ventricle is responsible for the systemic blood flow and pulmonary blood flow is achieved via cavopulmonary connections.

| What are the 4 surgical components of a stage 1 Norwood procedure? | 1. Atrial septectomy
2. Aortic arch reconstruction
3. Creation of pulmonary atresia, and anastomosis of the proximal PA to the aorta
4. Pulmonary blood flow established via modified Blalock-Taussig shunt, central shunt, or RV to PA conduit |

POSTOPERATIVE CARE

| What are the guiding principles of postoperative care after heart surgery in children? | Maintenance of oxygen delivery and adequate tissue perfusion with early interventions BEFORE hemodynamic instability occurs |

| What are 7 methods of postoperative monitoring? | 1. Skin temperature
2. Urine output
3. Heart rate
4. Blood pressure
5. Mixed venous oxygen saturation
6. Serum lactate level
7. Acid-base balance |

| During what period would CO be considered at its nadir after heart surgery for congenital defects? | 6 to 12 hours |

| What is the acceptable rate of urine output after surgery? | 1 mL/kg/hr |

| How much bleeding is too much in a child? | More than 200 mL/m^2/hr |

OXYGEN DELIVERY AND CARDIAC OUTPUT

| What are 3 methods to increase oxygen delivery? | Oxygen delivery = CO × hemoglobin × (difference between arterial sat and venous sat) + small contribution from dissolved arterial oxygen. Therefore:
1. Increase CO. |

2. Transfuse to increase hemoglobin
3. Improve oxygenation

How can you augment CO after surgery?

CO = stroke volume × heart rate
Think: Rate, rhythm, preload, after-load, contractility, mechanical.
Fix the heart rate and rhythm.
Give volume to achieve an optimum Starling curve (neonates have stiff hearts, and CO is more dependent on heart rate).
Begin afterload reduction to decrease the work of the heart.
Add an inotrope to increase contractility.
Consider mechanical support.

What are 3 causes of a postoperative elevated left atrial pressure?

1. Increased (systemic) ventricular end-diastolic pressure because of decreased ventricular function
2. Myocardial hypertrophy
3. Volume overload

What are 3 common afterload reducers used in the pediatric cardiac ICU?

1. Sodium nitroprusside
2. Nitroglycerin
3. Milrinone (is also an inotrope)

What are 3 common inotropic agents used in the pediatric cardiac ICU?

1. Dopamine
2. Dobutamine
3. Epinephrine

MANAGING COMPLICATIONS

What 5 things are done during an unexpected postoperative course?

1. Bedside evaluation
2. CXR
3. ECG
4. Echocardiogram
5. Cardiac catheterization with or without intervention

What are 4 common infections after cardiac surgery in children?

1. Pneumonia
2. Intravascular catheter infection
3. Urinary tract infection
4. Wound infection

Arrhythmias

What are 5 common postoperative arrhythmias in children?	1. Junctional rhythm 2. Sinus node dysfunction (SND) 3. Ventricular tachycardia 4. Junctional ectopic tachycardia (JET) 5. Heart block
What is the workup for a postoperative arrhythmia?	If the patient is hemodynamically stable, get a 12-lead ECG. If P waves are not apparent on the 12-lead ECG, perform an atrial electrogram from atrial wires or a transesophageal ECG recording.

Describe the management of the following:

Postoperative heart block?	If acute, perform ventricular pacing or AV sequential pacing. A chronotropic agent (e.g., isoproterenol) should be used if pacing wires are not available. Consider permanent pacing if AV conduction has not returned by 1 week.
Postoperative SVT?	Atrial overdrive pacing if atrial wires are available; adenosine infusion if they are not. Correct electrolyte disturbances.
Postoperative JET?	Increase sedation. Wean inotropes if possible. Provide IV amiodarone, mild cooling to 34°C, or both.
Postoperative ventricular tachycardia?	Cardioversion if the patient is hemodynamically unstable. Use antiarrhythmics if the patient is stable. Procainamide infusion and IV amiodarone appear to be more efficacious than lidocaine.

Postoperative Surgical Complications

What are 7 potential surgical complications of pediatric heart surgery?	1. Bleeding 2. Pericardial tamponade 3. Pneumothorax 4. Infection (line sepsis, pneumonia, urinary)

5. Phrenic nerve paralysis
6. Recurrent laryngeal nerve paralysis
7. Chylothorax

How do you diagnose and treat the following?

Acute postoperative pulmonary hypertension?

Diagnosis: elevated pressures measured with echo and/or catheterization

Treatment: alkalosis, hyperventilation, sedation, nitric oxide, milrinone, prostaglandin E_1

Pericardial tamponade?

Diagnosis: echo demonstrates pericardial fluid compressing the heart. Pericardial tamponade should be suspected with sudden cessation of chest tube drainage, decreased urine output, and hypotension. Get a stat echocardiogram in almost any child with acute deterioration in the early postoperative period.

Treatment: pericardiocentesis

Coagulopathy?

Diagnosis: Elevated PT/PTT, elevated heparin level, and/or abnormal thromboelastogram

Treatment: protamine, platelets, and/or fresh frozen plasma, depending on the cause

Pneumothorax?

Diagnosis: decreased breath sounds on exam, pleural air visible on CXR

Treatment: chest tube

Diaphragmatic paralysis?

Diagnosis: lack of diaphragmatic movement on CXR or ultrasound. Occurs more commonly in reoperations.

Treatment: supportive care

Recurrent nerve paralysis?

Diagnosis: laryngeal palsy seen with flexible laryngoscopy. Occurs following coarctation repair, PDA, and reoperations on left side of the heart (RV outflow tract reconstruction).

Treatment: supportive care or surgical reapproximation of the vocal cords.

Chylothorax?

Diagnosis: pleural fluid with elevated triglycerides and cell count of greater than 80% lymphocytes

Treatment: chest tube drainage, no-fat diet, nothing through the mouth, thoracic duct ligation

Catheterization and Interventional Procedural Complications

What are 10 complications associated with diagnostic catheterization?

1. Perforation of heart or vessel
2. Pericardial effusion/tamponade
3. Pleural effusion
4. Myocardial (contrast) stain
5. Arrhythmia, including heart block
6. Embolic stroke
7. Bleeding/anemia: blood loss, dilutional
8. Osmotic diuresis/renal failure secondary to contrast load
9. Contrast allergy
10. Nerve traction injuries secondary to positioning

What are 6 potential complications associated with arterial access following cardiac catheterization?

1. Arterial spasm with transient loss of distal pulses
2. Arterial thrombotic occlusion
3. Vessel tear or avulsion
4. Retroperitoneal hematoma
5. Arterial venous fistula
6. Arterial aneurysm

What is the treatment of loss of arterial pulse?

Systemic heparin

Thrombolytic therapy (threatened limb)

Surgical thrombectomy or vessel repair (threatened limb)

What are 5 complications associated with device closure of the PDA?

1. Embolization of the device to the pulmonary or systemic circulation: occlusive and nonocclusive
2. Left PA stenosis

3. Residual leak
4. Hemolysis
5. Infection

What are 4 complications associated with percutaneous pericardiocentesis?

1. Cardiac perforation
2. Coronary artery laceration
3. Pneumopericardium or pneumoperitoneum
4. Infection

What are 3 complications associated with PA angioplasty?

1. PA rupture: hemoptysis, tamponade, hemothorax
2. Pulmonary edema to previously underperfused vascular bed: immediate or delayed (24 hours)
3. RV dysfunction in a prolonged procedure secondary to decreased CO and increased afterload

Complications from Specific Operations

What are the specific complications of following?

Stage I palliation?

Low CO, pulmonary overcirculation, restrictive atrial septum, arch obstruction, shunt stenosis, thrombosis, low CO, tricuspid regurgitation

Bidirectional cavopulmonary anastomosis?

Cyanosis, hypertension, stenosis at SVC/PA anastomosis, chylothorax, diaphragmatic paralysis, venous arterial collaterals, irritability (high SVC pressure producing headache), SND

Fontan?

Stenosis of Fontan pathway, low CO, venous/arterial collaterals, early arrythmias (including JET and SND), pleural peritoneal effusions, late SND, atrial flutter

Tetralogy of Fallot?

Systolic and diastolic RV dysfunction (manifested by high CVP/RAP and low CO), arrhythmias (including JET and heart block), residual RV outflow tract

	obstruction (RV, PA, branch PAs), residual VSD, left ventricular dysfunction (injury to left anterior descending artery)
Coarctation?	Incomplete relief coarctation, recurrent coarctation, chylothorax, recurrent nerve injury, hypertension in older children, mesenteric arteritis
Arterial switch operation?	Low CO syndrome, myocardial ischemia
VSD closure (including truncus repair, AV canal repair)?	Low CO syndrome, pulmonary hypertension, heart block

30

Trauma Patients

The initial phase of trauma care in the United States follows what widely accepted protocol?	The Advanced Trauma Life Support (ATLS) precepts of the American College of Surgeons
What are the 3 main elements of the ATLS protocol?	1. Primary survey/resuscitation 2. Secondary survey 3. Definitive care

PRIMARY SURVEY

What are the 5 steps of the primary survey? *(You MUST know these!)*	
A	Airway
B	Breathing
C	Circulation
D	Disability
E	Exposure
What principle is followed in the primary survey?	Address life-threatening problems before proceeding to the next step.

AIRWAY

What are the 2 goals during assessment of the airway?	1. Securing the airway 2. Protecting the spinal cord. Spinal immobilization during intubation is essential if spinal injury is suspected.
What constitutes adequate spinal immobilization?	Use of a full backboard and a rigid cervical collar

In an alert patient, what is the quickest test for an adequate airway?	Ask a question. If the patient can speak, the airway is intact.
What is the first maneuver used to establish an airway?	Chin lift and/or jaw thrust. If successful, an oral or nasal airway often can be used to temporarily maintain the airway.
If these methods are unsuccessful, what is the next maneuver used to establish an airway?	ET intubation via the nasal or oral route
What is a contraindication to nasotracheal intubation?	Maxillofacial fracture!
If all other methods are unsuccessful, how should an emergent airway be established?	Cricothyroidotomy, either by percutaneous placement of a needle through the cricothyroid membrane or by surgical placement of a tube through the cricothyroid membrane (i.e., "surgical airway").
In what population is a surgical cricothyroidotomy NOT recommended?	Any patient younger than 12 years. Instead, perform needle cricothyroidotomy or tracheostomy.
What 2 factors must always be kept in mind during difficult attempts at establishing an airway?	1. Spinal immobilization 2. Adequate oxygenation If possible, patients must be adequately ventilated with 100% O_2 using a bag and mask before any attempt at establishing an airway.

BREATHING

What are the 2 goals in assessing breathing?	1. Securing oxygenation and ventilation 2. Treatment of life-threatening thoracic injuries
What comprises adequate assessment of breathing?	1. Inspection: for respiratory rate, cyanosis, tracheal shift, symmetric

chest expansion, use of accessory muscles

2. Auscultation: for upper airway and lower airway sounds (stridor, wheezing, gurgling)
3. Percussion: for hyperresonance or dullness
4. Palpation: for SQ emphysema, flail segments

What are 5 life-threatening conditions to address during Breathing stage of the survey?

1. Airway obstruction
2. Tension pneumothorax
3. Open pneumothorax
4. Flail chest
5. Massive hemothorax

Name 7 signs and symptoms of pneumothorax.

1. Dyspnea
2. Tachypnea
3. Anxiety
4. Pleuritic chest pain
5. Unilateral decreased or absent breath sounds
6. Tracheal shift away from the affected side
7. Hyperresonance on the affected side
Remember, tension pneumothorax is a clinical diagnosis, not a radiologic diagnosis!

What is the treatment of a pneumothorax?

Immediate decompression by needle thoracostomy in the second intercostal space, midclavicular line, followed by tube thoracostomy in the anterior/ midaxillary line in the fourth intercostal space (level of the nipple in males)

How is an open pneumothorax, also known as sucking chest wound, diagnosed?

The presence of an open pneumothorax usually is obvious, with air movement through a chest wall defect.

How is an open pneumothorax treated?

In the emergency room by intubation with positive-pressure ventilation, tube thoracostomy (chest tube), and occlusive dressing

Why is an open pneumo-thorax potentially lethal?	If the chest wall defect is greater than $^2/_3$ of the diameter of the trachea, air will preferentially enter the chest through the defect rather than the airway during inspiration, and the patient will be unable to breathe.
How is flail chest diagnosed?	The "classic" picture is that of multiple fractured ribs, resulting in a segment of the chest wall that moves paradoxically and produces hypoventilation. The real culprit, however, often is an underlying pulmonary contusion that results in progressive respiratory failure.
How is flail chest treated?	Intubation with positive-pressure ventilation and PEEP
How is massive hemothorax diagnosed?	Hypotension, unilaterally decreased or absent breath sounds, dullness to percussion. If massive, the diagnosis is obvious on CXR, but if under 500 mL, it may be largely hidden by the diaphragm on upright films.
How is massive hemothorax treated?	1. Volume replacement and tube thoracostomy: large chest tube 2. Use of a cell saver if available 3. Removal of the blood, which allows apposition of the parietal and visceral pleura, which often will seal the defect and slow the bleeding

CIRCULATION

What are the 2 goals in assessing circulation?	1. Securing adequate tissue perfusion 2. Treating external bleeding
What is the initial test for adequate circulation?	Palpation of pulses. If a femoral or carotid pulse is palpable, systolic pressure is at least 60 mm Hg. If a radial pulse is palpable, systolic pressure is at least 80 mm Hg.

Is systolic BP a good estimate of organ perfusion?

No. MAP is a better estimate.

What 5 elements comprise adequate assessment of circulation?

1. Heart rate (HR)
2. BP
3. Peripheral perfusion: capillary refill, skin temperature
4. UOP
5. Mental status

Beware of relying only on BP, especially with young patients, in whom autonomic tone can maintain BP until cardiovascular collapse is imminent.

How is cardiac tamponade diagnosed?

Beck's triad of decreased heart sounds, jugular venous distention, and decreased pulse pressure. The full triad is present only in $1/3$ of patients with this diagnosis. Also, tachycardia, pulsus paradoxus, and Kussmaul's signs may be present. Hypotension caused by tamponade implies imminent cardiac collapse. Cardiac tamponade is more common with penetrating than with blunt trauma.

How is cardiac tamponade treated?

1. Immediate IV fluid bolus and pericardiocentesis.
2. Subsequent surgical exploration with subxiphoid pericardial window often is necessary.

How are sites of external bleeding treated?

By direct pressure. Avoid tourniquets and blind clamping of bleeding sites, because both lead to increased limb loss.

What is the preferred IV access in the trauma patient?

Two large-bore (14–16 gauge) IV catheters in the upper extremities

What are the alternate sites of IV access?

Percutaneous and cutdown catheters in the lower leg saphenous (cutdown) and femoral veins (percutaneous). Avoid subclavian and jugular lines if possible because of the increased morbidity of placement and the smaller diameter of the catheters.

How does one remember the anatomy of the groin for insertion of a femoral vein catheter?

Mnemonic: **IVAN**
Inside
Vein
Artery
Nerve
Vein is medial to artery.

What is the resuscitation fluid of choice in trauma patients?

Lactated Ringer's solution, which is isotonic. The lactate helps to buffer the metabolic acidosis caused by poor perfusion.

Why is normal saline not as appealing as lactated Ringer's solution?

The high chloride content of normal saline can lead to metabolic acidosis.

DISABILITY

What is the goal in assessing disability?

Determination of neurologic injury. (Think neurologic disability.)

What comprises adequate assessment of disability?

1. Mental status: GCS.
2. Pupils: a blown pupil reflects an intracranial mass lesion (blood) as the CN III is compressed (mass lesion is on the same side as blown pupil 90% of the time).
3. Motor/sensory: screening exam for extremity movement, sensation.

EXPOSURE

What are the goals in obtaining adequate exposure?

Complete disrobing to allow a thorough visual inspection and palpation of the patient during the secondary survey

Examination of what part of the trauma patient's body often is forgotten?	The patient's back. Logroll the patient, and examine! (This is especially pertinent in penetrating trauma.)

SECONDARY SURVEY

What principle is followed in completing the secondary survey?	Complete head-to-toe physical examination including all orifices: ears, nose, mouth, vagina, rectum
What are 4 typical signs of a basilar skull fracture?	1. Raccoon eyes 2. Battle's sign: mastoid hematoma 3. Clear/bloody otorrhea or rhinorrhea 4. Hemotympanum
What must not be missed on the eye exam?	Traumatic hyphema (anterior chamber bleeding)
What potentially destructive lesion must not be missed on the nasal exam?	Nasal septal hematoma. If left unevacuated, the hematoma will result in pressure necrosis of the septum.
What is the best indication of a mandibular fracture?	Dental malocclusion. Ask, as the patient bites down, "Does that feel normal to you?"
What 4 signs of thoracic trauma often are found on the neck exam?	1. Crepitus or SQ emphysema from tracheobronchial disruption 2. Tracheal deviation from tension pneumothorax 3. Jugular venous distention from cardiac tamponade 4. Carotid bruit heard with carotid artery injury from seatbelt trauma
What must be considered in every penetrating injury of the thorax at or below the level of the nipple?	Concomitant injury to the abdomen. Remember, the diaphragm rises to the level of the nipples in males on full expiration. This can be evaluated with DPL, laparoscopy, or ultrasound.

What is the proper technique for examining the thoracic and lumbar spine?

Logrolling the patient to allow complete visualization of the back and palpation of the spine to elicit pain or detect a deformity over a fracture

What must be documented from the rectal exam?

1. Sphincter tone: as an indication of spinal cord injury
2. Presence of blood: as an indication of colon or rectal injury
3. Prostate position: as an indication of urethral injury secondary to a pelvic fracture

What is the best technique for detection of pelvic and hip fractures?

Lateral compression of the iliac crests and greater trochanters and AP compression of the symphysis pubis to elicit pain

What 4 physical signs indicate possible urethral injury, thus contraindicating placement of a Foley catheter?

1. High-riding, ballottable prostate on rectal exam
2. Presence of blood at the penile meatus
3. Scrotal or perineal ecchymosis
4. Inability of the patient to spontaneously void

What is the standard diagnostic test for suspected urethral injury?

First, a retrograde urethrogram. If this is normal, a Foley catheter can be placed and a voiding cystogram obtained to evaluate the bladder.

How is the bladder drained in the case of a urethral injury?

Suprapubic catheter

What 2 types of hollow-organ decompression must the trauma patient receive?

1. Gastric decompression with an NGT
2. Foley catheter bladder decompression after a normal rectal exam

In the presence of a maxillofacial fracture, how should gastric decompression be accomplished?

NOT with an NGT. The tube may perforate the cribriform plate and move into the brain if maxillofacial fracture/ skull fracture is present. Place an OG tube.

What must be documented from the extremity exam?	Fractures and injuries, open wounds, and a motor and sensory exam (particularly distal to any fractures, pulses, and peripheral perfusion)
What complication often is seen after prolonged ischemia to an extremity, and must be treated immediately to save the extremity?	Compartment syndrome
What is the treatment of compartment syndrome?	Fasciotomy

ABDOMINAL CAVITY

What conditions must exist for a patient's abdominal physical exam to be pronounced normal?	An alert patient without head or spinal cord injury, drug/alcohol intoxication, or distracting injuries elsewhere in the body.
What 5 physical signs may indicate intra-abdominal injury?	1. Guarding 2. Tenderness 3. Distension 4. Absent bowel sounds 5. Rebound or other signs of peritoneal irritation
What is DPL?	Diagnostic peritoneal lavage
When is DPL indicated?	In blunt trauma patients who are unstable and have suspected intra-abdominal hemorrhage
What is the only absolute contraindication for DPL?	An existing indication for laparotomy
How is DPL performed?	1. Decompress the bladder and stomach. 2. Anesthetize an area below the umbilicus.

3. Make a small, vertical incision through the skin and SQ fat to the peritoneum.
4. Lift the peritoneum with forceps, and incise.
5. Insert a peritoneal dialysis catheter into the abdomen.
6. If no gross blood is aspirated, infuse 1 L of warmed lactated Ringer's.
7. After 5 to 10 minutes, drop the empty lactated Ringer's bag on the floor, and allow the intra-abdominal fluid to siphon out into the bag.
8. Send the fluid for analysis (see below).

What should be done differently when performing DPL in the presence of a fractured pelvis or pregnancy?

A supraumbilical approach should be taken.

What constitutes a positive DPL?

1. Gross blood, bile, or particulate matter
2. RBCs greater than 100,000 cells/mm^3
3. WBCs greater than 500 cells/mm^3
4. Gram stain positive for bacteria
5. Amylase greater than 175 units/L

What is FAST?

Focused abdominal sonography for trauma; a test that is replacing DPL as a modality for detecting blood in the abdomen of unstable patients

What is the rationale behind FAST?

Ultrasound is used to detect free blood in specific locations where it is likely to collect.

What 4 areas are inspected during FAST?

1. Pericardium
2. Hepatorenal fossa: Morrison's pouch
3. Splenorenal fossa
4. Pelvis: pouch of Douglas

What are 4 advantages of FAST compared to DPL?

1. Less invasive
2. Rapid
3. Repeatable
4. Equal sensitivity in experienced hands

List 3 disadvantages of FAST compared to DPL.

1. The results are more operator and patient dependent: bowel gas and obesity may decrease sensitivity.
2. It is sensitive but not as specific: there may be a non-bloody fluid collection.
3. Misses GI and pancreatic injuries.

List 5 findings that would require a celiotomy in a blunt trauma victim.

1. Peritonitis
2. Free air on radiograph
3. Positive DPL/FAST
4. Refractory hypotension
5. Suspicion/evidence of certain injuries on CT scan

In a patient with severe intra-abdominal bleeding and hypotension refractory to fluid resuscitation, what can be done to increase perfusion to the vital organs?

Emergency thoracotomy with cross-clamping of the aorta preserves perfusion to the brain and heart. If the patient loses his or her pressure while on the operating table, the surgeon can simply apply pressure to the abdominal aorta at the diaphragm.

Coagulopathy and low filling pressures after laparotomy for trauma indicate what process?

Continued bleeding. It often is impossible to correct coagulopathy in the face of continued traumatic hemorrhage. Re-exploration often is necessary. Hypothermia should also be suspected in continued coagulopathy.

What are 3 common intra-abdominal injuries associated with use of seatbelts?

1. Intestinal injuries
2. Fracture of 2nd lumbar vertebra
3. Pancreatic injury

What is abdominal compartment syndrome?

Abdominal organ dysfunction caused by increased intra-abdominal pressure.

Causes include bleeding, bowel edema, and bowel gas. Renal and intestinal blood flow are compromised, causing ischemia and low UOP. High abdominal pressure also decreases pulmonary compliance and worsens respiratory status.

How is abdominal compartment pressure measured?

100 mL of fluid are instilled in the bladder through a Foley catheter and the tubing filled with fluid and clamped. The sampling port is entered with a needle connected to a calibrated pressure transducer, and the intra-abdominal pressure is measured. A value greater than 25 to 35 mm Hg requires decompression of the abdomen.

How is the abdomen decompressed?

The abdomen is surgically opened and closed without tension. A vacuum closure relieves tension by not reapproximating fascia or skin. The bowel is covered with a nonadherent dressing and blue towels. Two Jackson-Pratt drains are placed over the towels, and then a large Ioban drape is placed over the entire abdomen and sealed to the skin. The drains are then connected to wall suction.

SOLID ORGAN INJURY

LIVER

Describe the liver's blood supply.

The liver has a dual blood supply. It receives approximately 75% of its blood from the portal vein and 25% from the hepatic artery.

How often can blunt liver injuries be managed nonoperatively?

Most liver injuries are low grade, and approximately 50% to 80% can be managed conservatively with observation in the ICU (95% success rate).

In conservatively managed patients, for what complication other than bleeding should physicians be alert?

A bile leak and formation of a bile collection

What study can be used to inspect the bile duct if an injury is suspected?

Endoscopy retrograde cholangiopancreatography

Name 5 surgical techniques that are used in controlling hepatic bleeding.

1. Suturing: hemostatic suturing using a blunt needle and chromic suture.
2. The Pringle maneuver: a noncrushing clamp is applied to the portal triad to cut off portal venous flow to the liver (possible because of the liver's dual blood supply).
3. Finger-fracture technique: finger dissection through the liver parenchyma to reach deep vessel injuries.
4. Perihepatic packing.
5. Omental patch.

Name 4 techniques for retrohepatic caval injuries.

1. Retrohepatic packing
2. Sequential clamping: vascular clamps are applied to the inferior vena cava (IVC), supradiaphragmatic IVC, and hepatoduodenal ligament.
3. Atriocaval shunt: usually a chest tube placed through the right atrial appendage to the subhepatic vena cava.
4. Balloon tamponade.

Following liver trauma, GI bleeding with normal upper endoscopy and colonoscopy could indicate what condition?

Hemobilia, which occurs from a fistula between branches of the hepatic artery and biliary duct. Treatment is embolization.

What is acute acalculous cholecystitis?	Severe acute cholecystitis without gallstones
Compare the natural history of acute acalculous cholecystitis with that of acute calculous cholecystitis.	The natural history of acute acalculous cholecystitis is worse, with a higher incidence of perforation, gangrene, morbidity, and mortality.
Who is at risk for acute acalculous cholecystitis?	Critically ill patients who are septic or recovering from trauma or surgery. It is associated with gallbladder stasis (i.e., nothing through the mouth and TPN) and poor perfusion.
Name the 4 most common causes of hepatocyte damage following trauma.	1. Direct trauma 2. Ischemic injury 3. Drugs 4. Sepsis
Why are patients with liver disease especially sensitive to hemodynamic changes?	Cirrhosis increases portal pressures; therefore, patients require higher systemic arterial pressures for perfusion. A normal liver receives approximately 50% of its O_2 from portal blood, whereas chronic portal hypertension reduces this to 20%. Thus, patients require adequate hepatic artery pressure for O_2 delivery.
Cirrhosis sets up what other complication?	Increased bleeding because of low clotting factors and platelets.

SPLEEN

What management options are available for splenic injury?	Depending on the grade of injury: 1. Observation alone 2. Splenorrhaphy 3. Partial splenectomy 4. Splenic artery ligation or embolization 5. Total splenectomy

Who is a candidate for nonoperative management?

Patients younger than 56 years with grade I, II, or III injuries diagnosed by CT who are hemodynamically stable and without other indications for celiotomy or injuries to preclude serial abdominal examinations

Describe the typical features of nonoperative management.

Admit for close observation and bed rest with frequent vital signs, Hgb/Hct levels (every 6 hours), and serial abdominal exams for the first 24 hours. Any changes in hemodynamic, laboratory, or physical exam findings indicate the need for more aggressive management.

Spenectomy patients are at high risk for what 5 postoperative complications?

1. Thrombocytosis
2. Infection and subdiaphragmatic abscess: patients should receive at least 5 days of broad-spectrum antibiotics after splenectomy.
3. Rebleeding: caused by failure to securely ligate splenic hilum or short gastric vessels.
4. Left lower lobe atelectasis and/or left pleural effusion.
5. Pancreatitis.

What is overwhelming postsplenectomy infection, and who is most susceptible?

After splenectomy, the immunologic function of the spleen must be carried out by the reticuloendothelial system of the liver. The liver does not effectively kill unopsonized bacteria, however, making patients vulnerable to encapsulated organisms. Overwhelming postsplenectomy infection occurs in 0.5% of adults and has a mortality rate of 80% to 90%. Therefore, pneumococcal, *Haemophilus influenza,* and meningococcal vaccines are indicated in splenectomy patients.

What is delayed rupture of the spleen?	Rupture up to several weeks after abdominal trauma. This probably is caused by bleeding from a lysed clot at the site of the original injury or by rupture of an undiagnosed splenic artery aneurysm.
Ten days after a splenectomy, a trauma patient develops fever, leukocytosis, and left upper quadrant pain. What is the likely diagnosis?	Subphrenic abscess

THORACIC TRAUMA

Name 5 intra-thoracic injuries.	1. Pulmonary and cardiac contusions 2. Pneumothorax and hemothorax 3. Tracheal and esophageal rupture or penetration 4. Cardiac tamponade 5. Trauma to the intrathoracic great vessels
When are emergency thoracotomies indicated?	In patients with penetrating chest injuries and signs of life at the scene who lose pulses in transit or in the ER.
Name 4 possible interventions during emergent thoracotomy.	1. Cross-clamping the aorta to increase vital perfusion. 2. Stop bleeding from heart or large vessels. 3. Relieve pericardial tamponade. 4. Direct cardiac compressions.
What is the significance of 1st or 2nd rib fractures?	Very little specific significance. These findings do indicate, however, that enough energy transfer occurred to possibly cause an intrathoracic injury (e.g., aortic disruption).

CHEST TUBE MANAGEMENT

What are the indications for thoracotomy after chest tube placement in trauma patients?

Initial output of 1,500 mL, or more than 200 mL/hr for more than 2 to 4 hours. These are guidelines only. Remember to account for blood left in the chest after tube placement, blood lost on the floor during the procedure, and rate of bleeding based on the amount of time between injury and initial drainage.

Name 3 reasons why is it important to obtain a CXR after tube placement.

1. To estimate how much blood may be left in the chest
2. To look for a residual pneumothorax
3. To check tube placement

Up to 1 L of blood may be difficult to see on the chest film of supine patients.

If a chest tube clots off, what should be done?

Place a second tube. Flushing or declotting with a Foley catheter is more likely to cause infection.

List 4 settings in which chest tubes should be left in the trauma patient.

1. Total drainage of more than 100 mL in 24 hours.
2. Recurrence of pneumothorax on water seal.
3. Patient is still on positive-pressure ventilation.
4. If any doubt about the need for the tube exists. Leaving chest tubes in too long is safer than pulling them too early.

How is a chest tube removed?

Have the patient take maximum inhalation, then pull the tube out rapidly while simultaneously holding Vaseline gauze over the incision. Upright chest films should be taken immediately and again in 12 hours.

Why is it important to thoroughly drain a traumatic hemothorax?

Complications of undrained hemothorax include fibrothorax, with subsequent loss of lung volume, and empyema (infection of the residual blood).

PULMONARY CONTUSION

What are the 2 major issues in treating patients with pulmonary contusions?

1. Avoidance of overhydration and volume overload
2. Maintenance of optimal pulmonary toilet

These patients may need ventilatory support.

What causes the greatest hypoxia in flail chest?

The underlying pulmonary contusion

What is the most effective treatment of pulmonary contusion and rib fractures in the awake, cooperative patient?

A vigorous pulmonary toilet (e.g., chest physiotherapy, nasotracheal suctioning). Intubation should be avoided if possible. Rib blocks are not very helpful, because they must be repeated every 6 to 8 hours. Epidural anesthesia can be considered.

CARDIAC CONTUSION

How are cardiac contusions diagnosed?

History of chest trauma or sternal fractures, with ECG changes, heart failure, increased MB isoenzyme of creatine kinase (CK-MB)/troponin, or arrhythmias. The gold standard is wall motion abnormality on echocardiogram.

What is the treatment of cardiac contusion?

The goal is to detect and treat malignant arrhythmias: O_2, analgesia, medication to treat dysrhythmias, fluids and inotropes for low CO. Avoid general anesthesia if possible.

Are CK-MB levels of prognostic value?

No

TRAUMATIC BRAIN INJURY

What is the GCS?	Glasgow Coma Scale; an objective assessment of neurologic function and impairment after head injury. A score of 15 is normal; a score of 13 or less is indicative of significant head injury.
How is the GCS calculated?	
Eye opening (E)	4 = opens spontaneously 3 = opens to voice (command) 2 = opens to painful stimulus 1 = does not open eyes
Motor response (M)	6 = obeys commands 5 = localizes painful stimulus 4 = withdraws from pain 3 = decorticate posture 2 = decerebrate posture 1 = no movement
Verbal response (V)	5 = appropriate and oriented 4 = confused 3 = inappropriate words 2 = incomprehensible sounds 1 = no sounds
How does ATLS define mild, moderate, and severe head injuries based on the GCS?	Mild: GCS score of 14 or 15 Moderate: GCS score of 9 to 13 Severe: GCS score of 3 to 8
Below what GCS score is considered to be a coma?	8
What should be done for any patient with a GCS score of 8 or less?	Intubation for airway protection
What is ICP?	Intracranial pressure. An ICP of greater than 20 mm H_2O is intracranial hypertension.

What is CPP?	Cerebral perfusion pressure (CPP = MAP - ICP)
How can you treat a sudden increase in ICP?	1. Elevation of the head of the bed 2. Hyperventilation to decrease P_{CO_2} ($\sim$30 mm Hg) 3. Mannitol infusion 4. Sedation and paralysis 5. Craniotomy
How does hyperventilation affect increased ICP?	Reducing P_{CO_2} causes vasoconstriction and temporarily reduces intercranial volume. A P_{CO_2} level of 25 to 35 mm Hg is considered to be acceptable during periods of increased ICP. Patients should be hyperventilated cautiously because of the risk of causing cerebral ischemia.
What is a pentobarbital coma?	Intentionally decreasing brain metabolism and the need for cerebral blood flow (CO_2 production) with high-dose pentobarbital
What physical exam signs are the best indicator of intracranial herniation?	Pupillary dilatation and response
Raccoon eyes (periorbital ecchymosis) and Battle's sign (retroauricular ecchymosis) are indicative of what?	A basilar skull fracture
Name and describe the 4 major injuries associated with blunt head trauma.	1. Epidural hematomas: middle meningeal artery ruptures ($^1/_3$ may be of venous origin) appears biconvex or "lenticular" (lens shaped) on CT because they are confined by dural attachments to skull. 2. Subdural hematomas: more common than epidural hematomas,

and typically originate from the rupture of bridging veins. Subdural blood may overlay an entire hemisphere and often is associated with severe underlying brain damage, thus worsening the prognosis.

3. Diffuse axonal injury or damage: brain injuries that result in prolonged low GCS scores but that are not associated with mass lesions or ischemic injuries.

4. Cerebral contusions: result from intraparenchymal bleeding. Most common in the frontal and temporal lobes after blunt trauma, they either resolve or coalesce to form an intracerebral hematoma.

Which head injury patients with normal neurological exams should undergo head CT?

Any patient who experiences loss of consciousness, posttraumatic amnesia, or severe headaches should undergo head CT without contrast enhancement.

What is the Monro-Kellie doctrine?

A concept that illustrates ICP dynamics:

1. Intracranial volume remains constant.

2. Any increase in mass (hematoma) must result in the squeezing-out of an equal volume (venous blood, CSF) to maintain normal ICP.

3. Once the compensatory threshold is reached, even small increases in mass result in large increases of ICP (herniation).

What 3 complications most frequently cause a sudden neurologic deficit in the ICU trauma patient?

1. Intracranial hematoma: epidural/subdural

2. Cerebral edema

3. Delayed intracerebral hemorrhage

ORTHOPEDIC TRAUMA

COMPARTMENT SYNDROME

What is compartment syndrome?

An increase in the intracompartmental pressure of an extremity with associated neurovascular compromise

What is the etiology of compartment syndrome?

1. Fractures
2. Tight fascial surgical closure
3. Tight cast/bandage application
4. Increased 3rd-space fluid secondary to ischemic/reperfusion injury or burns
5. Crush injury
6. Electrical injury

Which 3 injuries have a high incidence of extremity compartment syndrome?

1. Burns and electrical injuries
2. Supracondylar elbow fractures: especially in children
3. Proximal tibial fractures

What are the 4 compartments in the lower leg?

1. Lateral
2. Anterior
3. Posterior, superficial
4. Posterior, deep

What are the 3 compartments in the forearm?

1. Extensor
2. Flexor, superficial
3. Flexor, deep

What are signs/symptoms of extremity compartment syndrome?

The **5 P's**:

Pain out of proportion to injury: especially with passive flexion/extension. This usually is the earliest indicator.

Pulselessness: inconsistent. May have a pulse with a compartment syndrome. Loss of pulses is the last effect of increasing compartment pressures.

Pallor: decreased capillary perfusion.

Paresthesia.

Paralysis.

How is the diagnosis of compartment syndrome established?	Measurement of compartment pressures and clinical exam. It is important to evaluate compartment pressure in relation to the diastolic BP. Compartment pressures greater than 30 to 40 mm Hg or within 30 mm Hg of diastolic BP are significant.
What is the treatment of compartment syndrome?	Fasciotomy. This often is done prophylactically.

FAT EMBOLISM SYNDROME

What is fat embolism syndrome?	Embolization of fat particles from bone marrow
What is the most common cause of fat embolism syndrome?	Long bone fractures
What is the usual time of presentation?	Usually within 24 to 72 hours after fracture
What are 3 risk factors for fat embolism syndrome?	1. Multiple long bone fractures 2. Delayed fracture immobilization 3. Delayed operative stabilization
List 5 signs/symptoms of fat embolism syndrome.	1. Petechiae: especially in upper trunk and arms 2. Irritability/confusion 3. Tachycardia 4. Hypoxia 5. Intravascular fat or fat in the urine: rare
What are the CXR findings of fat embolism syndrome?	Fluffy infiltrate and interstitial/alveolar pattern resembling adult respiratory distress syndrome (ARDS). CXR findings often lag behind the clinical picture.
How is fat embolism syndrome managed?	1. Immobilize the long bone fracture

2. Provide supportive care, and monitor ABG.
3. Provide ventilatory support if necessary.

CRUSH SYNDROME

What is crush syndrome?

Renal failure associated with compression injuries to the extremities

What are the causes of crush syndrome?

Combined effects of myoglobin precipitation in renal tubules, hypoxia, hypotension, hyperkalemia, and circulating cytokines

What is a risk factor for crush syndrome?

Prolonged compression/crush of an extremity

Name 3 signs/symptoms of crush syndrome.

1. Pale
2. Hypotensive
3. Hypovolemic

What is the appearance of the patient's urine?

Red to blackish brown because of myoglobin

What is the management of crush syndrome?

1. Monitor for cardiac effects of hyperkalemia, which can kill these patients.
2. Release the crushed extremity's compartments early.
3. Replace fluids, and treat hyperkalemia.
4. Resect necrotic tissue.
5. Use mannitol to keep UOP high.
6. Alkalinize urine to keep myoglobin soluble.

Identify 4 complications associated with crush syndrome.

1. Compartment syndrome
2. Extremity infection/sepsis: necrotic tissue
3. Potential lethal arrhythmias: secondary to elevated potassium released from crushed tissue

4. Systemic inflammatory response syndrome (SIRS) and multisystem organ failure if soft-tissue injury is extensive

CRITICAL CARE OF TRAUMA PATIENTS

What is SIRS?

Systemic inflammatory response syndrome; an overactivation of the immune system in response to an insult (trauma, burn, infection) that causes damage to tissues by overwhelming the body's natural ability to buffer the effects of its own noxious substances (O_2 metabolites, proteolytic enzymes)

Compare SIRS to sepsis and septic shock.

SIRS: fever and leukocytosis
Sepsis: SIRS and infection
Septic shock: sepsis with volume-resistant hypotension and organ dysfunction

What is multiorgan dysfunction?

Functional abnormalities in two or more in a patient with SIRS.

Describe the pathophysiology of organ dysfunction.

Activated circulating neutrophils adhere to endothelium, where they release toxic granules. The damaged endothelium facilitates infiltration of inflammatory mediators into the tissue parenchyma, resulting in organ injury.

Name 4 substances associated with SIRS.

1. Interleukin-1
2. Tumor necrosis factor
3. Nitric oxide
4. O_2^-

Is it important to complete all diagnostic studies before admitting a trauma patient to the ICU?

No. Patients can be better warmed and more closely monitored in the ICU setting. It usually is best for the patient to be moved to the ICU as soon as the need for surgery has been excluded.

What is the "deadly triad"?

The combination of hypothermia, acidosis, and coagulopathy

How is "damage-control" surgery used in the setting of the deadly triad?

With unstable patients, an initial, short damage-control operation is used to correct life-threatening injuries (e.g., severe bleeding). The patient is then stabilized and warmed in the ICU before a second operation is undertaken to definitively address further surgical issues.

Should ETTs be removed from the nasal passages of chronic ICU patients?

Yes. These tubes often impede drainage from the sinuses, leading to stasis and bacterial infection. This is a source of infection that must be investigated in the trauma victim. Large NGTs should also be replaced as early as possible with feeding tubes.

At what point should tracheostomy be performed in the ICU trauma patient?

The general consensus is that early tracheostomy decreases both ventilator days and mortality and allows for easier ventilator weaning. Tracheostomy is indicated if the patient is ventilated for at least 10 days or has failed extubation twice. Some say that a tracheostomy is almost always overdue by the time the clinician has thought of it.

FLUIDS, HYPOVOLEMIA, AND RESUSCITATION

What percentage of blood loss can be tolerated without a change in resting vital signs?

Up to 30%

How does the American College of Surgeons define categories of hemorrhage?

Class I: up to 15% blood loss; minimal symptoms
Class II: 15% to 30% blood loss; HR greater than 100 bpm, normal BP, UOP of 20 to 30 mL/hr, agitated

Class III: 30% to 40% blood loss; HR greater than 120 bpm, decreased BP, UOP of 5 to 15 mL/hr, confused

Class IV: greater than 40% blood loss; HR greater than 140 bpm, decreased BP, UOP of 5 to 15 mL/hr, lethargic

Is Hct a good indication of blood loss in acute hemorrhage?

Absolutely not. It takes 8 to 12 hours to conserve enough sodium to expand our intravascular volume, making a low blood volume and a normal Hct possible. Furthermore, aggressive volume resuscitation with crystalloids has a dilutional effect.

What is the lowest acceptable UOP for an adult trauma patient?

0.5 mL/kg/hr

Which are better resuscitating fluids, colloids or crystalloids?

Crystalloids. It takes 3-fold more volume to reach the same goals with crystalloids because of their tendency to redistribute into the interstitial space, but they have equal survival benefit and much lower cost than colloids.

If a patient fails to respond to the first 2-L bolus of fluids, what action is indicated?

Transfusion of type O whole blood

What is the goal of volume resuscitation?

To maintain a CO sufficient for tissue oxygenation and aerobic metabolism

How do we know when a patient is resuscitated?

Patients are resuscitated when they have normal tissue perfusion. This can be assessed in various ways, including hemodynamic parameters, UOP, base deficit, and lactate level.

What is base deficit?

An easily accessible parameter that is calculated by most blood gas analyzers. Like blood lactate levels, it correlates with tissue hypoxia in hypovolemia. A base deficit between − 3 and +3 mmol/L is desirable.

What are some lab tests that indicate poor perfusion?	Elevated lactate. Trends in lactate values are better indicators than single values. High mortality is reported for patients with lactate greater than 2 mg/dL at 24 hours after admission.

RENAL

Why are trauma patients at risk for acute tubular necrosis?	Acute tubular necrosis is a subtype of acute renal failure that results from prolonged hypovolemia and poor kidney perfusion (shock) or exposure to nephrotoxic agents (e.g., contrast dyes, aminoglycosides, myoglobin).
List 4 indications for hemodialysis in oliguric acute renal failure (ARF).	1. Hyperkalemia: most deadly complication of ARF 2. Metabolic acidosis 3. Complications of uremia: pericarditis or encephalopathy 4. Refractory pulmonary edema
Name 2 ways to minimize the risk of contrast material–induced nephropathy in high-risk patients.	1. Fluid administration to maintain brisk, high UOP for 12 hours before and after administration of contrast material 2. *N*-acetylcysteine

HEMATOLOGY/INFECTIOUS DISEASE

Why do trauma patients become coagulopathic?	In addition to the consumption of platelets and clotting factors in hemorrhagic states, acidosis, hypothermia, and transfusion of blood products lacking clotting factors all contribute to coagulopathy.
What is the workup for fever in the ICU patient after trauma?	1. CXR 2. CBC with differential 3. Blood cultures 4. Urine analysis and culture

5. Thorough physical exam and review of pertinent history
6. CT of the sinuses in patients with long-standing NGTs.

Always change or remove indwelling venous lines, especially those with sugar in them.

NUTRITION

Name 5 laboratory values used to assess nutrition.

1. Albumin: half-life of 18 to 21 days
2. Prealbumin: half-life of 3 to 5 days
3. Transferrin: half-life of 7 to 10 days
4. Total iron-binding capacity
5. Retinol binding protein

What is the primary rule about routes of nutrition?

If the gut works, use it!

Which 2 groups of patients should receive enteral tube feeding?

1. Those who are unable to take adequate nutrition by mouth for 5 days
2. Those with high risk for translocation of gut bacteria: burn victims

Which type of feeding decreases infectious complications in ICU trauma patients?

Enteral feeding decreases incidence of nosocomial pneumonia, ICU days, and ventilator days after trauma. TPN has an increased rate of sepsis compared to enteral feeding.

How are basal energy expenditures calculated in trauma patients?

Trauma = hypercatabolic state
Therefore,
25 to 35 kcal/day nonprotein + 1.5 to 2 g/kg/day protein
Alternatively, use the Harris-Benedict equation, and multiply by 1.5 for major trauma and by 2 for major burns.

Are predictive equations good estimates of energy expenditure in trauma patients?

NO! These equations tend to overestimate by up to 60%.

How can protein requirements be determined?	24-hour nitrogen balance. Nitrogen excreted in urine, plus a coefficient of 4 to 6, is subtracted from the total amount of nitrogen administered by feeding in 24 hours. The goal is a positive balance of approximately 5 g. A negative balance indicates that protein intake is inadequate. Alternatively, serial prealbumin levels may be used.
How can energy expenditure be directly measured?	Indirect calorimetry measures O_2 consumption and CO_2 production.
Which patients should receive parenteral supplementation?	Patients who cannot meet nutritional requirements with tube feeding alone
Why is it important to use an enteral route when possible?	Enteral feeding prevents degenerative changes in the bowel mucosa, which in turn helps to prevent bacterial translocation and subsequent sepsis of bowel origin.
What amino acid is the principal fuel for enterocytes?	Glutamine
Is glutamine an essential or a nonessential amino acid?	Glutamine is made by skeletal muscle (nonessential), but adequate amounts of it are not produced in hypermetabolic states, thus making it conditionally essential in stressed patients.
Why are branched-chain amino acids important for trauma patients?	Metabolized in muscle, they are a good fuel source for skeletal muscle, and they prevent degradation of muscle proteins.

TRAUMA RADIOLOGY

What 3 views should be included in a typical radiographic series for blunt trauma?	1. Lateral C-spine 2. AP chest 3. AP pelvis
What other views may be appropriate in addition to the trauma series?	1. AP and odontoid C-spine 2. Views of any area in which the patient is tender
Name 6 CXR findings for traumatic aortic disruption.	1. Wide mediastinum 2. Apical cap 3. Depression of left mainstem bronchus 4. Loss of aortic knob 5. Deviation of trachea or esophagus (NGT) to the right 6. Obliteration of AP window
What radiologic modality is most useful in diagnosing vascular injuries?	Angiography is the "gold standard." It can be both diagnostic and even therapeutic in areas that are hard to reach surgically (e.g., pelvis, subclavian artery).
What film should be obtained if a tension pneumothorax is suspected?	None! This is a clinical diagnosis based on physical exam. Do not x-ray; instead, decompress.
Name 4 CXR findings that suggest splenic injury.	1. Fracture of the 9th, 10th, or 11th rib on the left 2. Displacement of gastric bubble to the right 3. Elevation of left hemidiaphragm with a pleural effusion 4. Impingement on the colon's splenic flexure
List 5 fractures that indicate the transfer of high kinetic energy and increased risk for internal injury.	1. Scapula 2. Sternum 3. 1st or 2nd rib 4. Pelvis 5. Femur

31   Burn Patients

SKIN BASICS: ANATOMY AND PHYSIOLOGY

What is the largest organ in the human body?

The skin. It comprises 16% of total body weight.

What are the 5 main functions of intact skin?

1. Barrier to infection
2. Barrier to moisture
3. Temperature regulation
4. Sensation
5. Absorption of ultraviolet light for vitamin D synthesis

List, from innermost to outermost, the 5 divisions of the epidermis.

1. Stratum basale
2. Stratum spinosum
3. Stratum granulosum
4. Stratum lucidum
5. Stratum corneum

List the 2 divisions of the dermis.

1. Papillary
2. Reticular

Which provides the barrier function, the dermis or the epidermis?

The epidermis

Which gives skin most of its strength, the dermis or the epidermis?

The dermis (because of the high collagen content)

Where are the cells that allow the skin to re-epithelialize?

In the stratum basale of the epidermis. In burns, epithelium regenerates from this layer surrounding sweat glands and hair follicles.

Where are the blood vessels that regulate temperature located?

The capillary loops in the papillary dermis

Identify the numbered items in the skin

1. 3rd-degree burn
2. 2nd-degree burn
3. 1st-degree burn
4. Epidermis
5. Reticular dermis
6. Hair follicle
7. Capillary loop
8. Papillary dermis
9. Blood vessels
10. SQ tissue

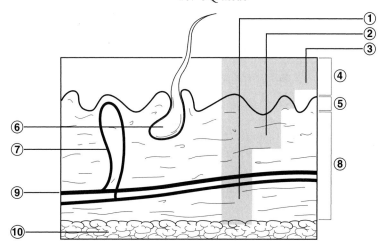

DEFINITIONS

List 5 categories of "burns."

1. Thermal: scald, flame, flash, contact
2. Frostbite
3. Chemical
4. Electrical
5. Exfoliative

What is a 1st-degree burn?

Injury limited to the epidermis

What is a superficial 2nd-degree burn?

Injury limited to the papillary dermis

What is a superficial partial-thickness burn?

A superficial 2nd-degree burn

What is a deep 2nd-degree burn?	Injury limited to the reticular dermis
What is a deep partial-thickness burn?	A deep 2nd-degree burn
What is a 3rd-degree burn?	Injury involving the entire dermis into the SQ tissue
What is a full-thickness burn?	A 3rd-degree burn
What is a 4th-degree burn?	Injury of the entire skin and SQ tissue, including deeper tissues (e.g., muscle and bone)
What is Acticoat?	An artificial, antibacterial coating used to cover excised areas before skin grafting
What is Accuzyme?	An enzymatic debridement
What is Adaptic?	A nonstick gauze
What is AlloDerm?	Freeze-dried human dermis for use as dermal replacement
What is an allograft?	A skin graft using cadaver skin
What is an autograft?	A skin graft using the patient's own skin
What is collagenase?	An enzymatic debridement (breaks down collagen)
What is Biobrane?	An artificial skin substitute consisting of a silicone outer layer, a nylon middle layer, and porcine collagen I to allow adherence to the wound
What is Carasyn?	A topical wound gel
What is a circumferential burn?	A burn that encircles the entire trunk or extremity

What is a cultured epithelial autograft?	A method for generating a graft from a patient's cells in the lab. A full-thickness skin graft is excised soon after injury and sent to a lab. Cells are cultured for 2 weeks. A cultured epithelial autograft is useful in large burns with limited donor sites.
What is early excision?	Surgical removal of burned tissue soon after the burn injury. This is usually done in less than 5 days but may be done up to 12 days.
What is eschar?	Thick, inelastic, unyielding coagulated skin/crust resulting from thermal or chemical injury
What is escharotomy?	Cutting through the eschar to relieve constriction
What is Exudry®?	An absorbent burn dressing
What is Ezyme®?	An enzymatic debridement
What is FTSG?	Full-thickness skin graft
What is Kaltostat®?	A calcium alginate (seaweed-based) wound dressing
What is Kerlix™?	Rolled gauze
What is an inhalation injury?	Pulmonary injury after breathing in toxic smoke from burning materials (e.g., plastics, synthetics, building materials)
What is Integra®?	A 2-layer, artificial skin consisting of acellular dermis covered by a layer of silicone sheeting. It is useful as a dermal replacement.
What is Neosporin®?	A topical antibiotic

What is the Parkland formula?

A formula developed at the Parkland Hospital (Dallas, TX) to estimate fluid requirements of adults during the first 24 hours:

24-hour fluid requirement = 4 mL $\times$ body wt(kg) $\times$ %TBSA burned where %TBSA is percentage of total body surface area burned.

What is Pluronic®?

A topical antibiotic blend in a carrier that offers good soft-tissue penetration

What is Polysporin®?

A topical antibiotic

What is primary contraction?

Shrinkage of a skin graft immediately after it is cut from the donor site. Primary contraction increases with increasing amount of dermis in graft.

What is secondary contraction?

Shrinkage of a skin graft over time as it heals, mediated by contractile fibroblasts. Secondary contraction increases with decreasing amount of dermis in graft.

What is scar contracture?

Limitation of movement because of restriction by hypertrophic scar formation across a joint or joints

What is Silvadene®?

Silver sulfadiazine; probably the most widely used topical antibacterial treatment for burn wounds

What is Sorbsan®?

An absorbent burn dressing

What is Sulfamyalon®?

Mafenide acetate; a topical antimicrobial for burn wounds (contains no sulfa)

What is STSG?

Split-thickness skin graft

What is TBSA?

Total body surface area

What is a xenograft?

A skin graft using nonhuman (usually pig) skin

STATISTICS

Approximately how many burns occur in the United States each year?	1.25 million
Approximately how many patients require hospitalization for burns in the United States each year?	50,000 to 70,000 ($\sim$5%)
Approximately how many people die from burns in the United States each year?	Approximately 4,000
What are the 4 most common mechanisms of burn injury?	1. Scald 2. Flame 3. Flash 4. Contact
What 4 factors most influence burn injury mortality?	1. Size of the burn: %TBSA 2. Age 3. Presence or absence of inhalation injury 4. Comorbid conditions: heart disease, diabetes
What 2 age groups are most at risk of mortality from burn injury?	1. Those younger than 10 years 2. Those older than 50 years
What size burns are associated with greater mortality?	10% for young and old 20% for others
How can you estimate mortality from a burn wound?	Age (years) + %TBSA burn This formula may overestimate mortality in large burns because of advances in care, especially for children.
What kinds of fires are most often associated with inhalation injury?	House fires. Inhalation injury should be suspected in all patients exposed to indoor fires. In addition, it may occur

with outdoor gasoline/flammable vapor fires on cloudy (low atmospheric pressure) days, because high concentrations of vapor are held close to the ground and, thus, can be inhaled.

IMMEDIATE CARE

What is the first treatment of the burn victim?	Stop the burning process.
How can you stop the burning process?	Irrigation with water
What should be removed from a burn victim as soon as possible?	All clothing, rings, watches, jewelry, belts, or anything that can retain heat near the patient
What is a complication of removing clothing and irrigation with water?	Hypothermia. Cover the patient with a clean blanket if possible.
What 2 cardiac complications are associated with hypothermia?	1. Ventricular fibrillation 2. Asystole
What hematologic complication is associated with hypothermia?	Coagulopathy
What are 4 causes of temperature instability in the burn patient?	1. Exposure 2. Increased evaporative fluid losses 3. Administration of large volumes of hypothermic fluids 4. Central temperature instability
What is the initial approach to the burn patient?	Mnemonic: **ABCDE** **A**irway **B**reathing **C**irculation **D**isability: mental status **E**xposure

What must a rescuer be aware of while helping a burn victim?	The risk of becoming a second victim from contact with the patient, clothing, or toxins in the environment. Wear universal precautions/safety gear.
List the 5 tubes required by severely burned patients.	1. 2 large-bore peripheral IVs 2. Foley catheter 3. ETT 4. NGT
Why are 2 IVs and a Foley required?	To deliver fluid and to measure the adequacy of resuscitation
Why do some patients need an ETT?	To control the airway in case edema develops
Why do patients need an NGT?	To decompress the stomach. Ileus and air swallowing are common.
List 8 initial labs or studies for burn patients.	1. CBC 2. Serum electrolytes 3. BUN 4. Creatinine 5. Glucose 6. ABG 7. CXR 8. Carboxyhemoglobin
Which exam should be included in the secondary survey of the patient with circumferential burns?	Examination of peripheral pulses to ensure adequate perfusion to distal limbs
Which exam should be included in the secondary survey of the patient with suspected inhalation injury?	Neurological exam. Hypoxic damage may be subtle.
What are the 10 criteria for referral to a designated burn center?	1. Partial-thickness burns greater than 10% TBSA at any age 2. Any full-thickness burn

3. Burns with the potential for serious long-term functional and/or cosmetic impairment, especially burns involving the face, hands, feet, genitalia, perineum, or major joints as well as circumferential burns to the extremities or chest
4. Inhalation injury
5. Electrical burns, including those from lightning
6. Chemical burns
7. Patients with pre-existing medical disorders that could complicate management, prolong recovery, or affect outcome
8. Burn patients sustaining other trauma
9. Children in hospitals without qualified personnel or equipment
10. Patients who will require special social, emotional, or long-term rehabilitative intervention, including suspected child/elder abuse, substance abuse, psychiatric conditions, etc.

What findings prompt escharotomy to be performed?

Reduced peripheral pulses or poor ventilation in the setting of circumferential burns

How is escharotomy performed?

Bedside electrocautery with sedation, scalpel, or enzymatically. Go through the eschar but NOT into the SQ tissues.

In what part of the body is enzymatic debridement more likely to be useful?

In the hands, because of the risk of injury to neurovascular structures with escharotomy to the fingers

Draw the locations of chest escharotomy.

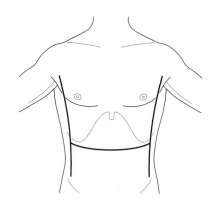

BURN SHOCK

What is burn shock?

Hypovolemic and cellular shock; inadequate blood delivery to support cellular needs secondary to fluid shifts from the intravascular to the interstitial space

What level of burn is associated with burn shock in adults?

Greater than 25% TBSA

What tissue state results from the fluid shifts following a burn?

Edema

When does edema peak after a burn injury?

Minor burns: 8 to 12 hours
Major burns: 12 to 24 hours

What 7 factors govern edema formation?

1. Capillary permeability
2. Plasma hydrostatic pressure
3. Interstitial hydrostatic pressure
4. Plasma oncotic pressure
5. Interstitial oncotic pressure
6. Oncotic reflection coefficient
7. Lymph flow

After a burn, what would you expect to happen to each of the following?

Intravascular volume	Decreases
Hct	Increases
SVR	Increases
CO	Decreases
End-organ perfusion	Decreases: ischemia
blood pH	Decreases: metabolic acidosis

FLUID RESUSCITATION

Why is fluid resuscitation so important?

It reduces mortality if done correctly.

What is the most common error made in burn resuscitation?

Underestimating fluid requirements

What is the best measure of fluid resuscitation?

Urine output via Foley catheter

Which vital sign is the best indicator of fluid resuscitation?

Pulse

Why is BP an unreliable measure in burn patients?

Peripheral edema

What is an adequate urine output for an adult?

0.5 mL/kg/hr

What is an adequate urine output for a child?

1 mL/kg/hr

What is the Parkland formula?

An estimate of the fluid resuscitation requirements for burn victims during the first 24 hours.
24-hour fluid requirement =
  4 mL $\times$ body weight(kg) $\times$
  %TBSA burn

Give half the volume during first 8 hours and the remaining half during the next 16 hours.

The Parkland formula is valid for which patient group?

Adults

Is the Parkland formula always right?

No. Always adjust fluid requirements according to urine output.

What time is the starting point for the purposes of fluid resuscitation?

The time of injury. If a patient has been in transport/transferred and has received fluid, add this fluid into your estimates.

What formula can be used for children?

$4 \text{ mL} \times$ body weight(kg) $\times$ %TBSA burn $+ 1,500 \text{ mL/m}^2 \times$ BSA

which represents the Parkland formula plus pediatric maintenance fluid requirements. This formula usually works out to

$6 \text{ mL} \times$ body weight(kg) $\times$ %TBSA burn

For what size burns do children require resuscitation?

Greater than 10% TBSA

What is the "Rule of 9's"?

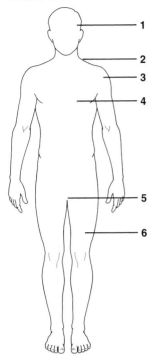

The method used to estimate BSA:
1. Head: 9%
2. Back: 18%
3. Arms: 9% each
4. Chest: 18%
5. Perineum: 1%
6. Legs: 18% each

The Rule of 9's is not accurate for what patient group?

Small children, because the head comprises a larger BSA and the legs a lower BSA. In this case, the head equals 18% and the legs 13.5% each.

What is the quickest way to estimate burn area?

The palm equals approximately 1% BSA.

What happens if a patient is under-resuscitated?

Inadequate perfusion to vital organs. The first organs to be affected will likely be the kidneys and GI tract.

What 3 things happen if a patient is over-resuscitated?

1. Cerebral edema
2. Pulmonary edema
3. Conversion of partial-thickness burns in the "zone of stasis" to full-thickness burns

How does pain correlate to burn-wound severity?	Inversely. Increasing depth of burn equals decreased pain.
Why should IM/SQ pain medications not be given to burn patients?	Variable/unpredictable absorption with fluid shifts
How do you treat a burn patient with myoglobinuria/hemoglobinuria?	Alkalinize the urine with sodium bicarbonate, and increase fluids.
What is the goal urine output for an adult patient with myoglobinuria/hemoglobinuria?	1 to 2 mL/kg/hr

INHALATION INJURY

What is the associated mortality of burn patients with inhalation injuries?	40% to 50% (as compared to 10% without)
What are some early complications of inhalational injury?	Barotrauma resulting in: 1. Pneumothorax 2. Pneumomediastinum 3. Pneumoperitoneum 4. SQ emphysema
What are 4 potential long-term effects of serious inhalation injury?	1. Restrictive lung disease 2. Bronchiectasis 3. Tracheomalacia 4. Tracheal stenosis
What is the most common cause of long-term effects?	Iatrogenic injury associated with intubation
What 3 anatomic regions of the airway can be injured by smoke and/or heat?	1. Supraglottic 2. Tracheobronchial 3. Lung parenchyma
What area is most susceptible to direct thermal injury?	The upper airways (especially the epiglottis)

Where does smoke inhalation cause the most injury?

The bronchial tree and alveolar membranes

What is a common cause of upper airway obstruction?

Edema of the laryngeal structures

Name 4 ways that smoke inhalation injures the respiratory tree.

1. Disrupts the epithelium.
2. Decreases mucociliary clearance.
3. Incites an inflammatory response with increased blood flow and airway edema formation.
4. Increases permeability of the alveolar–capillary membrane with subsequent interstitial edema and alveolar flooding.

What is the best treatment of upper airway injury?

Endotracheal intubation

List 7 symptoms that suggest inhalation injury.

1. Tearing
2. Coughing
3. Wheezing
4. Hoarseness
5. Disorientation
6. Obtundation
7. Shortness of breath

List 5 signs that suggest inhalation injury.

1. Carbonaceous sputum
2. Facial burns
3. Singed nose hairs
4. Stridor
5. Conjunctivitis

What are 7 vital pieces of information to obtain in the history for inhalation injury?

1. Closed/open space
2. Type of burning materials
3. Duration of exposure
4. Time to hospital
5. Administered O_2 at scene/ en route
6. Mental status
7. Intoxication

How big is the alveolar surface area?	A tennis court!
What is the best way to establish the diagnosis of inhalation injury?	Bronchoscopy
How frequent are major complications with bronchoscopy in acute inhalation injury?	Very rare (<0.5%)
Are pulmonary function tests (PFTs) useful in the early diagnosis of inhalation injury?	No. Most patients cannot cooperate to do forced expirations; however, normal PFTs rule out inhalation injury.
What 4 labs/studies should be ordered if you suspect inhalation?	1. ABG 2. CXR 3. ECG 4. Carboxyhemoglobin
When is the peak of upper airway inflammation?	Approximately 24 hours
How much extra fluid do patients with inhalation injury need compared to patients with the same %TBSA burn but without inhalation injury?	40% to 75% during first 24 hours
What maneuvers can be used to decrease upper airway edema?	Elevate the head of the bed to 30°.
What is the maximum cuff pressure to use in an intubated patient?	20 mm H_2O
In an intubated patient, how can the resolution of airway edema be assessed?	Deflate the ETT cuff. If passage of air around the tube is audible, consider extubation.

What other signs are useful to help judge the resolution of airway edema?	Decreased facial and periorbital edema. Direct laryngoscopy can assess the supraglottic region.
List 2 important toxic compounds frequently found in smoke.	1. Carbon monoxide 2. Hydrogen cyanide
Why is carbon monoxide dangerous?	It displaces O_2 from hemoglobin
How much greater affinity does carbon monoxide have for hemoglobin than O_2?	200-fold greater
What is the blood test for carbon monoxide?	Carboxyhemoglobin
What is the treatment for carbon monoxide poisoning?	1. 100% O_2 2. Intubation if mental status changes 3. Hyperbaric O_2 if available
What is the half-life of elimination for carbon monoxide with room air?	250 min
What is the half-life of elimination for carbon monoxide with 100% O_2?	40 to 60 min
What is the half-life of elimination for carbon monoxide with hyperbaric O_2 at 3 atm?	30 min
What are the effects of carbon monoxide poisoning with the following levels of carboxyhemoglobin?	
Less than 10%	None
10%	Headache

30%	Increased headache
	Vision changes
	Nausea
	Vomiting
	Collapse
60%	Coma
90%	Death in minutes

What is the characteristic odor of cyanide?

Bitter almonds

Name 5 signs and symptoms of cyanide poisoning.

1. Lethargy
2. Nausea
3. Headache
4. Coma
5. Metabolic acidosis

How is cyanide lethal?

Reversible inhibition of mitochondrial cytochrome oxidase leads to tissue anoxia.

What is a normal serum level of cyanide?

Nonsmokers: 0.02 μg/mL
Smokers: 0.04 μg/mL

What is a toxic level of cyanide?

0.1 μg/mL

What is the treatment for cyanide poisoning?

1. 100% O_2
2. Sodium thiosulfate
3. Hydroxocobalamin

INFECTION CONTROL

What is the goal of prophylactic topical therapy?

To minimize colonization of burn wound

What is burn-wound colonization?

Less than 10^5 organisms/g tissue. Bacteria in wound are from the environment or the patient's flora.

Are all burn wounds colonized?

Yes

What is a septic burn wound?	When the colonization is **greater** than 10^5 organisms/g tissue and/or there is bacterial invasion into viable tissue
What is burn-wound sepsis?	When the patient is symptomatic and has systemic (blood or lymphatic) spread of microorganisms or their toxic products and greater than 10^5 organisms/g in the burn wound
List 9 cardinal signs of Gram-positive burn-wound sepsis.	1. Septic burn wound 2. Gradual onset of symptoms 3. Fever greater than 40°C 4. WBC greater than 20,000 cells/mm³ 5. Decreased Hct 6. Wound macerated with soupy exudate 7. Ileus 8. Reduced urine output with hypotension 9. Reduced appetite
List 8 cardinal signs of Gram-negative burn-wound sepsis.	1. Septic burn wound 2. Rapid onset of symptoms 3. Slight or no fever 4. Satellite lesions distant from burn wound 5. Wound with focal gangrene 6. Mental obtundation 7. Ileus 8. Reduced urine output with hypotension
What is the treatment of burn-wound sepsis?	Start broad-spectrum double coverage with systemic antibiotics. Specific treatment should follow based on wound/blood culture isolates.
What is the name of the satellite lesion in Gram-negative sepsis?	Ecthyma gangrenosum

How are *Pseudomonas* sp. frequently detected?	"Sniff test." *Pseudomonas* sp. have a characteristic odor.
List 3 other common causes of sepsis in a burn patient.	1. Pneumonia 2. Urinary tract infection 3. Line infection
What is the best method of infection control in a burn patient?	Early closure of wounds
What 4 common, Gram-positive pathogens are found in burn patient infections?	1. Streptococci 2. *Staphylococcus aureus* 3. *S. epidermidis* 4. Enterococci
What 4 common, Gram-negative pathogens are found in burn patient infections?	1. *Pseudomonas aeruginosa* 2. *Escherichia coli* 3. *Enterobacter cloacae* 4. *Klebsiella pneumoniae*
What is the most common fungal infection in the burn patient?	*Candida* sp.
What 3 viruses are common in burn patients?	1. Cytomegalovirus 2. Varicella zoster virus 3. Herpes simplex virus
How well does silver sulfadiazine (Silvadene®):	
Penetrate eschar?	Poorly
Cover *Staphylococcus aureus*?	Well
Cover other Gram-positive organisms?	Well
Cover Gram-negative bacteria?	Well
Cover *Pseudomonas* sp.?	Well
Cover *Candida* sp.?	Well

What is a common reaction to silver sulfadiazine?	Transient leukopenia
How well does mafenide acetate (Sulfamyalon⁴):	
Penetrate eschar?	Well
Cover *Staphylococcus aureus*?	Not well
Cover other Gram-positive organisms?	Well
Cover Gram-negative bacteria?	Well
Cover *Candida* sp.?	Not well
What is a common, unpleasant reaction to mafenide?	Pain on application
What acid-base imbalance is created by treatment with mafenide?	Hyperchloremic metabolic acidosis. Mafenide is a carbonic anhydrase inhibitor, so it causes increased respiratory rate (to blow off CO_2) and acidosis.
How well does silver nitrate:	
Penetrate eschar?	Poorly
Cover *Staphylococcus aureus*?	Well
Cover other Gram-positive organisms?	Well
Cover Gram-negative bacteria?	Well
Cover *Pseudomonas* sp.?	Well
Cover *Candida* sp.?	Well
What does silver nitrate do to sheets and anything it comes in contact with?	Turns it black (think tarnish)

What side effects does silver nitrate have?	It may leach electrolytes and cause methemoglobinemia.
Should tetanus prophylaxis be given to all burn victims?	Yes, except those patients who were actively immunized within the preceding 12 months.

BURN-WOUND MANAGEMENT

How is burn depth assessed?	Clinically. Currently, no invasive or noninvasive procedure/technique/device is in common use that augments a careful physical exam.
List 3 general depths of burns.	1. Superficial: 1st degree 2. Partial thickness: 2nd degree 3. Full thickness: 3rd degree
The severity of which type of burn is difficult to determine?	Partial-thickness burns between superficial and deep. These are the "indeterminate" burns.
How reliable is an experienced surgeon's initial assessment in predicting the need for grafting of an "indeterminate" burn?	50% to 70%
Name 4 signs of a superficial partial-thickness burn.	1. Blisters: may form later 2. Very painful 3. Blanches with pressure 4. Red/pink: secondary to increased blood flow
Name 4 signs of a deep partial-thickness burn.	1. Blisters 2. Discomfort more than pain 3. Often mottled pink/white 4. Slow/no capillary refill
Name 4 signs of a full-thickness burn.	1. Often charred areas 2. No pain 3. Clotted SQ vessels 4. No capillary refill

Which burns will heal well on their own?

Superficial and some partial-thickness burns, both of which can heal in less than 3 weeks

Which burns require surgical excision and grafting?

All full-thickness wounds and any partial-thickness wound that is deemed unlikely to heal in less than 3 weeks

If you cannot tell initially which burns will and will not need grafting, how do you plan surgery?

Reassess questionable areas and wound healing over the course of hospital admission, including at dressing changes and in the OR.

Identify the 3 burn zones of blood flow around partial-thickness burns.

1. Zone of coagulation
2. Zone of stasis
3. Zone of hyperemia

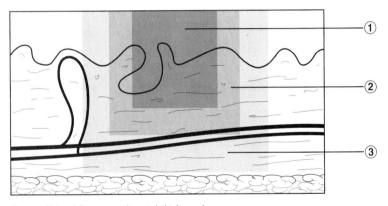

Zones of blood flow around partial-thickness burns.

Describe the blood flow in each of the 3 zones.

Zone of coagulation: dead tissue, no flow
Zone of stasis: microvascular sludging
Zone of hyperemia: excess flow

Which zone is "tissue in danger"?

Zone of stasis

What is the importance of managing the zone of stasis properly?

If the patient is not over- or under-resuscitated, tissue in the zone of stasis may survive. The %TBSA of full thickness burns can therefore be kept to a minimum.

What are the 3 advantages of early wound closure in burn patients?	1. Reduced mortality 2. Shortened hospital stay 3. Reduced costs
How is early wound closure accomplished?	Excision and grafting
List 2 types of excision	1. Tangential: sequential excision of thin layers of burn eschar until a viable bed is encountered. 2. Fascial: flap of eschar is raised and dissection extended until all dead tissue down to the fascia level has been excised.
In what situations is tangential excision appropriate?	In *most* burns, in which you can reasonably expect viable tissue above the level of the fascia.
Where is fascial excision appropriate?	In *very deep* burns or burns so massive that quicker fascial excision is necessary to keep the procedure to a reasonable time
What is the complication associated with fascial excision?	Contour defects that result from removal of the SQ fat and deeper tissues
How are the excised areas covered?	Split-thickness skin graft is the norm. These can be either allograft (cadaver skin) or autograft (patient's own skin). The choice depends an the availability of donor sites and the surface area of the burn. Cultured skin and other skin substitutes are available as well.
How do skin grafts survive without a blood supply?	Nutrients diffuse from the wound into the graft until blood vessels grow in.
List 4 factors that can cause a skin graft not to take.	1. Inadequate debridement 2. Shearing 3. Hematoma/seroma formation 4. Infection

What is the physiology behind graft failure because of:

Inadequate debridement?

Results in inadequate blood supply to nutritive surface of the wound bed.

Shearing?

Early manipulation of the graft site causes the graft to slide, shearing new tissues and disrupting the ingrowth of new blood vessels.

Hematoma/seroma formation?

Separates the graft from its source of nutrition, the wound bed.

Infection?

Halts wound healing. In addition, bacterial enzymes may actually dissolve the graft.

WOUND HEALING AND WOUND CARE

List the 3 main ways that skin may repair a wound.

1. Re-epithelialization
2. Scar formation
3. Contraction

Which burns heal by:

Re-epithelialization?

1st-degree and superficial 2nd-degree burns

Scar formation and contraction?

Deep 2nd-degree burns as well as 3rd- and 4th-degree burns

What kind of wound bed will help keratinocytes to migrate rapidly?

Moist, viable tissue. Cells have to "cut" their way through hardened tissue.

What are the 3 phases of scar formation?

1. Inflammatory (lag) phase
2. Proliferative phase
3. Maturation phase

How long does each phase of scar formation last?

Inflammatory: 4 to 5 days
Proliferative: 2 to 3 weeks
Maturation: months to years

What happens in each phase of scar formation?

Inflammatory

Neutrophils enter the wound and kill bacteria, followed by macrophages that phagocytose tissue and secrete factors that stimulate fibroblast migration.

Proliferative

Fibroblasts secrete collagen and other extracellular matrix components in a disorganized manner, providing a matrix for epithelium and strength for the wound.

Maturation

Fibroblasts secrete and dissolve collagen to reorganize it so that it is more compact.

What is the most important WBC regulator of wound healing?

Macrophages

Which cells are responsible for collagen deposition (and strength gain) in a healing wound?

Fibroblasts

Which cells are responsible for contraction of healing wounds?

Myofibroblasts

What is the difference between a hypertrophic scar and a keloid?

Hypertrophic scars stay within the margin of the wound. Keloids expand beyond the wound margins.

METABOLIC RESPONSES TO BURNS

What happens to energy expenditure following a burn?

Energy expenditure increases by 60% to 100%

What is the "ebb and flow" response to burn injury?

Decrease in metabolic rate during the first 12 to 24 hours, followed by a prolonged period of hypermetabolism that lasts for months.

What is the result of prolonged hypermetabolism?

Weight loss and depletion of protein stores. This leads to immunosuppression, delayed wound healing, and death.

Name 2 ways to reduce energy expenditure.

1. Increased room temperature
2. Early excision and grafting

What is diabetes of injury?

Insulin resistance and blood sugar from increased stress hormones (glucagon, epinephrine, and cortisol)

Is TPN or enteral nutrition preferred?

Enteral nutrition. TPN has increased mortality.

How many calories do burn patients need?

This must be constantly reassessed, but the starting point should be 20% to 50% more than normal.

What is the preferred major source of calories for burn patients?

Carbohydrate

Does feeding extra protein help burn patients?

Yes. These patients show better immune function, less bacteremia, and improved survival.

What is the importance of each of the following micronutrients?

Vitamin A

Helps wound healing and epithelial growth.

Vitamin C

Essential for normal synthesis and cross-linking of collagen.

Iron

Important in hemoglobin and myoglobin
Essential cofactor for many enzymes
(There is a lot of iron in blood transfusions.)

Zinc	Helps wound healing DNA and RNA synthesis Lymphocyte function Essential cofactor for metalloenzymes
Selenium	Important in the function of lymphocytes
What happens to a patient's body temperature following a burn?	Body temperature increases by 1 to 2°C secondary to circulating cytokines and increased metabolism.
What is SIRS?	Systemic inflammatory response syndrome
How is SIRS defined?	The presence of 2 or more of the following: 1. Body temperature greater than 38°C or less than 36°C 2. Heart rate greater than 90 bpm 3. Respiratory rate greater than 20 breaths per minutes, or an arterial partial pressure of carbon dioxide ($PaCO_2$) less than 32 mm Hg 4. WBC more than 12,000 cells/μL, less than 4,000 cells/μL, or greater than 10% bands
What is the most frequent change involving bone after a burn?	Osteoporosis from bed confinement, immobilization, hyperemia, and adrenocortical hyperactivity
Name 2 effects of major burns on the GI tract.	1. Adynamic ileus and gastric dilatation (place an NGT in all patients with burns greater than 20% TBSA) 2. Curling's ulcer
What is a Curling's ulcer?	A gastric ulcer in burn patients resulting from loss of mucus and increased acid
How is a Curling's ulcer prevented?	1. H_2-blockers, carafate, and/or antacids.

2. Keep gastric pH above 4.
3. Provide early enteral feedings (within 24 hours).
4. Do not use both antacid medications and carafate.

CHEMICAL EXPOSURE

List the 2 main types of chemical "burns."

1. Acid
2. Alkali

What is the initial treatment of both types of chemical burns?

Remove all clothing and irrigate with water.

Why must health care workers be especially careful with chemical burns?

Possibility of contact with caustic substance when treating the patient. Wear all precautions!

Are acid or alkali burns usually deeper?

Alkali burns usually are deeper.

Why is neutralization of acid/base not indicated?

The reaction is likely to be exothermic and will worsen the wound by the addition of thermal injury.

Where might a mechanic come into contact with a strong acid?

Car batteries, which contain hydrochloric acid

What is a common household strong base?

Drain opener

Hydrofluoric acid is used in industry and seen in industrial accidents. Name 1 of its major deleterious effects.

It scavenges calcium from affected parts, causing severe pain and cellular dysfunction. Large exposures are lethal.

What is the "almost magical" treatment for hydrofluoric acid exposure?

Calcium infusion into the exposed limb

ELECTRICAL INJURY

What is the incidence of deaths from electrical injury?

Approximately 1% of all accidental deaths (25% are caused by lightning)

What are the 2 major types of electrical burn injuries?

1. Electrical arc injuries, in which the current passes external to the body, thus causing local burns
2. Injuries in which the current passes through the body.

What 7 factors determine the magnitude of electrical injury?

1. Type of current
2. Amount of current
3. Pathway of current
4. Duration of contact
5. Area of contact
6. Resistance of the body
7. Voltage

Which layer of the skin is responsible for most resistance to electrical current?

Stratum corneum, which acts as an insulator of deeper tissues (note that surface resistance drops dramatically if wet)

Why are electrical burns so dangerous?

Most of the destruction is internal, because the route of least electrical resistance follows nerves, blood vessels, and fascia. Injury is far worse than external burns indicate. Cardiac arrhythmias, myoglobinuria, acidosis, and renal failure are common.

What is Ohm's law, and what is its significance?

Current = voltage/resistance
Current is directly responsible for injury; therefore, the higher the voltage and the lower the resistance, the greater the current and resultant injury.

What is "let-go" current?

The amount of current above which involuntary muscle contractions prevent the victim from escaping the current's source ($\sim$15 mA).

What effect does electrical current have on the respiratory system?

If the amount of current exceeds approximately 20 mA, it can cause tetany of the respiratory muscles and result in asphyxia if the source of the current is not removed.

Name 3 considerations in the management of electrical burns.

1. Cardiac monitoring
2. Cardiac enzymes
3. Treatment of myoglobinuria

What effect does electrical current have on the cardiac system?

If the current exceeds 30 to 40 mA, ventricular fibrillation may be induced. Current is dependent on the duration of shock and on the weight of the individual. At very high currents, however, complete depolarization occurs; once the source is removed, the heart will convert to normal sinus rhythm (i.e., defibrillation).

What is the treatment for a low-voltage burn victim who is without vital signs once removed from the source of the current?

Initiation of CPR and ACLS protocols

What determines the path of a high-voltage electrical current passing through the body?

The current will follow the shortest path between contact points and involve the structures in its path.

What is the significance of entrance and exit wounds?

They signify local destruction to deeper tissues, which often is grossly underestimated.

What is the significance of underlying muscle tissue injury?

Tissue damage with extravasation of fluid and subsequent swelling may result in fascial compartment syndromes.

What are the symptoms and signs of a developing compartment syndrome?

The **5 P's**:
Pain
Paresthesias
Pallor
Paralysis
Pulselessness

What other complications can significant muscle necrosis cause?

Renal failure and hyperkalemia secondary to rhabdomyolysis

What is rhabdomyolysis?

Injury to muscle causing myoglobin release into the bloodstream and filtration in the urine; often seen in electrical or crush injuries

How is the diagnosis of rhabdomyolysis established?

1. Presence of dark, tea-colored urine
2. Urine positive for myoglobin and other hemochromogens: dipstick positive for blood, but no RBCs on microscopic examination

What is the treatment of myoglobinuria?

1. Maintain urine output greater than 100 mL/hr with vigorous IV fluids and mannitol.
2. Alkalinize urine with IV bicarbonate to prevent precipitation of myoglobin in renal tubules.

What are 2 common GI complications associated with electrical injuries?

1. Adynamic ileus
2. Stress ulcers: Curling's ulcers

FROSTBITE

What 2 factors predispose to frostbite injuries?

1. Alcoholism
2. Psychiatric illness

What are the 3 mechanisms of frostbite injury?

1. Cellular dehydration
2. Ice crystal formation within the tissue: both intracellular and extracellular
3. Microvascular occlusion

How is the vasculature affected?

1. On thawing, increased permeability occurs, with subsequent plasma fluid leaking into the interstitium.
2. Hemoconcentration in the microvascular beds results in platelet aggregation and thrombosis.

What is the Hunting reaction?

Alternating peripheral vasodilatation and vasoconstriction that occurs when extremity temperatures decrease to less than 10°C. This response is an effort to slow the freezing process; however, preservation of core temperature is sacrificed.

How are frostbite injuries classified?

By the appearance of the extremity after thawing:
1. 1st degree: hyperemia, edema, superficial freezing of the epidermis
2. 2nd degree: hyperemia, edema, vesicle formation (cutaneous sensation remains intact)
3. 3rd degree: necrosis of all skin layers that extends into SQ tissues
4. 4th degree: full-thickness injury that extends into the underlying bone and muscle

Is motor function always impaired in severe frostbite injuries?

No. Proximal muscles and tendons may remain intact, thus allowing movement of distal extremities.

What is the treatment of frostbite injuries?

1. Rapid rewarming in a 40°C water bath.
2. Narcotics to relieve pain.
3. Leave vesicles intact, because they protect underlying tissue.
4. Daily wound care and whirlpool therapy
5. Avoidance of further trauma to the injured extremity: bed rest, foot cradles, sheepskins
6. Surgical intervention/debridement. This must be delayed until demarcation is clear, however, and may take several weeks. Early estimates of tissue damage often overestimate the extent of nonviable tissue. Note, however, that progression to wet gangrene requires early debridement.

Is rapid rewarming of the extremity indicated?	Yes. It provides a chance for marginal tissues to recover. Immersion in a 40°C water bath with adequate circulation is optimal.
Are fasciotomies indicated in severe injuries?	No. Vessels are already thrombosed rather than merely constricted by tissue swelling.

HYPOTHERMIA

What is the hallmark of hypothermia?	Core body temperature less than 34°C
What is the most common symptom of hypothermia?	Altered mental status
List 3 other signs of hypothermia.	1. Decreased heart rate 2. Decreased BP 3. Decreased respiratory rate
What is the most important therapeutic intervention?	Rapid initiation of rewarming
What is the treatment of hypothermia?	Warm IV fluids and "passive" rewarming (warm blankets, warming lights, increase room temperature, etc.) if core temperature is greater than 28°C and the patient is shivering
In what 2 situations is "active" rewarming indicated?	1. Asystole 2. Core temperature less than 28°C 3. Failure of passive rewarming
What are 3 methods of active rewarming?	1. Total body immersion in a 40°C water bath 2. Warm lavage via chest tube thoracostomy 3. Cardiopulmonary bypass
What 2 forms of monitoring are essential during rewarming?	1. ECG: for development of arrhythmias, most of which are supraventricular

2. Monitoring of electrolytes: tendency toward hypokalemia

EXFOLIATIVE CONDITIONS

List 2 important exfoliative conditions.

1. Stevens-Johnson syndrome
2. Toxic epidermal necrolysis (TEN)

List 2 ways that exfoliative diseases are similar to burns.

1. They compromise the normal integrity of the skin, often over a large surface area.
2. They often are treated in a burn center.

List 3 drugs/classes of drugs that can cause epidermolytic reactions.

1. Phenytoin
2. Sulfonamides
3. Nonsteroidal anti-inflammatory drugs

What are the signs and symptoms of Stevens-Johnson syndrome?

Raised, target-like lesions on the skin that can coalesce AND mucous membrane ulceration at 2 or more sites (conjuntiva, mouth, pharynx, urethra)

What are the signs and symptoms of TEN?

Sheets of skin sloughing off

What are 8 steps in treating TEN?

1. Stop all suspected drugs
2. Administer pain medication and antipyretics
3. Debridement and closure with biologic or synthetic dressing
4. Empiric antibiotics if neutropenic
5. IV diphenhydramine
6. Stress ulcer prophylaxis
7. Oral nystatin
8. Avoid steroids

PAIN MANAGEMENT

How is pain management different in burn patients?

Burn patients have more interventions. Pain management must cover procedures (dressing changes, visits to tank/tub), activity (physical therapy), and baseline pain.

What are 2 general components of pain management in burn patients?

1. Pain control
2. Anxiolytics

What 4 principles should be followed in pain management for burn patients?

1. Patient report guides management.
2. Scheduled/patient-controlled analgesia is better than as-needed.
3. Use an established IV rather than injecting each time medication is needed (each needle stick causes new pain).
4. Re-evaluate dose and type frequently.

What are 3 major advantages of fentanyl over morphine?

1. Fentanyl is shorter acting, so it is easier to avoid oversedation.
2. Fentanyl does not cause itching from histamine release.
3. Fentanyl is available in a lollipop for kids.

What are 2 major advantages of lorazepam over diazepam?

1. Lorazepam (Ativan) is cleared faster than diazepam, so effective doses are easier to maintain.
2. Lorazepam is not metabolized by the P450 system, so it has no interactions with H_2-blockers (commonly used in the ICU).

REHABILITATION

When should rehabilitation begin?

With the initial care plan for the patient

What are major complications to avoid in the acute setting?

Shearing newly placed grafts, shortening of tendons due to prolonged nonweight-bearing, improper positioning of joints (not allowing maximum return to mobility)

PSYCHOLOGICAL AND SOCIAL ISSUES

Name 6 causes of delirium in burn patients.	1. ICU psychosis 2. Sepsis 3. Electrolyte imbalance 4. Hypertension 5. Hypoglycemia 6. Pain
What 5 patient groups are more likely to experience psychosis/delirium?	1. Males 2. Those with burns greater than 30% TBSA 3. Those with previous substance abuse 4. Teens 5. Elderly
What is the proper approach to psychosis?	Check organic causes including: 1. Vital signs 2. Blood chemistries 3. Glucose 4. O_2 saturation 5. Sepsis investigation 6. Pain management Then, consider adding an antipsychotic (e.g., Haldol).
List 4 symptoms of posttraumatic stress disorder (PTSD)?	1. Sleep disorder 2. Intrusive memories of the injury 3. Anxiety 4. Hypervigilance
What are 8 symptoms of depression?	1. Sleep changes 2. Interest (loss of) 3. Guilt 4. Energy (decreased) 5. Concentration (inability to) 6. Appetite (loss of) 7. Psychomotor slowing 8. Suicidal ideation
How is depression/PTSD treated?	1. Check pain control

2. Consider a selective serotonin-reuptake inhibitor (e.g., Prozac) or a tricyclic (e.g., imipramine).

What are 2 goals in psychiatric management of the burn inpatient?

1. To assist in managing pain and acute psychiatric disorders
2. To maximize participation in therapy and care

Do the majority of burn survivors suffer long-term, major psychiatric disorders?

No. $1/3$ develop PTSD within 2 years of injury. There is no increase in suicidality, and fewer than 50% suffer a major depressive episode. Self-esteem is normal, although appearance is often a concern.

Injuries in children and the elderly should always make you think of what?

Potential child/elder abuse

ETHICAL ISSUES

Who is Donald "Dax" Cowart?

Mr. Cowart suffered a 65% TBSA burn injury in a propane tank explosion in 1973. At the scene of the accident and repeatedly during treatments, Mr. Cowart refused further care so that he might be allowed to die. His treatments were continued, and he survived.

What challenges do burn centers face regarding costs of treatment?

Burn treatment can be expensive, but up to 70% of the costs may be for materials and equipment. It is important to attempt to control costs so that effective care of burn patients can be achieved while minimizing the strain on limited health care resources.

32

Vascular Surgery Patients

CAROTID ARTERY DISEASE

What are the 2 main types of stroke?	1. Ischemic: 85% 2. Hemorrhagic: 15%
What are the 3 mechanisms of ischemic stroke?	1. Embolic 2. Thrombotic 3. Hypoperfusion secondary to arterial stenosis or systemic hypotension
Define transient ischemic attack (TIA).	Temporary focal brain or retinal hypoperfusion events resolving in less than 24 hours
What is a stroke or cerebrovascular accident?	A neurologic deficit of more than 24 hours' duration without complete resolution
What are crescendo TIAs?	Repeated, focal neurologic events with a return to baseline in between.
What is a stroke in evolution?	Repeated neurologic events with actively deteriorating neurologic status
What is cerebral hyperperfusion syndrome?	Post-CEA, unilateral head, face, and eye pain. This can progress to seizures, intracerebral hemorrhage, and death.
What is the etiology of cerebral hypoperfusion syndrome?	Chronic, high-grade stenosis of the carotid artery leads to maximal dilatation of the intercerebral arteries, thus leading to loss of autoregulation after CEA.

Is cerebral hypoperfusion syndrome common?

Unknown. The mild form probably is more common than is currently recognized. The incidence of post-CEA hemorrhage ranges from 0.4% to 2%.

When does intracranial hemorrhage occur?

Postoperative days 2 to 4

How does intracranial hemorrhage occur?

Rupture of a maximally dilated, hyperperfused cerebral vessel

List 5 risk factors for intracranial hemorrhage.

1. Recent stroke
2. High-grade stenosis
3. Severe operative and perioperative HTN
4. Anticoagulant use
5. Chronic cerebral ischemia

Name 5 symptoms of intracranial hemorrhage.

1. Unilateral migraine
2. Vomiting
3. Neurologic deficits
4. Seizures
5. Obtundation

What is the etiology of post-CEA HTN?

Unclear. Post-CEA HTN is speculated to result from impaired cerebral autoregulation and/or baroreceptor dysfunction.

How common is post-CEA HTN?

As much as $^2/_3$ of all postoperative CEA patients

What are 5 risk factors for post-CEA HTN?

1. History of HTN
2. Stenosis greater than 50%
3. Cardiac arrhythmias
4. Renal insufficiency
5. Shunting

How do you treat post-CEA HTN?

1. Home medications
2. IV nitrates
3. β-Blockade
4. Adequate analgesics

What is the target systolic BP?	Between 90 and 160 mm Hg
What is the average perioperative stroke rate in experienced hands?	1% to 2%
What is the most common cause of perioperative stroke?	Technical error (90%)
What is the best course of action if neurologic deficit is seen after CEA?	If in the OR or in recovery: re-exploration If delayed: anticoagulation and diagnostic imaging
What is the treatment of acute neck swelling and stridor following CEA?	Re-explore the wound.

EXTREMITY ISCHEMIA

What are the 5 mechanisms of extremity ischemia?	1. Embolism 2. Thrombosis of pre-existing stenosis 3. Trauma: loss of arterial continuity 4. Compartment syndrome 5. High-grade venous thrombosis
What are 3 early signs and symptoms of extremity ischemia?	1. Pain 2. Discoloration 3. Pulselessness
What are 3 late signs of extremity ischemia?	1. Paresthesias 2. Paralysis 3. Necrosis
Which embolus to the upper extremity is more limb-threatening: proximal to profunda brachii, or distal?	Proximal to profunda brachii
Why is this so?	Lack of distal collateralization proximal to the profunda brachii

What percentage of emboli originate in the heart?

90%

What are 6 risk factors for arterial emboli?

1. Atrial fibrillation
2. MI: mural thrombus
3. Myxoma
4. Vegetations
5. Aneurysm proximal to occluded vessel: thromboemboli
6. Diffuse large vessel disease: atheroemboli

What are the 5 most commonly occluded vessels?

1. Common femoral artery
2. Common iliac artery
3. Popliteal artery
4. Aorta
5. Superior mesenteric artery, just distal to the middle colic artery

What is the treatment of acute occlusion?

1. Anticoagulation: immediate
2. Thrombectomy
3. Bypass: if acute thrombosis of pre-existing stenosis
4. Thrombolysis

What is the mortality rate following acute extremity arterial occlusion?

10% (most commonly from cardiac causes)

What is included in the workup for acute arterial occlusion?

1. Arteriogram
2. Echocardiogram
3. CT or ultrasound of the abdomen
4. Hypercoaguable workup

What is included in a hypercoagulable workup?

1. Protein C and protein S
2. Factor V Leiden
3. Homocysteine level
4. Prothrombin
5. Antithrombin III
6. Lupus anticoagulant
7. Anticardiolipin antibody
8. Fibrinogen level
9. Evaluation for malignancy

What are 6 causes of acute arterial thrombosis?

1. Indwelling catheters
2. Atherosclerosis
3. Trauma
4. Aneurysms
5. Adjacent tissue injury: infection, missile
6. Extrinsic compression: 1st rib compression of the subclavian artery in thoracic outlet syndrome

What is compartment syndrome?

Elevated pressure within a fascial compartment that impedes arterial flow, thus resulting in ischemia to tissues within the compartment

What are 5 causes of compartment syndrome?

1. Trauma: most common
2. Reperfusion after revascularization procedures
3. Snakebite
4. Cardiopulmonary bypass
5. Anticoagulation and bleeding into a compartment

What are 5 signs of compartment syndrome?

1. Pain
2. Pressure
3. Paresthesia
4. Intact pulses
5. Tense compartment

What is "pain with passive movement"?

Patients with compartment syndrome will have extreme pain with stretch of an affected compartment.

What is the most commonly affected compartment?

Anterior compartment of the leg

What is the long-term deficit from delay in treatment of anterior compartment symptoms?

Foot drop from peroneal nerve injury

What is the therapy for compartment syndrome?

Fasciotomy

What is a normal compartment pressure?	Less than 10 mm Hg
At what pressure does compartment syndrome occur?	There is no universally agreed on pressure. The diagnosis is a clinical one.
What should be included with fasciotomy if muscle necrosis has occurred?	Renal protection from rhabdomyolysis: aggressive hydration, mannitol, and alkalization of the urine (pH > 6).

HIT AND HITTS

What is HIT?	Heparin-induced thrombocytopenia
What is HITTS?	HIT associated with thrombosis
What is the causative agent?	Anti-heparin immunoglobulin G directed against the heparin–platelet factor 4 complex.
How is HIT diagnosed?	Decrease in platelet count to less than the normal range or a 50% or greater decrease
What is the diagnostic lab test?	Antiheparin antibody
What is the incidence?	1% to 31% of patients receiving heparin in any form
What is the treatment?	Stop all heparin.
Can you use LMW heparin?	No. There is an approximately 92% cross-reactivity with LMW heparin.
What are 2 other options for anticoagulation?	1. Coumadin 2. Thrombin inhibitors: hirudin, argatroban, dextran
When does it occur?	3 to 10 days after administration of the initial heparin dose
What is the morbidity and mortality?	60% and 25%, respectively

AORTIC DISSECTION

What is aortic dissection?

Hemorrhage within the layers of the wall of the aorta

How are aortic dissections classified?

Type A: involves the ascending aorta and/or aortic arch; 90% involve the entire aorta.
Type B: involves the descending aorta.

Which type is more common?

Type A

Between what layers does aortic dissection occur?

An intimal tear extends through to the plane of dissection, usually between the inner $^2/_3$ and outer $^1/_3$ of the media (95%), and creates a "false lumen."

What is a "double-barrel" aorta?

When the dissection, or false lumen, tears back into the true lumen

How do patients normally present?

1. Ripping or tearing chest and back pain that radiates to the interscapular space
2. Tamponade
3. Paraplegia
4. Mesenteric ischemia
5. Other signs of aortic branch occlusion

What disease process is most commonly associated with dissection?

HTN (present in 80%–90% of all patients with aortic dissection)

What is the mortality rate of aortic dissection?

50% if associated with complications from involvement of branch vessels

Which lumen is larger, the true or the false lumen?

The false lumen

How are branch vessels affected?

1. Static obstruction: the dissection flap enters and narrows a vessel lumen.
2. Dynamic obstruction: the dissection flap prolapses across the vessel lumen.

3. Static and dynamic obstruction: combination of item 1 and item 2.

Which vessels can be affected?

Any branch of the aorta

How is aortic dissection evaluated?

1. History & physical
2. ECG
3. CXR

What are 4 findings on CXR?

1. Wide mediastinum
2. Cardiomegaly
3. Pulmonary edema
4. Dilated aorta

CXR is normal in 10%.

What are 4 findings ECG?

1. Left-axis deviation
2. Left ventricular hypertrophy
3. Possible ischemic changes
4. Conduction defects

Do ECG changes and elevated troponin levels rule out dissection?

No. If the dissection involves a coronary artery, it will cause MI.

What are 6 findings on the physical exam?

1. Tamponade: Beck's triad
2. Weak peripheral pulses
3. Differing upper extremity BP
4. Signs of end-organ ischemia
5. Pulmonary edema
6. Murmur of aortic insufficiency

What is Beck's triad?

1. Hypotension
2. Muffled heart sounds
3. Distended neck veins

What 5 medical conditions place someone at greater risk for dissection?

1. Marfan's syndrome
2. Ehlers-Danlos syndrome
3. Coarctation of the aorta
4. Syphilitic aortitis
5. Pregnancy: pregnancy-induced HTN and hyperkinetic heart

What is the initial management of aortic dissection?

BP control with β-blockers and nitrates

What are the surgical indications in a type A aortic dissection?

The presence of a type A dissection is an indication for repair.

What are 4 possible sequelae of type A dissections?

1. Dissection of coronary arteries and MI
2. Cardiac tamponade
3. Stroke
4. CHF

Describe the management of a type B aortic dissection.

BP control. The goal is to convert from an acute to a chronic dissection.

Name 7 indications for repair of a type B aortic dissection.

1. Failure to control HTN
2. Continued pain
3. Expansion of the aneurysm
4. Pleural effusion
5. Signs of rupture
6. Development of neurologic deficit
7. Compromise of visceral or extremity arteries

What is the target BP and CO in acute dissection?

The lowest possible level while still maintaining adequate cerebral, coronary, and renal perfusion (80–90 mm Hg systolic)

What is the success rate of converting an acute to a chronic dissection?

Approximately 85% at 1 year

THORACOABDOMINAL ANEURYSM

What are the 4 Crawford classifications of thoracoabdominal aortic aneurysms (T-AAAs)?

Type I: left subclavian artery to below the visceral vessels
Type II: left subclavian artery to below the renals
Type III: midthoracic aorta to below the renals
Type IV: diaphragm to bifurcation or "total abdominal aortic aneurysm"

At what size should repair be recommended?	Types I–III: 6 cm Type IV: 5 cm
What percentage of patients have synchronous aneurysms in the ascending aorta or arch?	Approximately 10%
What percentage of patients have had previous abdominal aortic aneurysm (AAA) repair?	Approximately 30%
What percentage of patients have some degree of associated visceral or renovascular occlusive disease?	30%
What test should be performed in all patients being considered for T-AAA repair?	Dipyridamole–thallium scan or echocardiogram (high incidence of synchronous coronary artery disease)
Should all T-AAAs that meet the size criteria be repaired?	Those with comorbidities that suggest a life expectancy of less than 2 years should probably be treated nonoperatively.
What is appropriate nonoperative therapy?	1. Aggressive β-blockade 2. HTN control 3. Smoking cessation
What is the perioperative mortality of T-AAA repair?	Approximately 10% (5% if considering only elective repairs)
What 2 postoperative complications most significantly increase mortality?	1. Renal failure 2. Paraplegia These increase mortality by factors of 6 and 16, respectively.
What is the incidence of postoperative spinal cord ischemic complications?	5% to 10%

What 4 factors significantly increase the risk of spinal cord ischemia?

1. Cross-clamp time
2. Extent of aneurysm
3. Emergency operation
4. Traumatic transection greater than dissection greater than T-AAA

What cross-clamp time is significantly associated with ischemic cord injury?

Incidence approaches 100% at 60 minutes. There is a steep increase in the incidence of neurologic deficit after 35 minutes of warm ischemia.

What artery is associated with spinal cord ischemia?

Anterior spinal artery (artery of Adamkewicz)

Where does the anterior spinal artery originate?

Most commonly from the intercostals in the T9 through L1 region. There can be multiple levels of collaterals, however, from the arch to the iliacs.

What is the spinal cord perfusion pressure?

MAP – CSF pressure (normal is at least 50 mm Hg)

How is spinal cord perfusion pressure commonly monitored and maintained at an optimal level?

Spinal cord drainage. Perioperatively, the CSF pressure is monitored and regulated by an intrathecal catheter.

How can spinal cord ischemia manifest clinically?

Complete paralysis to lower extremity paraperesis

What are 2 other neuroprotective adjuncts?

1. Hypothermia
2. Pharmacologic adjuncts

What 2 types of pharmacologic agents are used in treatment?

1. Nonspecific neuroprotectors: steroids, prostaglandins, magnesium, barbiturates
2. Excitatory neurotransmitter inhibitors: naloxone, calcium-channel blockers, free-radical scavengers

How is hypothermia protective?

Hypothermia decreases tissue metabolism.

What 2 methods are available to produce hypothermia?

1. Complete cardiopulmonary bypass and hypothermic circulatory arrest
2. Selective hypothermic perfusion of end organs

Is either method proven to be clinically effective?

No adjuvant therapy has been proven clinically efficacious. Hypothermia is associated with severe cardiac arrhythmias.

What is the most common postoperative complication?

Respiratory failure

How common is respiratory failure as a postoperative complication?

25% to 45% of patients

What are 3 risk factors for thoracoabdominal aneurysm?

1. Chronic obstructive pulmonary disease
2. Preoperative tobacco use
3. Radial division of the aortic hiatus intraoperatively

What is the incidence of postoperative renal failure?

8% to 10%

How is postoperative renal failure defined?

Doubling of the preoperative creatinine level, or an absolute creatinine level of greater than 3 mg/dL

What are 3 predictors of postoperative renal failure?

1. Preoperative renal insufficiency: most predictive
2. Cross-clamp time
3. Failure of renal artery reconstruction

What is the long-term survival rate?

60% at 5 years

What is the most common cause of late mortality?

Cardiac events

ABDOMINAL AORTIC ANEURYSMS

What is an infrarenal AAA?	Dilatation of the aorta by more than 3 cm
What is the most important factor in predicting an aneurysm rupture?	Size of the aneurysm
What is the annual risk of rupture for aneurysms of the following sizes?	4 to 5 cm: 0.5% to 5% 5 to 6 cm: 3% to 15% 6 to 7 cm: 10% to 20% 7 to 8 cm: 20% to 40% Greater than 8 cm: 30% to 50%
What 6 types of aneurysms require repair?	1. Ruptured aneurysms: emergent 2. Aneurysms larger than 5.5 cm 3. Aneurysms that have enlarged more than 0.5 cm in 6 months 4. Symptomatic aneurysms: painful 5. Aneurysms with focal ulceration 6. Aneurysms with distal atheroemboli
Are there patient factors that influence elective repair?	Yes. Patients with a life expectancy of less than 2 years because of comorbidities probably should be observed. In the face of endovascular repair of aneurysms, however, these recommendations are changing somewhat.
What is the perioperative mortality rate of open repair?	5%
What is the perioperative mortality rate of endovascular repair?	1% to 8% (new and evolving data)
What is the most common cause of perioperative and late mortality following AAA repair?	Coronary artery disease

What percentage of late deaths are attributable to CAD?	50% to 60%
What percentage of patients will have a nonfatal myocardial ischemic event?	3% to 16%
What percentage of patients with AAA have normal coronary arteries?	10%
What measure can be taken to significantly reduce the incidence of postoperative cardiac events?	β-Blockade and subsequent reduction of myocardial work
What is the rate of postoperative renal failure?	6% (because of acute tubular necrosis)
How does renal failure affect mortality?	Increases 50% to 70%

COLONIC ISCHEMIA

What is the most serious GI complication following AAA repair?	Left colon ischemia
What is the cause?	Lack of sufficient collateralization
What condition increases the risk?	Previous partial colon resection
How can this complication present?	1. Bloody diarrhea 2. Abdominal distension 3. Frank peritonitis
When does it occur?	Within 48 hours
What test confirms the diagnosis?	Flexible sigmoidoscopy

What is seen on endoscopy?	Findings can range from limited to mucosal involvement to transmural necrosis and gangrene
What 3 lab tests can help to confirm the diagnosis?	1. Serum lactate 2. ABG 3. CBC: leukocytosis Do not wait for lab results before performing endoscopy if the diagnosis is suspected.
What is the incidence?	1% to 6%
What is the treatment?	Limited mucosal involvement: observation; will usually resolve Transmural necrosis: reoperation and resection
How does bowel ischemia affect perioperative mortality?	Bowel ischemia increases the incidence of perioperative mortality by 70% to 90%.

RUPTURED AAA

What is the mortality rate of patients with a ruptured AAA?	Approximately 50% of all patients with a ruptured AAA die before reaching a hospital. Approximately 25% of those patients who do reach a hospital do not survive.
How do ruptured AAAs present?	1. Abdominal or back pain 2. Hypotension 3. Pulsatile abdominal mass
Should aggressive fluid resuscitation be undertaken in the emergency room first?	No. Mild, permissive hypotension may be beneficial in preventing blood loss through the rupture site. The goal is a systolic BP of approximately 90 mm Hg.
If the patient is hemodynamically stable, can other studies be performed?	Yes. A stable patient can be taken for emergent CT or ultrasound to rule out other pathology.

In the case of stable patients with the above symptoms and a large, intact aneurysm, should they go straight to the OR?

No. Symptomatic aneurysms can have improved outcomes with pulmonary artery catheterization and hemodynamic optimization before urgent repair.

What is the incidence of major complications after ruptured AAA repair, and how does it compare to elective repair?

1. Renal failure: 16%
2. Ischemic colitis: 60% ($\sim$13% benign transmural necrosis)
3. Cardiac complications (arrhythmias and ischemic episodes): 50%
4. Respiratory failure: 53%

The incidence of all major complications is increased compared to those associated with elective repair.

Of those patients who survive to discharge, what percentage survive 5 years?

Approximately 65%

DEEP-VEIN THROMBOSIS

What is Virchow's triad?

1. Stasis
2. Hypercoagulability
3. Endothelial injury

How many factors of Virchow's triad need be present for thrombosis to occur?

2

Where does venous thrombosis most commonly occur?

The deep veins. 90% of cases occur in "proximal veins," or those from the popliteal vein up to and including the inferior vena cava (IVC).

What is the prevalence of DVT?

1 million patients per year.

How many deaths are caused by PE per year in the United States?

200,000

What are the 2 sequelae of DVT?	1. Pulmonary embolism (PE) 2. Chronic venous insufficiency
What percentage of patients with DVT eventually develop chronic venous insufficiency or post-thrombotic syndrome?	50%
What is the cause of chronic venous insufficiency?	Valvular reflux and residual venous obstruction
What are 4 areas of risk factors for DVT?	1. Demographics: age older than 60 years; pregnancy or less than 1 month postpartum 2. Immobilization: bed confinement for 72 hours or longer; confining travel for more than 4 hours 3. Medical conditions: CHF, chronic obstructive pulmonary disease, MI, nephrotic syndrome, malignancy, hypercoagulable state, previous DVT, previous PE 4. Surgical conditions: prolonged surgical procedure, severe trauma, pelvic surgery, total joint replacement, pelvic or long bone fracture, neurosurgery
What is the recommended prophylaxis for each of the following risk groups?	
Low risk	No specific measures
Moderate risk	Low-dose unfractionated (LDU) heparin every 12 hours, LMW heparin, or intermittent pneumatic compression (IPC)
High risk	LDU heparin every 8 hours or LMW heparin (plus IPC)
Very high risk	LDU heparin every 8 hours, LMW heparin (plus IPC), or warfarin

What is the difference between LDU heparin and LMW heparin?	LMW heparin is produced through depolymerization and fractionation of standard heparin sodium.
Does activated PTT need to be monitored with LMW heparin therapy?	No. The effects of LMW heparin mainly are on factor X_A.
Are the bioavailabilities of LMW heparin and heparin sodium equal?	No. LMW heparin is 90% bioavailable; heparin sodium is only 20% bioavailable.
How is this difference in bioavailability important clinically?	LMW heparin is more effective at DVT prophylaxis.
How are LDU heparin and LMW heparin administered for prophylaxis?	LDU heparin: 5,000 U SQ BID or TID based on risk factor evaluation LMW heparin: 30 mg SQ BID
What are 4 symptoms of DVT?	1. Unilateral swelling of an extremity 2. Calf pain 3. Venous distension 4. Homan sign Often, the diagnosis is not suspected until after the patient has suffered a PE.
What is the Homan sign?	Pain on manual dorsiflexion of the foot
How is the diagnosis of DVT established?	1. Clinical suspicion. 2. Venous duplex scan. 3. Venogram is the gold standard.
What is the treatment of DVT?	Anticoagulation (thrombectomy and thrombolysis for iliofemoral DVT)
How is anticoagulation achieved?	1. IV heparin: goal activated PTT of 55 to 85 seconds 2. LMW heparin: 1 mg/kg SQ every 12 hours 3. Warfarin: should be started after or in conjunction with items 1 and 2.

What is the therapy for calf-vein DVT?	Controversial. The risk for complication is less than 5% at 5 years. For patients in whom the thrombotic risk has not been eliminated, anticoagulation can be justified.

How long is therapy indicated for each of the following?

Idiopathic DVT	6 months
Recurrent DVT (1st instance)	6 months
Recurrent DVT (2nd instance)	1 year
Recurrent DVT (3rd or later instance)	Lifelong
Cancer(with DVT) or hypercoaguable state	Lifelong

Name 6 indications for vena caval filters.	1. Contraindication to anticoagulation in patients with proximal DVT 2. Complications from anticoagulation 3. PE while on therapeutic anticoagulation 4. Prevention of PE in very-high-risk patients 5. History of poor compliance 6. Pulmonary embolectomy (in conjunction with)
Name 6 relative indications for a vena caval filter.	1. DVT in patients with poor pulmonary reserve 2. Free-floating IVC thrombus 3. DVT/PE in the presence of a right-to-left shunt 4. Prophylaxis in high-risk trauma patients 5. Patients requiring prolonged immobilization and thus at high risk for DVT

6. Protection during venous thrombolytic therapy with large thrombus burden

Name 8 complications of vena caval filter placement.

1. Access-site thrombosis
2. Recurrent DVT
3. Filter-associated IVC thrombosis
4. Recurrent PE
5. Filter migration
6. Mechanical failure
7. IVC penetration with secondary internal organ injury
8. Filter infection

TRACHEO-INNOMINATE FISTULA

What is a tracheo-innominate fistula?

A fistula between the trachea and the innominate artery

How does a tracheo-innominate fistula develop?

Erosion of a cuff balloon through the trachea into the artery

What increases the risk of development?

Innappropriately low placement of a tracheostomy

How does a tracheo-innominate fistula present?

Sudden, exsanguinating hemorrhage. Patients usually will have 1 or more sentinel hemorrhages.

How is a tracheo-innominate fistula evaluated?

Bright red blood from a tracheostomy warrants fiberoptic evaluation.

How is a tracheo-innominate fistula managed?

Immediate tamponade with a finger or balloon and emergent exploration.

33

Transplant Patients

DEFINITIONS

What is an autograft?

When the same individual is both the donor and the recipient

What is an isograft?

When the donor and the recipient are genetically identical (i.e., identical twins)

What is an allograft?

When the donor and the recipient are genetically dissimilar but of the same species

What is a xenograft?

When the donor and the recipient belong to different species

What is an orthotopic transplant?

When the donor organ is placed in the anatomic position (liver, heart)

What is a heterotopic transplant?

When the donor organ is placed in a different anatomic position (kidney, pancreas)

What is a paratopic transplant?

When the donor organ is placed close to the original organ.

IMMUNOSUPPRESSION

Which transplant patients need to be immunosuppressed?

All recipients except auto- or isograft recipients

When is rejection most common (any organ)?

Within the first 1 to 2 months

IMMUNOSUPPRESSIVE AGENTS

How do the following immunosuppressive agents work?

Cyclosporine (CSA)?	Inhibits release of interleukin (IL)-2 from activated T-helper cells.
Tacrolimus (FK-506)?	Inhibits release of IL-2 from activated T-helper cells.
Sirolimus (Rapamycin)?	Inhibits cytokine-driven T-lymphocyte activation and proliferation
Azathioprine	A precursor to 6-mercaptopurine, it inhibits purine incorporation of both DNA and RNA.
Corticosteroids	Inhibit production of IL-2 from T lymphocytes and release of IL-1 from macrophages.
Daclizumab?	Monoclonal antibody to the IL-2 receptor.
Monoclonal OKT-3?	Blocks CD-3 receptors on T cells, thus preventing antigen recognition.
Polyclonal antithymocyte γ-globulin (ATGAM)/ antilymphocyte globulin?	Fixes complement, and lyses T lymphocytes.

COMMON USES

What is "three-drug therapy"?	1. CSA 2. Azathioprine 3. Prednisone
Some transplant centers use which 2 drugs in place of CSA?	1. Tacrolimus 2. Sirolimus
What is induction therapy?	Early use of antilymphocyte drugs to prevent rejection

What 2 drugs are used to treat acute organ rejection?	1. Glucocorticoids 2. OKT-3: for steroid-resistant rejection

SIDE EFFECTS AND DRUG INTERACTIONS

What 4 medications lower CSA levels?	1. Dilantin 2. Phenobarbital 3. Rifampin 4. Isoniazid
What 4 medications raise CSA levels?	1. Macrolides: erythromycin 2. Ketoconazole, itraconazole, fluconazole 3. Diltiazem 4. Amiodarone
What 3 medications may potentiate renal dysfunction when used with CSA?	1. Aminoglycosides 2. Amphotericin 3. Nonsteroidal anti-inflammatory agents
Name 6 side effects of steroids.	1. Glucose intolerance 2. Adrenal insufficiency: if acutely withdrawn 3. Cataracts 4. Osteoporosis 5. Cushingoid appearance 6. Skin fragility
What is the most common life-threatening complication of OKT-3 therapy?	Severe pulmonary edema
What are the most common side effects of the following agents that require a change in dose or agent?	
Azathioprine	1. Leukopenia 2. Thrombocytopenia 3. Pancreatitis

CSA	1. Nephrotoxicity
	2. Hypertension
	3. Tremulousness
Antithymocyte globulin	1. Thrombocytopenia/leukopenia.
	2. May cause anaphylaxis or pulmonary edema.
OKT-3	Pulmonary edema

TRANSPLANT INFECTION

What 2 groups of infections are more common in transplant patients than in other ICU patients?

1. Fungi
2. Viruses

When are infections most common after any transplant?

During the first 3 to 6 months

What 5 type of infections (other than a "cold") are most common after any transplant?

1. Bacterial: common
2. Atypical bacterial
3. Viral
4. Fungal
5. Protozoal

What process can masquerade with fever and an infiltrate following organ transplantation?

Transplant-associated B-cell lymphoma, which occurs in 1% to 5% of patients over time. (The frequency depends on the organ transplanted.)

What is the test of choice to evaluate serious infiltrates?

Bronchoalveolar lavage (BAL)

What foreign body is a common cause of sepsis in liver transplant patients?

IV catheters

VIRAL INFECTION

What is the most common cause of viral pneumonia in transplant patients?	Cytomegalovirus (CMV)
What is the treatment of choice for CMV?	Ganciclovir
What is the most common complication of ganciclovir?	Leukopenia
What antiviral agent can be used if ganciclovir toxicity (usually bone marrow suppression) occurs?	Foscarnet (acyclovir can also be used)
What organ systems are most frequently affected with CMV infections?	GI: stomach, colon Lung: pneumonitis Other: heart CMV infections can also stimulate the immune system and, therefore, are frequently associated with rejection.
What virus most commonly causes encephalitis in transplant patients?	Herpes simplex virus (HSV)
What is the treatment of choice for HSV infection?	High-dose IV acyclovir

FUNGAL AND PROTOZOAL INFECTION

When is prophylactic amphotericin B indicated in the transplant patient?	After re-explorations or retransplants, secondary to the high incidence of postoperative fungal infections
What fungus usually is fatal in transplant patients if isolated from the brain?	*Aspergillus* sp.

What 4 organisms cause nonspecific pulmonary infiltrates in transplant patients?	1. *Legionella* sp. 2. *Aspergillus* sp. 3. *Histoplasma* sp. 4. *Cryptococcus* sp.
Why is Bactrim used in transplant patients?	For prophylaxis against *Pneumocystis carinii*

KIDNEY TRANSPLANT

What are the 2 major causes of immediate nonfunction of a cadaveric renal transplant?	1. Hyperacute rejection 2. Technical problem with anastomosis
Does cold ischemic time affect the degree of acute tubular necrosis (ATN) in a cadaveric renal transplant?	Yes. The longer the time of cold ischemia, the greater the degree of ATN may be. Living related donors have less ATN because of the lack of cold ischemic time.
What is the best measure of postoperative renal function?	UOP. BUN and creatinine also may be helpful.
What CVP generally is maintained in a post-operative renal transplant?	12 to 15 mm Hg
How can one estimate the amount of IV fluid needed to maintain adequate CVP in a transplant patient?	Input = output + 50 mL/hr in adults
If CVP is adequate and UOP is low, what is the next step in management, diuretics or vasopressors?	Diuretics: Lasix (100 to 200 mg IV); Bumex (3 to 5 mg IV); metolazone (10 to 30 mg IV)
Why should vasopressors be avoided?	Vasospasm and decreased renal perfusion may lead to vascular thrombosis and loss of graft.

Even with good UOP (>30 mL/hr), what are 2 reasons why fluids must be given to the postoperative kidney transplant patient to keep CVP at 10 mm Hg or greater?

1. The denervated transplant kidney is solely dependent on pressure for perfusion.
2. Intraoperative diuretics (mannitol and Lasix) may cause spuriously high UOP.

What radiographic test should be obtained if the kidney does not have adequate UOP despite adequate CVP and diuretics?

Doppler ultrasound to assess vascular flow

If the Doppler ultrasound confirms adequate flow and there is still no UOP, what is the next step?

1. A trial of diuretic therapy.
2. Hemodialysis may be required.

How can you differentiate ATN from rejection?

Transplant kidney biopsy

What 4 immunosuppressive agents are used during the immediate postoperative period in the cadaveric transplant recipient?

1. OKT-3
2. Azathioprine
3. Corticosteroids
4. ATGAM: antilymphocyte preparations

Why is CSA not generally used immediately after cadaveric renal transplant?

CSA causes arteriolar vasoconstriction, especially in the kidney. This may accentuate vasospasm, ATN, and poor graft function.

If a renal biopsy shows acute cellular rejection, what treatment is initiated?

Corticosteroid bolus with taper

If the kidney fails to respond to steroids, what is the next step?

OKT-3

What 2 clinical and laboratory signs are suggestive of a urine leak?

1. Clear fluid leakage from the wound
2. Increase in serum creatinine

How can a urine leak be diagnosed?	1. Send wound fluid for BUN and creatinine. 2. Ultrasound can show fluid collections or outlet obstruction. 3. Isotope (MAG-3) renogram scan for perfusion and excretion.

PANCREAS TRANSPLANT

What organ typically is transplanted concurrently with a pancreas?	Kidney
What group of patients typically receives pancreas/ kidney transplants?	Type I diabetics with end-stage renal disease
Name 2 types of exocrine pancreas drainage.	1. Enteric drainage to small bowel: currently preferred 2. Bladder drainage
What 3 parameters are followed in pancreas transplant recipients?	1. Blood glucose 2. Urinary amylase: if bladder drainage used 3. Parameters for kidney transplant: if the recipient is having a combined pancreas/kidney transplant
What 2 vessels provide the blood supply to the transplanted pancreas the majority of the time?	1. Iliac artery 2. Iliac vein
What should you do if the UOP is zero and clots are seen in the Foley bag with bladder-drained transplants?	Irrigate the Foley every hour to avoid ongoing obstruction, because this may cause bladder distension and lead to an anastomotic leak.
What CVP should be maintained in a pancreas transplant patient?	12 to 15 mm Hg (the same as for a cadaveric renal transplant patient)

What fluid rate should be maintained in a pancreas transplant patient?

When CVP is greater than 10 mm Hg: input = output + 50 mL/hr
When CVP is greater than 10 mm Hg: input = output

Is glucose placed in the maintenance fluid during the immediate postoperative period?

No

What is the most common cause of early graft loss?

Thrombosis

What 2 additional agents can be infused to attempt to prevent graft thrombosis?

1. LMW dextran: 20 mL/hr
2. Low-dose heparin drip

What 2 laboratory studies are suggestive of graft failure in a pancreas transplant?

1. Increased blood glucose
2. Decreased urinary amylase
(in U/hr, if the pancreas is bladder drained)

How is the diagnosis of graft thrombosis established?

Liberal use of magnetic resonance angiography (MRA)

Why not use CT scan or conventional arteriography to establish the diagnosis of graft thrombosis?

Iodinated contrast material often is contraindicated because of coexisting renal failure.

What surgery is required after graft thrombosis?

Transplant excision (thrombectomy usually fails)

What is the most common indication for surgery after a pancreas transplant?

Intra-abdominal infection

How is the diagnosis of pancreatic rejection established?

Biopsy of the associated kidney. If no kidney was transplanted with the pancreas, rejection is the presumptive diagnosis based on blood glucose and (if the pancreas is bladder drained) urinary amylase. The transplanted pancreas rarely is biopsied.

Which organ usually rejects first in the combined procedure, the kidney or the pancreas?

The kidney

Is there better long-term graft survival with pancreas transplant alone or with combined pancreas–kidney transplantation?

With combined pancreas–kidney transplantation

Would fluid requirements tend to be higher for a cadaveric renal transplant or for a combined pancreas–kidney transplant?

A combined pancreas–kidney transplant generally is done through an open abdominal procedure and has much higher 3rd-space losses.

LIVER TRANSPLANT

What 4 parameters are used to assess intravascular volume in a postoperative liver transplant patient?

1. CVP
2. PAD pressure
3. PCWP
4. UOP

What is the primary clinical measure of adequate postoperative perfusion?

UOP

In what subset of patients is UOP not an adequate measure of postoperative perfusion?

Patients with hepatorenal syndrome

What UOP is the lowest acceptable output?

Adults: 0.5 mL/kg/hr
Children: 1 to 2 mL/kg/hr

What unusual fluid loss is replaced during the immediate postoperative period in a liver transplant patient?

The fluid from three Jackson-Pratt drains is replaced milliliter for milliliter with 5% albumin during the first 48 hours.

When is FFP transfused in the early postoperative period?

If the patient is bleeding. Otherwise, correction may interfere with assessing the synthetic function of the new liver.

What is primary nonfunction?

Unexplained factors that cause the transplanted liver not to function, requiring emergent retransplantation

What is the most common hematologic disorder in postoperative liver transplant patients?

Thrombocytopenia

What is the workup for increased liver enzymes, increased PT, and increased bilirubin?

1. Doppler ultrasound to ensure hepatic arterial flow and intraductal dilation, which are technical problems
2. Liver biopsy to rule out rejection
3. Cholangiogram to evaluate biliary obstruction

Name 2 ways in which a posttransplant cholangiogram is obtained.

1. Endoscopic retrograde cholangiopancreatography
2. Percutaneous cholangiopancreatography: if the liver is drained into a Roux-en-Y anastamosis

What 3 parameters are followed to assess postoperative liver transplant function?

1. Lactic acid levels
2. PT/PTT: coagulation studies
3. Ammonia levels

What is the most common indication for early re-exploration of liver transplant patients?

Bleeding

What is the main indication for later re-exploration of liver transplant patients?

Sepsis

CARDIAC TRANSPLANT

How is the diagnosis of acute rejection in a cardiac transplant established?

Endomyocardial biopsy

What medication should not be used to treat bradycardia following heart transplantation?

Atropine

What 2 medications should be used to treat brady-cardia following heart transplantation?

Either:
1. Epinephrine
2. Isoproterenol

What medication should not be used to treat SVTs following heart transplantation?

Digoxin. Long-term use of β-blockers also generally is discouraged, because these agents reduce exercise tolerance.

Why are tachy-, brady-, and dysrhythmias treated differently in heart transplant recipients?

The heart is denervated; therefore, vagolytic (atropine) and vagotonic (digoxin) agents are not effective (as stated previously).

Can a heart transplant patient have a heart attack?

Yes. Coronary artery disease (CAD) is a manifestation of chronic rejection. Approximately 50% of heart transplant patients have some evidence of CAD at 5 years; this is usually significant in only 5% of transplant patients.

Does reinnervation ever occur?

Yes. 75% of heart recipients show some sympathetic reinnervation after 1 year.

Does reinnervation have any practical implication?

Yes. Patients who reinnervate have improved exercise performance (faster heart-rate response). Also, some recipients who develop CAD complain of chest pain.

How long can a heart or lung remain ischemic?	Approximately 4 hours (which determines how far you can travel to retrieve organs)
What is the most common arrhythmia?	Bradycardia
What is the treatment of bradycardia?	1. Chronotropes 2. Pacing
What 2 factors are most important for successful heart, lung, and heart–lung transplantation?	1. ABO compatibility 2. Approximate size match
In a heart–lung transplant recipient, is it possible to reject a lung without con-comitant heart rejection?	Yes. Either lung may show evidence of rejection without involvement of the opposite lung or the heart.

LUNG TRANSPLANT

What are 5 common indications for lung transplantation?	1. Chronic obstructive pulmonary disease (COPD) 2. Pulmonary fibrosis 3. Cystic fibrosis 4. α_1-Antitrypsin deficiency 5. Primary pulmonary hypertension
Why do patients with cystic fibrosis receive double-lung transplants, whereas patients with COPD commonly receive only single-lung transplants?	Patients with cystic fibrosis uniformly have chronic bacterial infection in both lungs. The remaining lung would serve as a nidus of infection.
What is the definition of rejection in a lung transplant?	Fever, infiltrate, and hypoxia that responds to antirejection medications

When seeing a patient after lung transplantation with dyspnea and a new lung infiltrate, what 2 situations should you consider?

1. Rejection
2. Infection

How can you determine if the infiltrate is caused by infection?

Bronchoscopy and BAL. The specimen is analyzed for WBC count and sent for culture and Gram's stain. High WBC counts in the BAL fluid are suggestive of infection.

How can you determine if the infiltrate is caused by rejection?

Bronchoscopy and transbronchial biopsy. A perivascular lymphocytic infiltrate is the hallmark of acute cellular rejection.

What is the differential diagnosis of lung recipients with dyspnea who wheeze?

1. Infection
2. Rejection
3. Anastomotic stenosis: bronchial
4. Disease of the nontransplanted lung: COPD, asthma
5. Cardiac disease

What is the differential diagnosis of lung recipients who are hypoxic?

1. Infection
2. Rejection: acute
3. Bronchiolitis obliterans: chronic rejection
4. Anastomotic stenosis: pulmonary artery
5. Cardiac disease

Index

Page numbers in italics (set in italics) denote figures; those followed by a t denote tables.

Brogan